Medicine and Western Civilization

Medicine and Western Civilization

EDITED BY DAVID J. ROTHMAN,
STEVEN MARCUS,
AND
STEPHANIE A. KICELUK

RUTGERS UNIVERSITY PRESS
New Brunswick, New Jersey, and London

Library of Congress Cataloging-in-Publication Data
Medicine and Western civilization / edited by David J. Rothman, Steven Marcus, and
Stephanie A. Kiceluk.
p.   cm.
Includes bibliographical references and index.
ISBN 0-8135-2189-0 (cloth : alk. paper) —
ISBN 0-8135-2190-4 (pbk. : alk. paper)
1. Medicine and the humanities. 2. Medicine—History—Sources.
3. Social medicine. I. Rothman, David J. II. Marcus, Steven.
III. Kiceluk, Stephanie A., 1950–
[DNLM: 1. History of Medicine. 2. Civilization. 3. Sociology, Medical.]
R702.M39   1995
306.4'61—dc20
DNLM/DLC
for Library of Congress   95-7203
                                                                            CIP

British Cataloging-in-Publication information available

Third paperback printing, 2003

Published by Rutgers University Press,
New Brunswick, New Jersey
All rights reserved
Manufactured in the United States of America

THE DIVINE IMAGE

To Mercy, Pity, Peace, and Love
All pray in their distress;
And to these virtues of delight
Return their thankfulness.

For Mercy, Pity, Peace, and Love
Is God, our father dear,
And Mercy, Pity, Peace, and Love
Is Man, his child and care.

For Mercy has a human heart,
Pity a human face,
And Love, the human form divine,
And Peace, the human dress.

Then every man, of every clime,
That prays in his distress,
Prays to the human form divine,
Love, Mercy, Pity, Peace.

And all must love the human form,
In heathen, turk, or jew;
Where Mercy, Love, & Pity dwell,
There God is dwelling too.

William Blake

Contents

Part 5 The Contaminated and the Pure

Part 6 The Healer

Part 7 The Experimenter

Part 8 The Institutionalization of Doctors and Patients

Part 9 The Construction of Pain, Suffering, and Death

Illustrations

Acknowledgments

In the course of researching, formulating, and teaching the materials that compose this book, we benefited greatly from an illuminating and lively exchange of ideas with Rita Charon and Peter Geller (Columbia University College of Physicians & Surgeons), Paul Edelson (Cornell-Methodist Hospital), and John Truman (Morristown Memorial Hospital).

Under the auspices of the National Endowment for the Humanities, a summer institute in Medicine and Western Civilization enabled us to teach and refine our original materials with faculty drawn from all over the country. We are especially grateful to those who taught the institute with us: Gert Brieger (Johns Hopkins University), Sander Gilman (University of Chicago), Regina Morantz-Sanchez (University of Michigan), and Katherine Park (Wellesley College).

Librarians were exceptionally generous with their knowledge and time, including Lois Black, Rachel Hansen, and Shaw Kinsley (New York Academy of Medicine), Clare Dunne (The Wellcome Centre Medical Photographic Library), Richard Hollinger (Augustus C. Long Health Sciences Library, Columbia University), and Richard J. Wolfe (Francis A. Countway Library of Medicine, Harvard Medical School). We would also like to thank Rebecca Behar for her help in identifying and securing French materials.

Nancy Lundebjerg, administrator of the Center, deftly oversaw every phase of this project. Aina Lakis and Helia Garcia fulfilled an almost dizzying array of tasks, and Martin Rivlin, our indefatigable research assistant, found no search too daunting to complete.

We are particularly pleased to acknowledge the support of this project by the National Endowment for the Humanities, Division of Education Programs and the Samuel and May Rudin Foundation. Our NEH program officer, Thomas Adams, demonstrated an enthusiasm for the project that was a constant source of encouragement. The readiness of both foundations to promote interdisciplinary innovations in curriculum design is deeply appreciated.

Finally, the spirit of inquiry and intellectual excitement that our students at Columbia College brought to these materials made it all the more important for us to publish this book.

In the interest of readability, deletions of full sentences or paragraphs in the selections that follow are not indicated, but omissions within sentences are marked by ellipses.

Medicine and Western Civilization

Introduction

This book aims to illustrate and to illuminate the many ways in which medicine and culture combine to shape our values and traditions. Medicine and culture are, in fact, inseparable entities and together make up a complex world, or set of worlds. Medicine itself is a culture and a world of its own, with institutions and subinstitutions peculiar to it, and with rites of passage, forms of education, standards of behavior, and sets of norms that have their own history and development and semiautonomous life—as anyone who has ever been hospitalized will immediately recognize. At the same time, however, medicine is an integral and indispensable part of larger social cultures as well—the culture of science, of religious and ethical beliefs, and of our changing society, with its own evolving values and attitudes. In their inseparability as practices that affect all of us in our daily lives and our ultimate fates, medicine and culture must, therefore, be considered together, both as they influence us in terms of our personal conduct and beliefs and as they function themselves through specific behaviors and institutions.

From Greco-Roman times to the present, medicine has been a vital source of authority in Western societies. It has affected and continues to affect everyday habits as well as our most elemental attitudes about the body, the proper ways to conduct life, and the fact and meaning of death. One cannot understand such massive and diverse cultural shifts in Western civilization as the decline of magic, the preoccupation with cleanliness, or the appreciation of the unconscious without recognizing medicine's extraordinary ability to intervene in—indeed, to shape—culture. Over time, medicine has acquired the power to demarcate the line between the normal and the abnormal, the biologically innate and the culturally determined, between male and female, life and death. In a more intimate sense, medicine affects what people will—or will not—eat, drink, touch, or embrace. It separates the clean from the dirty, the wholesome from the noxious.

However impressive this power may be, medicine is certainly not the exclusive arbiter of values in our culture. Since the dawn of Western civilization, religious doctrine has offered its own distinctive answers to what is clean (in its language, sacred) as against dirty (profane), what may or may not be eaten (for example, the elaborate Jewish dietary codes as described in the Bible), and what constitutes the moral or honorable life. Inevitably, cultural assumptions about and definitions of morality, sexuality, and gender influence physicians' own attitudes and practices; indeed, such assumptions and definitions themselves become part of the inner fabric of medical discourse and practice. In point of fact, as this book will make clear, the lines of influence run in both directions: from medicine to culture and from culture to medicine. The relationship is at once dynamic, intricate, and, in all its parts and details, fascinating and highly consequential.

There is no better method for sorting out this complex interplay than by examining notable literary, medical, and social texts from classical antiquity to the present. The range of relevant materials is enormous, and includes Roman treatises on the body, medieval treatises on witchcraft, and an eyewitness account of public anatomy lessons in the early Renaissance. In addition, fictional narratives, whether of a sixteenth-century plague, a nineteenth-century nervous breakdown, or a twentieth-century surgical procedure, are especially revealing of links between medicine and culture—as, of course, are the pioneering articles on vaccination, antisepsis, and germ theory. These later writings, too, are to be read not only as scientific treatises but as the expressions of a particular culture, time, and place.

The relationships between medicine and culture have only recently begun to attract wide attention. The growing interest in this new field of study expresses, in the first instance, developments within the disciplines of the humanities, particularly comparative literature and history. The history of the body, the semiotics of pathology, and the social construction of medical knowledges have all recently become an integral part of research and teaching in the humanities. Scholars now take as problematic—and hence as material for inquiry and analysis—phenomena that only recently had been perceived as inevitable or natural. The body, once assumed to be a biological constant independent of history or culture, is today the subject of investigation by historians and literary analysts. They ask not only who is privileged to cut or to intrude forcefully into the body, but also how different cultures at different times have understood how the body works, what has appeared to differentiate the female body from the male body, and what appeared and still appears to demarcate the mind from the body. In other words, the human body today has a history, and the comprehension of this history requires a combination of medical and cultural perspectives.

In this same spirit, scholars once presumed that the phenomena of disease made up a fixed and immutable class of characteristics and events. Tuberculosis, for example, was an entity that appeared to exist outside of culture; after all, the bacillus was real and specific enough, and so were the symptoms and the grim fate of its victims. The very acts of grouping a series of symptoms into a disease, naming the disease, explicating its causes, and attempting to treat it, are not only medical but social activities. The fluidity of disease categories, in fact, reflects a variety of cultural notions. In our culture, for example, tuberculosis was preceded by consumption. The older designation drew on what happened to the patient (the disease consumed her) and not on what the then invisible agent did (the tubercle bacillus caused the disease). Indeed, from a cultural-historical perspective, consumption and tuberculosis are two different diseases. They were attributed to different causes, invoked different treatments, and provoked over time different public responses. In another instance, if we think of sexually transmitted diseases, what we find, typically, is that the English called syphilis the French disease, the French ascribed it to the Italians, the Italians . . . and so on. This process of constructing a disease has its counterparts today: Is alcoholism to be labeled a moral failure or a congenital weakness? Is mental illness a myth or a reality? Only when medicine and culture are brought together can the varying interpretations of the causes of illness, the strategies created for its prevention, and the tactics deployed for its cure be fully understood.

The growing attention currently directed to these questions also expresses the new prominence of feminist studies. In many ways, feminist scholars were among the first to distinguish social from biological facts. They were drawn to this endeavor by their efforts to separate considerations of gender from sex, to ask whether the social roles ascribed to women were the outcome of cultural definitions (which could be changed) or biological facts (which were less tractable). It was not always as apparent as it is now that Sigmund Freud's readiness to assert that anatomy is destiny reflected a global cultural assumption and not an empirical finding from physiology.

Finally, the readiness to recognize how cultural considerations affect medical ideas and attitudes refers to a certain recent disillusionment with medicine in particular and with science more generally. Medical and scientific authority command less deference today than they did fifty years ago; to a post–atomic age generation, the equation of scientific breakthroughs with the advances and improvement of civilized life seems dubious. In a culture that is sensitive to the environmental impact of new technologies, an unmodified commitment to the slogan "Better living through chemistry" seems naive, if not actually mischievous. When patients can and do linger on respirators for weeks or months after they have lost and will never recover consciousness, it is not surprising that the ranks of those ready to question the authority of medical discourse are steadily growing.

The organization of this book is in part an extension of these intellectual and cultural developments. This work is not a survey of the history of medicine or a compendium of literary accounts of medicine. The groupings of materials are not in any conventional sense historical or literary. Rather, the materials are presented in ways or forms that facilitate the analysis of critical conceptions in the ongoing dialogue between medicine and culture.

Thus, the opening section, "The Human Form Divine," examines the body not simply as a biological and natural entity, but as a cultural construct. It introduces the three major traditions that have shaped Western ideas and beliefs about the body. Conceptions and representations of the body are influenced by a variety of meanings and values that are integral to, and yet apart from, the world of medicine. Thus, the classical body was represented by Greek and Roman physicians as naturally or inherently perfect; the Roman physician Galen considered the body to be a flawless example of the Creator's universal design. In turn, the Jewish and Christian traditions generally regarded the body as a sacred object, not only created by but belonging to God. In the Bible, God seals the covenant with his people by literally inscribing that covenant on the flesh of every male through circumcision.

This notion of the body as a kind of text that is written on for divine purposes survived well into medieval Christianity. Sister Chiara's body was opened up so that it could be searched for anatomical evidence of sainthood, while Sister Carlini's was minutely examined for the visible presence of Christ's stigmata. Medieval theorists imagined and described a magical body and were fascinated by the ways in which the body could serve as a vehicle for supernatural forces that worked unpredictable and incredible effects on its organs and functions. This same sense of profound mystery pervades the writings of the remarkable Renaissance physician Paracelsus.

The second section, "The Body Secularized," examines how the body came to be understood in naturalized and more mechanical terms, a process of change that illuminates the connections between early and modern medical theory and cultural change. The decline in magic was at once fostered by and expressed in new medical knowledge. Without a fundamental change in social values, the search for more precise anatomical knowledge, as conducted by the great anatomist Andreas Vesalius, would not have been allowed and could not have gone forward. The integrity or sacredness of the body no longer posed insurmountable barriers to the would-be investigator of anatomy. The deliberate search for regularity, order, laws and causes—in contradistinction to the belief that the natural world is controlled by miracles and by the forces of magic—was critical to a new understanding of the body in relation to the natural processes of health and disease. The domain in which such exploration was carried out was devoid of any deity and was characterized by the absence of any such intervening powers; knowledge and explanation were sought not in the discovery of divine purposes but in the complex fluids, organs, and functions of the body itself.

Even within this naturalistic orientation, however, there were always important differences at work. Plato and Hippocrates had been content to assist nature in redressing the disease-causing imbalance of the "humors," fluid substances that made up the constituent elements of the body; Paracelsus called for a more aggressive therapeutic strategy that would counteract toxins in the body by fighting poison with poison. As we approach the modern era, ever more radical explorations and interventions in the pursuit of knowledge begin, inexorably leading the investigator into the interior of the body itself. What we can call the visual imperative—the desire and the necessity to see in order to know—becomes dominant and supersedes the knowledge encoded in the once privileged treatises of ancient and medieval medicine. As Vesalius and William Harvey asserted and demonstrated, the visible, readable, decodable text of the naturalized body displaced all others as the compendium of what was to be known and mastered.

The third section, "Anatomy and Destiny," examines the variety of ideas from medicine and culture that attempt to conceptualize and represent the male and the female body. The sexual parts and reproductive organs of the body have always been sites of intense speculation and highly charged meaning. Thus, in almost every instance, ideas about the body become critical to defining the roles and functions ascribed respectively to the male and the female. From the classical to the modern era, the sex of men and women—the ascribed and asserted biological and anatomical differences between them—can be ascertained to be as much a cultural construction as are the more easily recognized social attributes of gender. The texts by Edward Clarke and Mary Putnam Jacobi illustrate how culture and medicine interacted to shape both sex and gender, in the process defining women's bodies and their functions as abnormal and even pathological. This interaction led to a secularized and scientific formulation that turned out to be not very different from the moral and religious notions expressed in such fifteenth-century texts on witchcraft as the *Malleus Maleficarum,* in which female sexuality was linked to evil and danger.

Modern medicine's secularization of sexuality took many forms, serving sometimes to destabilize—and sometimes to bolster—prevailing values and concepts. Freud's theories clearly did both. Although Freud vigorously affirmed the essential healthiness and normality of female sexuality, he also defined it as a lesser version of, or complement to, male drives and desires. At the same time, he designated the reproductive organs as the determinants of what he believed to be the moral and psychological destinies of each sex. Alfred Kinsey's and Mary Jane Sherfey's studies, in contrast, served to undermine traditional views. Drawing upon, among other things, research in animal behavior, Kinsey argued for the inherent naturalness and normalcy of homosexual behavior among human primates; so, too, Sherfey brought modern findings in embryology to bear on medical science's phallocentric notions about the biological development of males and females. How developments of this kind affected the cultural debate on sex and gender is made manifest in Simone de Beauvoir's pathbreaking book, which challenged the ideology of sexism and the status of women as the inferior "second" sex. Moreover, all of these materials make abundantly clear that separating medical findings from cultural values is not only a futile but a simplistic undertaking, and may end up by endowing medical "fact" with unwarranted authority.

The fourth section, "Psyche and Soma," explores the persistent effort to understand the connections between psyche and soma, the ongoing mystery of how mind, body, and "soul" are related. The Greek physician Hippocrates, for example, focused on demystifying the sacred disease of epilepsy, transforming it into a disorder that could be explained in natural and empirical terms; by contrast, St. Augustine, as a Christian philosopher, strove to anchor the ontological implications of the mind/body question within the revelations of Genesis. The enigmatic operations and natural influencings of mind and body upon each other fascinated the French essayist Montaigne and the English poet Wordsworth. These relations are just as relevant to William Styron's extraordinary effort to write about the terrifying physical and psychological burdens of deep depression.

The pioneer figures in psychoanalysis, Sigmund Freud and Josef Breuer, were no less determined to solve the mind/body puzzle, and their *Studies on Hysteria* uncovered many of the psychological mechanisms that underlay seemingly somatic illnesses and symptomatologies. Freud's own work carried a debt to the nineteenth-century French physician Philippe Pinel. As one of the first advocates of "moral" or psychological therapy for the insane, Pinel defined the mentally disturbed patient as someone whose story was clinically relevant to his illness, a notion that came to later fruition in Freud's theoretical elaboration and application of the "talking cure." Like Pinel, Freud grappled with questions fundamental to the study of psychopathology: Can the mind be diseased in the same way as the body is? Can disease be purely psychological? How does one locate, conceptualize, and treat such disease? It is impossible to understand or evaluate current cultural attitudes without reckoning with some of his answers to these questions.

The fifth section, "The Contaminated and the Pure," illustrates how moral connotations are embedded in the social and medical construction of disease. Disease is associated with that which is taboo, contaminated, and filthy, particularly when it is supposed that disease poses a danger to the public health. The report of the English reformer Edwin Chadwick, founder of the public health movement, is an outstanding case in point. His investigations of the dismal sanitary conditions of the laboring classes of mid-nineteenth-century England make clear that the effort to eliminate the "filthiness" of the poor was inseparable from the simultaneous effort to control their potentially radical and disruptive political tendencies. Cleanliness is linked not only to godliness but to political stability. By the same token, healthy behavior folds into a special and capitalistic definition of moral behavior. Implicit in the accounts that Chadwick includes is the idea that the poor are in general responsible for both their poverty and their diseases; were it not for their wasteful and corrupt habits and lax morals, they would as a group be both prosperous and healthy.

Not until the development of the germ theory did the moral rehabilitation of those suffering from contagious diseases begin. The discoveries of Ignaz Semmelweis, Joseph Lister, and Louis Pasteur all worked to transform once again cultural notions of disease and the ways by which modern society perceives, represents, and responds to its threat. Their writings are examples of how medical findings and theories can have the most profound impact on social perceptions. At the same time, a close reading of these selections yields critical insights into the making and writing of scientific texts, for modern society shapes not only the research agenda but also the ways its findings are presented and received. Although not literary productions in the common sense of the term, scientific reports nonetheless have a distinctive tone, style, and format that marks them as belonging to a genre all their own.

The intersection of values and medicine is nowhere more apparent than in the expectations and norms that are supposed to guide the behavior of the physician. The sixth section, "The Healer," demonstrates how the values and qualities that the good doctor should embody have shifted dramatically over time; nevertheless, a number of critical themes recur. From the time of Hippocrates down through the twentieth century, the physician has been peculiarly privileged to examine the body of the patient and to pry into any and all of its secrets; but this exceptional privilege also brings ethical responsibilities that place a special burden on physicians. Medical oaths have no precise counterpart among the other professions; in these oaths, the distinction between the private and the professional life of the doctor disappears, and virtue—or virtuous behavior—has ascribed to it both exceptional emphasis and importance. As the selections by Zora Neale Hurston and Sara Lawrence Lightfoot demonstrate, actual practice, whether it concerns patient care or medical school admissions policies, often falls short of the ideal.

The seventh section, "The Experimenter," makes clear that it is not always apparent to whom physicians owe their ultimate allegiance: Is it to the patient, or is it to the wider society in its search for useful knowledge? Balancing this dual allegiance to the patient and to society through medical science has not always been easy or successful. This dilemma is exemplified by Edward Jenner's experimental research into the efficacy of smallpox vaccination. His combined social standing and medical authority allowed him to convert his rural community into a virtual laboratory. We should note what passed at that time as an individual's consent to be the subject of medical experimentation, but we should note as well how Jenner "impartially" used his own family as part of his investigations.

This section also demonstrates how the role of innovation has been steadily foregrounded as medicine increasingly comes to be perceived as a scientific discipline. The nineteenth-century French physician Claude Bernard struggled heroically to balance a commitment to scientific method with the ethical requirements that are owed to patients. Others were less certain that the balance could be sustained. As is shown in section 6, the first great American woman physician, Elizabeth Blackwell, warned repeatedly about the dehumanizing sides of the ideology of modern science and the price that would be paid for medicine's wholesale adoption of it. In the terms we have been using here, acute tensions continue to exist between cultural values and scientific values, and such tensions will be periodically resolved in different ways at different times.

The eighth section, "The Institutionalization of Doctors and Patients," reveals that what might be thought of as the quintessential medical institution, the hospital, occupies not only a medical but a social space as well. How this space was formed and structured, who occupied it, and what rules and values governed it, form the focus of these readings. The essay by Philippe Pinel makes clear how the hospital, once among the most despised of social institutions, became a temple of science. The new hospital embodied a new way of seeing the patient as the carrier of the disease, of constructing medical knowledge, and of training physicians. As the French moralist and philosopher Michel Foucault powerfully indicated, these advances were made at the expense of the sick poor. Those who were both poor and very ill struck an implicit bargain with their doctors and their society: They gave their bodies over to medical science and teaching in exchange for "free" care. George Orwell's experience in a Paris hospital in the 1930s dramatically illustrates the extent to which this clinical and social objectification of the poor continued into our own time to dehumanize both physician and patient.

On the other hand, however, two mid-nineteenth-century hospital reformers, Dorothea Dix and Florence Nightingale, offered far more benign views of the hospital. Dix pleaded for the confinement of the insane on the grounds that an institutional asylum would be a curative as well as a more human setting for them. Nightingale argued that the hospital could be converted into a moral and efficient environment, and she set forth measures to purify and restructure it to this end. Throughout these discussions it is palpably evident that considerations of social status as well as of medical science shape the place, the style, and the function of the hospital in society. In virtually identical fashion, the U.S. Senate hearings on the Tuskegee experiments make clear the extent to which considerations of class, race, and gender determine the practice of medicine in our own society.

The concluding section, "Pain, Suffering, and Death," surveys the subjective experiences of patients, which are all too often filtered out of medical discourse and overlooked in medical practice. Both Frances Burney's and Jean Stafford's accounts of their surgeries, although separated in their composition by some 125 years, convey in vivid detail the intense physical suffering incurred when bodily integrity is violated. Together with William Cowper's account of his mental illness and the writings of Paul Monette on AIDS, such readings demonstrate the impossibility of separating psychological from physical pain. Just how difficult it is for physicians to respond to patients' pain is apparent both in James Simpson's account of how physicians reacted to the discovery of anesthesia in the mid–nineteenth century and in Ernest Hemingway's brilliant short story "Indian Camp." Physicians must interpret as well as empathize with patients' pain, and the two goals are often at cross-purposes.

Moreover, anyone who would doubt the profound effects that cultural attitudes have on medical practice need do nothing more than consult, examine, and analyze the arguments that doctors presented against the use of anesthesia to relieve pain.

Medicine's ability to filter out—or even to deny and negate—subjective meaning is seen at its extreme in the Harvard Medical School Committee's effort to establish the cessation of brain activity as the moment of death. The Harvard statement presents an image of the body as essentially constructed by medical technology, an object whose primary value is located in its reusable parts for organ transplantation. In contrast, Pius XII's pronouncement addresses the moral and religious concerns that are evoked by the body, and continues a dialogue that runs through the entirety of this volume.

The relationship between medicine and culture as it unfolds here involves us directly in the core beliefs and values that shape both our individual lives and our collective responses. Those beliefs and values, as we grow more conscious of them, become part of an important and engrossing story, a history that is only now beginning to be told.

PART 1

The Human Form Divine

The Bible (6th Century B.C.)

The Pentateuch, or the first five books of the Bible, was codified in the late sixth century B.C., shortly after the return of the Hebrews to Palestine from their exile in Babylon. To a degree that does not hold for any other text, these writings can be said to have inaugurated and shaped an entire civilization. The Pentateuch, or Chumash, is, above all else, the story of the evolution of a people, beginning with the creation of the first human beings. Throughout this record, the relationship between creator and creature, the divine and the human, is seen as the single most important element in history. The primary medium through which this ineluctable relationship makes itself felt is the human body. Fashioned in the image of the creator, Adam and Eve become the parents of a nation that inscribes its covenant with God on the bodies of its male children, conceding God's dominion over the processes of human procreation and the bringing forth of successive generations. A history of this covenant in the flesh, these five books stand as an originative moment in Western civilization's construction of the human body as divine artifact. The site of wounding and of regeneration, of the abominable and of the holy, the body exists as the semiological canvas of the creator, the inscribed text that gives witness to his signature in all things.

GENESIS

1.26 Then God said, "Let us make man in our image, after our likeness; and let them have dominion over the fish of the sea, and over the birds of the air, and over the cattle, and over all the earth, and over every creeping thing that creeps upon the earth." 27 So God created man in his own image, in the image of God he created him; male and female he created them. 28 And God blessed them, and God said to them, "Be fruitful and multiply, and fill the earth and subdue it; and have dominion over the fish of the sea and over the birds of the air and over every living thing that moves upon the earth." 29 And God said, "Behold, I have given you every plant yielding seed which is upon the face of all the earth, and every tree with seed in its fruit; you shall have them for food. 30 And to every beast of the earth, and to every bird of the air, and to everything that creeps on the earth, everything that has the breath of life, I have given every green plant for food." And it was so. 31 And God saw everything that he had made, and behold it was very good. And there was evening and there was morning, a sixth day.

From *The Oxford Annotated Bible with Apocrypha* (Revised Standard Version), ed. Herbert G. May and Bruce M. Metzger (New York: Oxford University Press, 1965). Copyright 1952 by the Division of Christian Education of the National Council of Churches of Christ in the U.S.A.

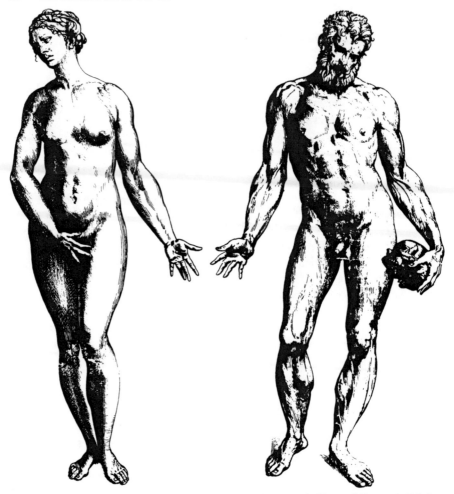

1. *Woodcut of female nude from Andreas Vesalius,* Suorum de Humani Corporis Fabrica Librorum Epitome *(Basle: Johannes Oporinus, 1543). Wellcome Institute Library, London.*

2. *Woodcut of male nude from Andreas Vesalius,* Suorum de Humani Corporis Fabrica Librorum Epitome *(Basle: Johannes Oporinus, 1543). Wellcome Institute Library, London. In portraying the male and female bodies, Jan Stefan von Kalkar drew on classical as well as Renaissance images and ideas of physical beauty. Behind these images stood a rich cultural heritage of iconography that centered on the figures of Adam and Eve as the embodiment of the Creator's handiwork, as the primordial emblems of the human form divine. Von Kalkar did, however, encode within the perfection of his figures the devastating consequences of the Fall. The mortality of the flesh is doubly signified by the female's gesture of concealment and the male's gesture of revelation, which leads the viewer to equate her genitalia with the skull he holds: What is hidden by the female is exposed by the male as the cradle of death.*

2.4 These are the generations of the heavens and the earth when they were created. In the day that the LORD God made the earth and the heavens, 5 when no plant of the field was yet in the earth and no herb of the field had yet sprung up—for the LORD God had not caused it to rain upon the earth, and there was no man to till the ground; 6 but a mist went up from the earth and watered the whole face of the ground— 7 then the LORD God formed man of dust from the ground, and breathed into his nostrils the breath of life; and man became a living being. 8 And the LORD God planted a garden in Eden, in the east; and there he put the man whom he had formed. 9 And out of the ground the LORD God made to grow every tree that is pleasant to the sight and good for food, the tree of life also in the midst of the garden, and the tree of the knowledge of good and evil.

15 The LORD God took the man and put him in the garden of Eden to till it and keep it. 16 And the LORD God commanded the man, saying, "You may freely eat of every tree of the garden; 17 but of the tree of the knowledge of good and evil you shall not eat, for in the day that you eat of it you shall die."

18 Then the LORD God said, "It is not good that the man should be alone; I will make him a helper fit for him." 19 So out of the ground the LORD God formed every beast of the field and every bird of the air, and brought them to the man to see what he would call them; and whatever the man called every living creature, that was its name. 20 The man gave names to all cattle, and to the birds of the air, and to every beast of the field; but for the man there was not found a helper fit for him. 21 So the LORD God caused a deep sleep to fall upon the man, and while he slept took one of his ribs and closed up its place with flesh; 22 and the rib which the LORD God had taken from the man he made into a woman and brought her to the man. 23 Then the man said,

> "This at last is bone of my bones
> and flesh of my flesh;
> she shall be called Woman,
> because she was taken out of Man."

24 Therefore a man leaves his father and his mother and cleaves to his wife, and they become one flesh. 25 And the man and his wife were both naked, and were not ashamed.

17.1 When Abram was ninety-nine years old the LORD appeared to Abram, and said to him, "I am God Almighty; walk before me, and be blameless. 2 And I will make my covenant between me and you, and will multiply you exceedingly." 3 Then Abram fell on his face; and God said to him, 4 "Behold, my covenant is with you, and you shall be the father of a multitude of nations. 5 No longer shall your name be Abram, but your name shall be Abraham; for I have made you the father of a multitude of nations. 6 I will make you exceedingly fruitful; and I will make nations of you, and kings shall come forth from you. 7 And I will establish my covenant between me and you and your descendants after you throughout their generations for an everlasting covenant, to be God to you and to your descendants after you. 8 And I will give to you, and to your descendants after you, the land of your sojournings, all the land of Canaan, for an everlasting possession; and I will be their God."

9 And God said to Abraham, "As for you, you shall keep my covenant, you and your descendants after you throughout their generations. 10 This is my covenant, which you shall keep, between me and you and your descendants after you: Every male among you shall be circumcised. 11 You shall be circumcised in the flesh of your foreskins, and it shall be a sign of the covenant between me and you. 12 He that is eight days old among you shall be circumcised; every male throughout your generations, whether born in your house, or bought with your money from any for-eigner who is not of your offspring, 13 both he that is born in your house and he that is bought with your money, shall be circumcised. So shall my covenant be in your flesh an everlasting covenant. 14 Any uncircumcised male who is not circum-cised in the flesh of his foreskin shall be cut off from his people; he has broken my covenant."

15 And God said to Abraham, "As for Sar'ai your wife, you shall not call her name Sar'ai, but Sarah shall be her name. 16 I will bless her, and moreover I will give you a son by her; I will bless her, and she shall be a mother of nations; kings of peoples shall come from her." 17 Then Abraham fell on his face and laughed, and said to himself, "Shall a child be born to a man who is a hundred years old? Shall Sarah, who is ninety years old, bear a child?" 18 And Abraham said to God, "O that Ish'mael might live in thy sight!" 19 God said, "No, but Sarah your wife shall bear you a son, and you shall call his name Isaac. I will establish my covenant with him as an ever-lasting covenant for his descendants after him."

24.1 Now Abraham was old, well advanced in years; and the LORD had blessed Abraham in all things. 2 And Abraham said to his servant, the oldest of his house, who had charge of all that he had, "Put your hand under my thigh, 3 and I will make you swear by the LORD, the God of heaven and of the earth, that you will not take a wife for my son from the daughters of the Canaanites, among whom I dwell, 4 but will go to my country and to my kindred, and take a wife for my son Isaac." 5 The servant said to him, "Perhaps the woman may not be willing to follow me to this land; must I then take your son back to the land from which you came?" 6 Abraham said to him, "See to it that you do not take my son back there. 7 The LORD, the God of heaven, who took me from my father's house and from the land of my birth, and who spoke to me and swore to me, 'To your descendants I will give this land,' he will send his angel before you, and you shall take a wife for my son from there. 8 But if the woman is not willing to follow you, then you will be free from this oath of mine; only you must not take my son back there." 9 So the servant put his hand under the thigh of Abraham his master, and swore to him concerning this matter.

EXODUS

13.1 The LORD said to Moses, 2 "Consecrate to me all the first-born; whatever is the first to open the womb among the people of Israel, both of man and of beast, is mine."

3 And Moses said to the people, "Remember this day, in which you came out from

Egypt, out of the house of bondage, for by strength of hand the LORD brought you out from this place; no leavened bread shall be eaten.

11 "And when the LORD brings you into the land of the Canaanites, as he swore to you and your fathers, and shall give it to you, 12 you shall set apart to the LORD all that first opens the womb. All the firstlings of your cattle that are males shall be the LORD's. 13 Every firstling of an ass you shall redeem with a lamb, or if you will not redeem it you shall break its neck. Every first-born of man among your sons you shall redeem. 14 And when in time to come your son asks you, 'What does this mean?' you shall say to him, 'By strength of hand the LORD brought us out of Egypt, from the house of bondage. 15 For when Pharaoh stubbornly refused to let us go, the LORD slew all the first-born in the land of Egypt, both the first-born of man and the first-born of cattle. Therefore I sacrifice to the LORD all the males that first open the womb, but all the first-born of my sons I redeem.' 16 It shall be as a mark on your hand or frontlets between your eyes; for by a strong hand the LORD brought us out of Egypt."

LEVITICUS

26.9 "And I will have regard for you and make you fruitful and multiply you, and will confirm my covenant with you.

14 "But if you will not hearken to me, and will not do all these commandments, 15 if you spurn my statutes, and if your soul abhors my ordinances, so that you will not do all my commandments, but break my covenant, 16 I will do this to you: I will appoint over you sudden terror, consumption, and fever that waste the eyes and cause life to pine away. And you shall sow your seed in vain, for your enemies shall eat it.

38 "And you shall perish among the nations, and the land of your enemies shall eat you up. 39 And those of you that are left shall pine away in your enemies' lands because of their iniquity; and also because of the iniquities of their fathers they shall pine away like them.

40 "But if they confess their iniquity and the iniquity of their fathers in their treachery which they committed against me, and also in walking contrary to me, 41 so that I walked contrary to them and brought them into the land of their enemies; if then their uncircumcised heart is humbled and they make amends for their iniquity; 42 then I will remember my covenant with Jacob, and I will remember my covenant with Isaac and my covenant with Abraham, and I will remember the land."

27.1 The LORD said to Moses, 2 "Say to the people of Israel, When a man makes a special vow of persons to the LORD at your valuation, 3 then your valuation of a male from twenty years old up to sixty years old shall be fifty shekels of silver, according to the shekel of the sanctuary. 4 If the person is a female, your valuation shall be thirty shekels. 5 If the person is from five years old up to twenty years old, your valuation shall be for a male twenty shekels, and for a female ten shekels. 6 If the person is from a month old up to five years old, your valuation shall be for a male five shekels of silver, and for a female your valuation shall be three shekels of silver. 7 And if the person is sixty years old and upward, then your valuation for a male shall be fifteen shekels, and for a female ten shekels. 8 And if a man is too poor to pay your valuation, then he shall bring the person before the priest, and the priest shall value him; according to the ability of him who vowed the priest shall value him.

28 "But no devoted thing that a man devotes to the LORD, of anything that he has, whether of man or beast or of his inherited field, shall be sold or redeemed; every devoted thing is most holy to the LORD. 29 No one devoted, who is to be utterly destroyed from among men, shall be ransomed; he shall be put to death."

DEUTERONOMY

28.49 "The LORD will bring a nation against you from afar, from the end of the earth, as swift as the eagle flies, a nation whose language you do not understand, 50 a nation of stern countenance, who shall not regard the person of the old or show favor to the young, 51 and shall eat the offspring of your cattle and the fruit of your ground, until you are destroyed; who also shall not leave you grain, wine, or oil, the increase of your cattle or the young of your flock, until they have caused you to perish. 52 They shall besiege you in all your towns, until your high and fortified walls, in which you trusted, come down throughout all your land; and they shall besiege you in all your towns throughout all your land, which the LORD your God has given you. 53 And you shall eat the offspring of your own body, the flesh of your sons and daughters, whom the LORD your God has given you, in the siege and in the distress with which your enemies shall distress you. 54 The man who is the most tender and delicately bred among you will grudge food to his brother, to the wife of his bosom, and to the last of the children who remain to him; 55 so that he will not give to any of them any of the flesh of his children whom he is eating, because he has nothing left him, in the siege and in the distress with which your enemy shall distress you in all your towns. 56 The most tender and delicately bred woman among you, who would not venture to set the sole of her foot upon the ground because she is so delicate and tender, will grudge to the husband of her bosom, to her son and to her daughter, 57 her afterbirth that comes out from between her feet and her children whom she bears, because she will eat them secretly, for want of all things, in the siege and in the distress with which your enemy shall distress you in your towns.

58 "If you are not careful to do all the words of this law which are written in this book, that you may fear this glorious and awful name, the LORD your God, 59 then the LORD will bring on you and your offspring extraordinary afflictions, afflictions severe and lasting, and sicknesses grievous and lasting. 60 And he will bring upon you again all the diseases of Egypt, which you were afraid of; and they shall cleave to you. 61 Every sickness also, and every affliction which is not recorded in the book of this law, the LORD will bring upon you, until you are destroyed. 62 Whereas you were as the stars of heaven for multitude, you shall be left few in number; because you did not obey the voice of the LORD your God."

GALEN (ca. A.D. 130–201)

"The Hand"

By the Middle Ages and up until the Renaissance, no body of medical writing carried greater authority than that of Galen. Born in Pergamum, Asia Minor, Galen was tutored in mathematics and natural science by his father, an engineer, while attending Pergamum's school of philosophy. At the age of eighteen, shortly after his father had a dream indicating that his son should become a physician, Galen undertook the study of medicine. For the next several years, he traveled from city to city, absorbing new ideas and methods, particularly in Alexandria, the site of the ancient world's famous center for the study of anatomy. Upon returning to Pergamum, Galen obtained the prestigious post of physician to the gladiators, and three years later, he found himself in the midst of imperial Rome, sought out by families of high rank. One of Galen's patrons, the consul Flavius Boethius, who shared Galen's fascination with anatomy, built him a suitable room for dissection and hired scribes to set down verbatim reports of Galen's procedures, thereby preserving many of his techniques and observations. It was, in fact, at the suggestion of Flavius that sometime around 165 Galen began *De usu partium,* a project that would take seventeen books and ten years to complete. In 168, Galen's work on it was interrupted when he was summoned to court and was invited to accompany Marcus Aurelius on a campaign against the Marcomanni in the region along the Danube River. Although tempted by the prospect of battlefields littered with enemy corpses, Galen thought better of the offer and persuaded the emperor that he would be more useful in Rome, which was then being overrun by immigrant "specialists" competing for patients. Having never joined any particular sect or guild, Galen often found himself embroiled in polemics with those who condemned his eclecticism and independence of mind. One of the underlying arguments of *De usu partium,* for example, is aimed at the Epicureans, the medical sect that disputed the claim that the body's perfection of design gave proof of divine craftsmanship. Refuting such blasphemy and upholding Plato's belief in the Demiurge, Galen framed his treatise as "a sacred discourse," a "true hymn of praise to our Creator."

Just as every animal is said to be one because, having a certain individual circumscription, it is manifestly not joined to other animals at any point, so also its parts, the eye, nose, tongue, or encephalon, are said each to be one, because each clearly has a circumscription of its own. But if it were not joined to the neighboring parts at some point, but were altogether separate, then it would not be a part at all, but

From *On the Usefulness of the Parts of the Body,* ed. and trans. Margaret Tallmadge May (Ithaca, N.Y.: Cornell University Press, 1968).

simply one. Therefore, all bodies that do not have their own circumscription at every point and are not everywhere joined to others are called parts. And if this is true, animals will have many parts, some large, some small, and some also not divisible at all into another form.

The usefulness of all of them is related to the soul. For the body is the instrument of the soul, and consequently animals differ greatly in respect to their parts because their souls also differ. For some animals are brave and others timid; some are wild and others tame; and some are, so to speak, members of a state and work together for it, whereas others are, as it were, unsocial. In every case the body is adapted to the character and faculties of the soul. The horse is provided with strong hoofs and adorned with a mane, for truly it is a swift, proud animal and not faint-hearted. The strength of the brave, fierce lion, however, lies in its teeth and claws. So, too, with the bull and boar; the one has horns as its natural weapons, and the other tusks. On the other hand, since the deer and hare are timid animals, their bodies are fleet, but entirely unarmed and defenseless; for swiftness, I think, befits the timid and weapons are for the brave, and so Nature did not arm the one at all or strip naked the other. Now to man—for he is an intelligent animal and, alone of all creatures on earth, godlike—in place of any and every defensive weapon, she gave hands, instruments necessary for every art and useful in peace no less than in war. Hence he did not need horns as a natural endowment, since, whenever he desired, he could grasp in his hand a weapon better than a horn; for certainly swords and spears are larger weapons than horns and better suited for inflicting wounds. Neither did he need hoofs, for clubs and rocks can crush more forcibly than any hoof. Furthermore, nothing can be accomplished with either horns or hoofs without coming to close quarters, but a man's weapons are effective at a distance as well as near by, javelins and darts excelling horns, and rocks and clubs excelling hoofs. But, you say, a lion is swifter than a man. Well, what then? With his skillful hands man tamed the horse, an animal swifter than a lion, and, using a horse, he both escapes and pursues the lion, from his lofty seat striking down at him below. Surely then, man is not naked, easily wounded, defenseless, or unshod, but, whenever he wishes, may have a corslet of iron (an instrument harder to damage than any kind of skin), and sandals, weapons, and vestments of all sorts are at his disposal. In fact, the corslet is not his only protection, since he also has houses, towers, and city walls. If he were born with a horn or some other defensive weapon of the kind growing upon his hands, he could not use them at all to build a house or tower, or to make a spear or corslet or other similar things. With these hands of his, a man weaves himself a cloak and fashions hunting-nets, fish-nets and traps, and fine-meshed bird-nets, so that he is lord not only of animals upon the earth, but of those in the sea and the air also. Such is the hand of man as an instrument of defense. But, being also a peaceful and social animal, with his hands he writes laws for himself, raises altars and statues to the gods, builds ships, makes flutes, lyres, knives, fire-tongs, and all the other instruments of the arts, and in his writings leaves behind him commentaries on the theories of them. Even now, thanks to writings set down by the hand, it is yet possible for you to hold converse with Plato, Aristotle, Hippocrates, and the other Ancients.

Thus man is the most intelligent of the animals and so, also, hands are the instruments most suitable for an intelligent animal. For it is not because he has hands that he is the most intelligent, as Anaxagoras says, but because he is the most intelligent that he has hands, as Aristotle says, judging most correctly. Indeed, not by his hands, but by his reason has man been instructed in the arts. Hands are an instrument, as the lyre is the instrument of the musician, and tongs of the smith. Hence just as the lyre does not teach the musician or tongs the smith but each of them is a craftsman by virtue of the reason there is in him although he is unable to work at his trade without the aid of his instruments, so every soul has through its very essence certain faculties, but without the aid of instruments is helpless to accomplish what it is by Nature disposed to accomplish. In observing newborn animals striving to exert themselves before their parts are perfected, we can see clearly that it is not the bodily parts that lead the soul to be timid or brave or wise. Now I have often seen a young calf butting before its horns have sprouted, a colt kicking with hoofs still soft, a shote, quite small, trying to defend itself with jaws innocent of tusks, and a newborn puppy attempting to bite with its teeth still tender. For every animal has, untaught, a perception of the faculties of its own soul and the virtues resident in its parts. Or why else, when it is possible for the small boar to bite with his little teeth, does he not use them for battle instead of longing to use those which he does not yet have? How, then, is it possible to say that animals learn the usefulness of their parts from the parts themselves, when they obviously know their usefulness even before they have them? Now if you like, take three eggs, an eagle's, a duck's, and a serpent's; warm them, and in due season hatch them out; and you will see two of the animals that have been formed making trial of their wings even before they are able to fly, and the other, though still soft and weak, wriggling and struggling to crawl. And if you raise them to maturity under one and the same roof and then take them out in the open and let them go, the eagle will fly up high in the air, the duck will fly down onto some marshy lake, and the serpent will creep away into the earth. Afterwards, without having learned, the eagle, I think, will hunt its prey, the duck will swim, and the serpent lurk in its den. "For," says Hippocrates, "the instincts of animals are untaught." So it seems to me that the other animals acquire their skills by instinct rather than by reason, bees, for example, molding [their wax], ants working at their treasuries and labyrinths, and spiders spinning and weaving. I judge from the fact that they are untaught.

Now just as man's body is bare of weapons, so is his soul destitute of skills. Therefore, to compensate for the nakedness of his body, he received hands, and for his soul's lack of skill, reason, by means of which he arms and guards his body in every way and equips his soul with all the arts. For if he had been born with a natural weapon, he would have that one alone for all time, and just so, if he had one natural skill, he would lack the others. But since it was better for him to make use of all weapons and all the arts, he was endowed with no one of them at birth. Indeed, Aristotle was right when he said that the hand is, as it were, an instrument for instruments, and we might rightly say in imitation of him that reason is, as it were, an art for arts. For though the hand is no one particular instrument, it is the instrument for all instruments because it is formed by Nature to receive them all, and similarly, although reason is no one of the arts in particular, it would be an art for the arts because it is naturally disposed to take them all unto itself. Hence man, the only one of all the animals having an art for arts in his soul, should logically have an instrument for instruments in his body.

Come now, let us investigate this very important part of man's body, examining it to determine not simply whether it is useful or whether it is suitable for an intelligent animal, but whether it is in every respect so constituted that it would not have been better had it been made differently. One and indeed the chief characteristic of a prehensile instrument constructed in the best manner is the ability to grasp readily anything of whatever size or shape that man would naturally want to move. For this purpose, then, which was better—for the hand to be cleft into many divisions or to remain wholly undivided? Or does this need any discussion other than the statement that if the hand remained undivided, it would lay hold only on the things in contact with it that were of the same size as it happened to be itself, whereas, being subdivided into many members, it could easily grasp masses much larger than itself, and fasten accurately upon the smallest objects? For larger masses, the hand is extended, grasping them with the fingers spread apart, but the hand as a whole does not try to grasp the smallest objects, for they would escape if it did; the tips of two fingers are enough to use for them. Thus the hand is most excellently constituted for a firm grasp of things both larger and smaller than itself. Furthermore, if it was to be able to lay hold of objects of many different shapes, it was best for it to be divided into many differing members, as it now is, and for this purpose the hand is obviously adapted best of all prehensile instruments. Indeed, it can curve itself around a spherical body, laying hold of and encircling it from all sides; it surrounds firmly objects with straight or concave sides; and if this be true, then it will also clasp objects of all shapes, for they are all made up of three kinds of lines, convex, concave, and straight. Since, however, there are many bodies whose mass is too great for one hand alone to grasp, Nature made each the ally of the other so that both together, grasping such a body on opposite sides, are in no way inferior to one very large hand. For this reason, then, they face toward one another, since each was made for the sake of the other, and they have been formed equal to one another in every respect, a provision suitable for instruments which are to share the same action. Now when you have considered the largest objects that man can handle with both hands, such as a log or rock, then give heed, pray, to the smallest, such as a millet seed, a very slender thorn, or a hair, and then, when you have considered besides how very many bodies there are that range in size from the largest to the smallest, think of all this and you will find that man handles them all as well as if his hands had been made for the sake of each one of them alone. He takes hold of very small objects with the tips of two fingers, the thumb and forefinger, and slightly larger objects with the same two fingers, but not with just the tips; those still larger he grasps with three fingers, the thumb, forefinger, and middle finger, and if there are any larger yet, with four, and next, with five. After that the whole hand is used, and for still larger objects the other hand is brought up. The hand could act in none of these ways if it were not divided into fingers differently formed; for it was not enough in itself for the hand merely to be divided. What if there had been no finger opposing the four, as there is now, but all five of them had been produced side by side in one straight line? Is it not very clear that mere number would be useless, since an object to be held firmly must be either encircled from all sides or at least laid hold of from two opposite points? The ability to hold an object firmly would be destroyed if all the fingers had been produced side by side in one straight line, but as it is, with one finger set opposite the rest, this ability is nicely preserved; for this one finger has such a position and motion that by turning very slightly it acts with each of the four set opposite to it. Hence it was better for the hands to act as they do now, and Nature therefore gave them a structure suited to such actions.

Now it was necessary not only that the tips of two opposed fingers should act in fastening upon small objects, but that the tips should also be such as they now are, soft, round, and provided with nails. Thus if the ends of the fingers were composed not of flesh but of bone, it would be impossible for them ever to lay hold of small articles such as thorns or hairs, nor would this be possible if, though they were fleshy, the flesh were too soft and moist.

Only nails that come even with the ends of the fingers will best provide the service for the sake of which they were made. It is for this reason that Hippocrates too has said, "The nails neither to project beyond, nor to fall short of, the finger tips." Thus, it is when they have a duly proportioned size that they best fulfill the uses for which they were made. Of course, they are also useful for many other purposes; for example, when it is necessary to scrape, scratch, skin, or tear something apart. In fact, in nearly all the circumstances of life and in all the arts, especially those requiring precise manual skill, we need some instrument of the sort, but it is as a prehensile instrument for seizing small, hard objects that the hand most needs the fingernails.

All the parts of the body are in sympathy with one another, that is to say, all cooperate in producing one effect. The large parts, main divisions of the whole animal, such as the hands, feet, eyes, and tongue, were formed for the sake of the actions of the animal as a whole and all cooperate in performing them. But the smaller parts, the components of the parts I have mentioned, have reference to the work of the whole instrument. The eye, for example, is the instrument of sight, composed of many parts which all cooperate in one work, vision; it has some parts by means of which we see, others without which sight would be impossible, others for the sake of better vision, and still others to protect all these. This, moreover, is also true of all the other parts, the stomach, mouth, tongue, and feet, and true of the hands too, concerning which I now propose to speak. Now everyone knows what the work of the hands is (for it is very clear that they were formed for the sake of grasping), but everyone does not yet perceive that all parts of the hand are of such a nature and size that they cooperate in the one work performed by the whole instrument. Hippocrates, however, perceived it, . . .

I shall explain further just this one point of all those set forth by him in the passage cited, a thing most necessary for a physician to learn, but impossible to discover without careful reflection on the usefulness of the parts. And what is this thing? It is the recognition of what is the best construction for the body. Now clearly the best construction is that in which all the parts [of the instruments] contribute services sufficient for the actions of the instruments as a whole. Thus Hippocrates says,

"A good shape for the fingers, a wide space between, and the thumb opposite the forefinger," and if you ask again why this is so, the answer he has written is at hand: "Taken as a whole, all the parts in sympathy, but taken severally, the parts in each part cooperate for its work." What, then, is the work of the hand, the part we are now considering? Obviously, it is grasping. But how will all the fingers cooperate for this effect? They will cooperate, if the spaces between them are wide, and the thumb is opposed to the forefinger, for then every action the fingers perform will be well done. And so, if you are seeking to discover the proper form for the eye or nose, you will find it by correlating structure and action. In fact, this is your standard, measure, and criterion of proper form and true beauty, since true beauty is nothing but excellence of construction, and in obedience to Hippocrates you will judge that excellence from actions, not from whiteness, softness, or other such qualities, which are indications of a beauty meretricious and false, not natural and true. Hence the qualities a slave dealer would value in a body are not the same ones that Hippocrates would commend. Perhaps you think that in Xenophon's story Socrates is jesting when he is arguing over beauty with those who were supposedly the most handsome men of their time. Now if he were speaking simply of beauty without reference to action and without using action as the one measure of beauty, then perhaps he would be only joking, but since in the whole discussion Socrates relates the beauty of construction of the parts to the excellence of their action, we must no longer believe that he is only joking, but that he is also very much in earnest. Of course it is characteristic of the Socratic muse constantly to mingle grave and gay. Well, what I have said thus far is amply sufficient to show the usefulness of my proposed task and to explain how the thoughts and sayings of the Ancients should be understood.

PARACELSUS (1493-1541)

Volumen Medicinae Paramirum

The son of a physician, Aureolus Theophrastus Bombastus von Hohenheim —better known as Paracelsus—was born in a small town near Zurich. At sixteen, he entered the University of Basle, but soon tired of it and left to study chemistry with the Abbot of Sponheim. Fascinated with chemistry, he visited the mines of the Tyrol, where he examined the properties of ores, metals, and mineral waters, as well as the diseases and occupational hazards of miners. After extensive travel across Europe, during which he often kept company with common vagrants and petty criminals to study their habits and living conditions, Paracelsus returned to Basle and, in 1526, was appointed its town physician. His experiences had convinced him that many chemicals—sulphur, antimony, mercury, and iron—had therapeutic properties, and he strove to introduce them into the physician's armamentarium. Breaking with tradition, he held his lectures in German, not Latin, grounding his commentaries in his own experiences and observations rather than in the writings of Galen and Avicenna. Demoting the theory of the four humors, Paracelsus subsumed it under a system based on the five *Entia*, or Powers, that held absolute dominion over body and mind. The *Volumen Medicinae Paramirum* is the manifesto that sets forth this new system and rails against the ignorance of those who continued to follow the old. In his effort to invent an adequate vocabulary for his revolutionary ideas about medicine, the cosmos, and the body, Paracelsus often resorted to a style and idiom that were mystifying, paradoxical, and provocative. Disturbed by his radical theories and his blatant attacks on colleagues, medical authorities forced Paracelsus to flee Basle, and after ten years as a wanderer, he died in Salzburg.

This *Parenthesis* has five *Tracts* and the subject of each *Tract* is one power (*Ens*). It behooves you to take note, that there are five powers (*Entia*) which constitute and bring forth all diseases. Five powers signify five origins. This is to be understood in this way that there are five origins the nature of each of which it is to bring about all diseases, to give birth to them mightily, however many diseases have ever and anon been in the world or are still with us or will appear in the future. You physicians should pay attention to these powers so [as not to fall into the error of believing] that all diseases come from one power only or are due to one cause. Rather, there are five, that is, five powers which produce potentially all diseases. Take as an example of this the following: You recognize in your practice a disease called pestilence. Now the question is where does it come from. You answer me and say, from a

---

From *Volumen Medicinae Paramirum*, trans. Kurt F. Leidecker, *Supplements to the Bulletin of the History of Medicine*, no. 11 (Baltimore: Johns Hopkins University Press, 1949).

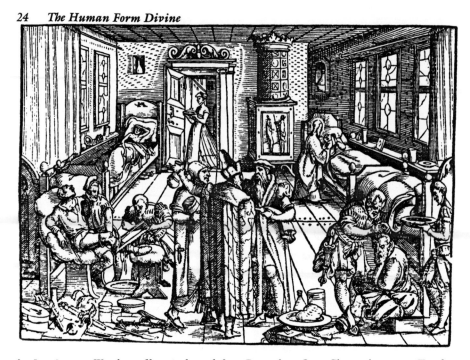

3. *Jost Amman, Woodcut of hospital ward, from Paracelsus,* Opus Chyrurgicum . . . *(Frank-furt: M. Lechler for S. Feyrabend & S. Huter, 1565). Wellcome Institute Library, London. Three doctors of medicine stand in the foreground flanked by several surgeons. The doctor on the right cradles an enema bag while the one in the center holds aloft a urine flask. As the elegantly dressed doctors stand arguing and theorizing, the surgeons, with their shirtsleeves up, vigorously pursue their craft. Amman depicts surgery and medicine within the terms of a pivotal Renaissance dichotomy—the active as opposed to the contemplative life—and reflects Paracelsus's iconoclastic preference for the "hands-on" approach of the surgeons as opposed to the "hands-off" approach of the physicians.*

breach of nature. There you are talking like the nature-healers. But the astronomer asserts that the course of the heavens brings about such a disease. Now, which one is correct? My decision would be that both of you are right. From nature is derived one [form of pestilence], from the heavenly bodies hails another, and others come from three additional quarters. For, nature is a power, also the heavenly body is a power. Thus you will recognize that there are five kinds of pestilence. We are not speaking of the character of these kinds of pestilence, their nature, form or shape, but of their origin, whence they are brought forth, let them be afterwards what they may. Accordingly we say that our body is subjected to five powers, and that each power has all diseases under it and with them holds sway over our body. For, there are five kinds of dropsy, five kinds of jaundice, five kinds of fever, five kinds of cancer; the same with other diseases.

Five powers (*Entia*) thus having been enumerated it behooves you medical practi-tioners to know what is recognized as a power. A power is a cause or a thing which has the ability to govern the body. But, your position, wherein you blunder, is that you are maintaining against us that all pestilence springs from the humors or from what is in the body. Here you are quite in error. Keep in mind what it is that poisons the body and not so much that the body lies there in a poisoned state. Do not imagine, furthermore, that all diseases, or any one of them originate exclusively in the body. The body must be in a virulent condition, or something there must be that makes it so. For, the body itself does not offer cause for any disease. With regard to this we lay it down that there are five things that corrupt body and dispose it to be diseased, a condition which it may not resist, but must suffer to be irritated by. They are the ones that lord it over man in the body which they vex according to their nature. Each power is thus so constituted that all diseases, without exception, are subject to it. There are, therefore, five fires that hold sway over the body, for the body must remain passive until some fire descends upon it and causes a disease in it. In dealing with a paralytic condition, the medical practitioner should consider which fire, which power, has provoked the paralysis. Because, there are five of them, as many as there are of diseases, based in five causes, that is, five origins. And, the practitioner who does not understand this is blind. For no power responds to the cure meant for another.

Having indicated the five powers, our next task is to recognize them. Although the ancients, our predecessors, would, if born again, be astonished and estranged by our medical science, that should be the least of our worries. Nevertheless we do not want to have their prescriptions discarded, but would like to extract their essence. To bring the book of introductory remarks to a close and impart to you an understanding of those powers that exercise control and violent coercion over our body, let us, then, begin with the *Parenthesis* as follows.

The *First Tract* of the *Parenthesis* tells how the heavenly bodies are endowed with a potency and a nature which have control over our body in such a manner that it must remain passive and accept whatever the heavenly bodies work in us. This potential of the heavenly bodies is called the *Ens Astrale* and is the first power which we are subjected to.

The second potential which governs us with an iron hand and brings on disease within us is the *Ens Veneni*. In this connection it is well to note that if the heavenly bodies do not cause us any harm and reside healthily within us, the *Ens Veneni* might dispatch us, since we are subject to it, must remain passive and are unable to ward it off.

The third is a force which diseases and weakens our body even though the two powers just mentioned dwell benevolently and happily within us. It is called *Ens Naturale*. This is the power which causes our very body to fall prey to disease in virtue of its aberrations and self-inflicted cleavages. Through it arise many other diseases and all diseases without exception even though all the other powers be benevolent.

The fourth power bears witness to the mighty spirits that disease and weaken and overpower our body. We must remain passive with respect to it and permit entrance into our body of those diseases that this power inflicts upon us.

The fifth power which exposes our body to diseases even though all the others lend us support with happiness and health, is the *Ens Dei.* Be sure to attend well to this power so you will be in a position to recognize the nature of every disease.

Having thus characterized and explained the different powers, you should remember that each one of them comprises all diseases under it so that we get five kinds of pestilence. In other words, one each from the *Ens Astrale,* from the *Ens Veneni,* from the *Ens Naturale,* from the *Ens Spirituale* and from the *Ens Dei.* All other diseases are of a like nature. Hence it is well to remember and ponder that the diseases are not due to one cause alone, but to five, whereas until now you have been getting along with only one power, and that one erroneously and wrongly, basically.

Lend us your ear further, if you will. The control over our body is apportioned among five princes who have to lord it over us and cause our body to fall ill. They are the *Ens Astrale,* the *Ens Veneni,* the *Ens Naturale,* the *Ens Spirituale* and the *Ens Dei.* This subject matter will be treated in the five *Tracts* of the *Parenthesis,* how the *Ens Astrale* has to govern man in his body, disease and kill it, the same as all other powers do. But before we begin the *Parenthesis* be warned that we intend to write as the pagans do, although we are born Christian. What moves us, however, in this is conviction. Were we to write as a Christian, the four *Entia Astrale, Veneni, Naturale* and *Spirituale* would have to be omitted and remain unrepresented. These are not in the Christian tradition, but are pagan. Yet, the last power with which we shall conclude, is a Christian conception. Even the pagan conception which we are describing in the four powers should not jeopardize faith. On the contrary, it should make our mental powers keener. We call it a pagan conception because it is foreign to belief in Christ; and we own that all of you who study and deal with the nature of the four powers are Christian by birth.

But what makes us call the first four powers pagan and the last one divine, will be explained to some extent in the same *Tract.* However, to be perfect in the right fundamentals of truth, we shall say the final and comprehensive words about this last power in the book of faith with which we conclude, where we shall apologize for the pagan conception and reaffirm the faith as one of the faithful who does not have a mind to push further into the pagan subject. This, we entreat you Christians, follow through with us and take proper cognizance of our book that is meant for those of faith.

TRACT CONCERNING THE "ENS ASTRALE"

. . . [Y]ou should understand by *Ens Astrale* the following. It is something we do not see, something which sustains life in us and in everything that is alive and sentient. This something derives from the heavenly bodies. To illustrate: A fire which burns must have wood. Otherwise there would be no fire. Thus you observe that fire is a vital thing, yet it cannot live without wood. Now for the application. Although this is too clumsy an illustration you must bear with it. The body is the wood, the life within it the fire. Now, life derives its substance from the body. Consequently, the body must possess something which prevents it from being consumed by life but, on the contrary, continues to exist. That is the thing concerning which we tell you as the *Ens.* It hails from the firmament. You say, and rightly so, if there were no air, all things would fall to the ground, and all that has life here below would stifle and die. By the same token remember that there is something else that sustains the body, the same body which sustains life. That you may do without as little as the air. The air is sustained in and by this something; this away, and the air would disappear. The firmament lives by virtue of this something, and if it were not in the firmament, the firmament would vanish. That something we call the M[YSTERIUM]. For there is nothing in the whole universe created above this, nothing higher, nothing is more important for the physician to bear in mind. Observe now carefully: This M[YSTERIUM], we say, does not originate in the firmament, nor has it sprung from it, nor does the firmament send it to us,—nothing of the kind. Nevertheless mark well that this M[YSTERIUM] is supporting all creatures, in heaven and on earth; and all elements live by and in it. But as to an explanation, take to heart what was said in *De Primo Creato* and what we are going to elaborate in the present discourse on the M[YSTERIUM].

As to the topic M[YSTERIUM], an example may be given to illustrate how the vapors of the planets cause damage to us. A pond, in the possession of its proper M[YSTERIUM], abounds in fishes. If the cold, however, becomes too severe, the pond freezes over and the fishes die because the M[YSTERIUM] is too frigid for the nature of the water. This frigidity does not originate with the M[YSTERIUM], but from the heavenly body which possesses this property and causes same. In the same way acts also the heat of the sun, so that the water becomes too warm and the fishes die for the reasons aforementioned. Just as these two, heat and cold, are two properties of some heavenly bodies bringing such things to pass, so there are others which make the M[YSTERIUM] sour, bitter, sweet, sharp, arsenic and the like to suit many hundred tastes and so forth. This great change of the M[YSTERIUM] is equivalent to changes in the body. Be on the lookout for the way in which the heavenly bodies pollute the M[YSTERIUM] causing us to fall sick and die, depending on the nature of their vapors. No physician should be surprised at that. For, however many kinds of poison there are on earth, there are as many and more in the stars. Let each physician be reminded that no disease is produced without a poison. For, poison is the origin of every disease, and all diseases are brought on by poison, be they of the body or a wound, nothing excluded.

TRACT CONCERNING THE "ENS VENENI"

Having explained above the *Ens Astrale,* we shall now expound the *Ens Veneni* which is the second power that diseases our body. Let us state right here the same thesis which we expressed in the *Ens Astrale,* that our body is coerced and made to suffer by five powers. But in order that you may understand us better and see our reasons, we let the discussion of these powers rest with the prefaces and shall proceed with an explanation of the thesis of the *Ens Veneni* as follows.

You know that man's body must have a sustenance, that is a driving force by which it is kept up and nourished; and where that is lacking, there is no life. Therefore, take to heart that he who created and made our body, made the food as well as the body, but not so perfect. Understand this to mean that the body has been given us without poison, and there is no poison in it. But in what we must offer the body as food, in that there is poison. In other words, the body has been created perfect, but not the other. Now, in that other animals and fruit are food for us, they may also be poison to us. However, as far as they themselves are concerned, they are neither poison nor food. In themselves they are creatures as perfect as we are. Yet, when they become food for us, they constitute a poison for us. What is not poison for itself is nevertheless poison for us.

Furthermore, it should be understood that everything is perfect within itself and well made in all its parts. But, if used as an end, it is either good or evil. Take a steer which eats grass: It eats his own poison as well as takes up healthy food. For, in the grass is contained poison and health stuff, nourishment and medicine. But in itself the grass is not poison. The food and drink that man takes up into himself is either poison or nourishment to him. But beyond that, understand, what he eats is not its own poison.

In what we are thus explaining know that we are referring to two different subjects: The one concerns man (barring the nature of animals and other growing things), the other concerns his intake. To make comprehension easier, note that the one thing that is in man is the great world of nature; the other is the poison that penetrates nature. In order to tell you all in the *Parenthesis,* we call your attention to the fact that God has created all things perfect in themselves, but imperfect if they serve one another's ends. This is the topic of our second *Ens,* that of *Veneni.* However, you should also be aware that we are not maintaining that God has appointed an alchemist to just watch over man or the creatures in their own functions. But he has appointed an alchemist for us to convert the imperfect which we have to utilize into something useful to us so that we may not consume the poison which we take in amongst the things that are good, as a poison, but eliminate it from the good.

What we are going to relate to you regarding this alchemist, mark it well.

Since every thing, in itself, is perfect but in relation to some other thing is either a poison or a good, our reasoning leads us to believe that God has appointed an alchemist for him who has to use the other for an end and which enters him, or is administered to him, as a poison or something beneficent. Such a great artist is he that he segregates the two, the poison in its proper bag, the good substance into the body. In the manner indicated it behooves you to understand and recognize well our thesis.

Once again it is well to take note that in every thing which man must needs take in, there is a poison hidden among what is good to wit: There is an *Essentia* and a *Venenum* in everything. *Essentia* is that which sustains man, *Venenum* that which makes him ill. The latter is contained in every foodstuff and is working against the animal that uses it, nothing excepted.

You physicians note in particular that so long as the body exists by food, has to have it, and is subject to it, it must take it as it is found under both aspects, good and ill, nothing separated, and let the alchemist analyze it.

Observe now with care: If the alchemist is not on the job and the poison is not eliminated perfectly from the good according to the rules of the art, there arises from the poison and the good ingredients combined a putrefaction and, subsequently, a product of digestion. It is that which indicates to us the disease of a person. For, all the diseases that a person may have from the *Ens Veneni* hail from the putrefied product of digestion. Digestion, to be sure, ought to be tempered with the alchemist not favoring either of the parties. But if the digestion is imperfect, the alchemist does not make full adequate use of his instrument. Decay is the consequence. This, then, becomes the mother of all diseases. As such it should be thoroughly impressed upon you physicians in favor of your extensive evasions. For, depending on its present state and course, decay will poison the body.

For example, water which is pure and clear may be tinctured with any color you desire. The body is thus like the water, and decay is the coloring matter. There is, indeed, no color except it have its origin in poison and is an indication and symbol of its poison.

TRACT CONCERNING THE "ENS NATURALE"

Since you physicians probably have developed an odd conception in your writings concerning the *Ens Naturale,* we shall not be bothered with that. Rather, we shall point out to you an *Ens Naturale,* the third *Ens* according to our *Parenthesis,* from which every disease might take its origin, . . . We are not employing in our interpretation of it your mother tongue nor the language you acquired while sitting in school and getting your first lessons, . . . Be reminded of the new order and the simplicity of the old men who are passé. The *Ens Naturale* is to be explained in this fashion. You are acquainted from astronomy with the problem of influences, the firmament and all heavenly bodies. . . . Just as you recognize the firmament in the heavens, so there is an identical constellation, firmament and the rest in man. We have nothing to be ashamed of as far as your doctrine is concerned according to which you call man a microcosm. The term is justly chosen. But you have never really understood it, and your explanations are obscure and guarded. Follow us in our interpretation of what we mean by microcosm. Similarly as the heavens are in themselves with their entire firmament and constellations, excepting nothing, so is man constellated mightily in and by himself. As the firmament is the heavens by itself and is not governed by any creature, so little is the firmament, that is in man, lorded over by other creatures. It just is a tremendous, free firmament without any ties whatsoever. Thus know two kinds of beings: Heaven and earth for one, and man for the other.

To begin with, let us fix our attention on the firmament regarding which you should first turn your mind to creation and predestination. These are beginning and end and whatever should happen in between. This with respect to the firmament.

In the body, take note, are embedded seven members. These seven members do not take in any food; they rather exist in themselves like the seven planets which feed on their own resources and none feeds off the other nor imbibes from other heavenly bodies. The explanation follows: Jupiter is a planet such as does not require fertilizer for the maintenance of its body. When created, it received sufficient endowment. Likewise the liver has no need of being fertilized, for it maintains its nature without any manure. However, if you object and speak of a fertilization of the liver, it strikes us funny just as when we hear a German poet speak of blue colors and mountains as if there were nothing behind. But, how the process of fertilization is to be interpreted, we shall leave to the alchemist, that is the farmer who dumps the manure on the field, for, these seven members do not produce any manure. The same as you have comprehended these things in the case of Jupiter and the liver, understand likewise that the brain is the Moon, the heart the Sun, the spleen Saturn, the lungs Mercury, the kidneys Venus. As the firmaments above have their course and aspect, identically the same understand to take place in these. In the event that you want to know the crisis of a disease you must recognize the natural cycle in the body. Should you be ignorant of that, you will be unable to determine the crisis of the *morbi naturales* that come from the *Ens Naturale.* For, of crises of diseases and celestial crises there are two, quite far apart as you are bound to observe.

TRACT CONCERNING THE "ENS SPIRITUALE"

Now let us explain the *Ens Spirituale.* It is also a perfect power which may disease the entire body and change it in all sicknesses. And though all sorts of criticisms will be made in the course of our discussions, we shall turn our backs on them, for we have no intention of bothering with objections which will nullify themselves in the end. For, the objections which they raise against us are not of such a nature as will be valid. However, if we are to speak about the *Ens Spirituale,* we are warning you that you give up the manner of thinking which you call theological. For not everything that is called theology is holy, neither are all blessed who profess it. Likewise, not all is true what those who do not comprehend theology, maintain. And though the theologians describe this *Ens* with all their persuasion, they do it not under the title or with what constitutes the text of what we call the fourth pagan element. Yet one thing we should be understood as saying that knowledge of this *Ens* does not proceed from Christian belief. For it is pagan. However, it is also not against the belief in which we shall die. This should make you realize that you ought by no means to regard an *Ens* as one of the spirits of whom you say: "They are all devils." There you would speak thoughtlessly and your words would carry no meaning were you to say: "The devil does it." Mark that in our *Ens Spirituale* there is neither any devil nor his handiwork, nor his abetting, because the devil is not a spirit. A spirit, moreover, is also not an angel. That is a spirit which issues from our thoughts, without any matter in a living body. What issues after we die, that is the soul.

. . . [We] want you to remember that there are two worlds that are absolutely essential: One is that of corporeality, the other that of spirit. Now, body and spirit are united, for the spirit is generated by the body through will. At the same time be assured, however, that spirits have their world the same as we, in which they live and exist as we do in the flesh, and bear against each other special favor, envy, hate, ire and the like without the body being implicated. Thus, mark our words that we humans may live amongst ourselves as we may, spirits do the same. It is not true that, should bodies injure each other, spirits do not harm each other, nor that if spirits deal each other injury, which they have the power to do as well as our physical bodies, the latter are similarly not affected or cajoled into behaving likewise. But, if spirits inflict injury upon each other, then the body of the spirit that is harmed must carry the burden which the spirit has assumed.

For the sake of better understanding, examine a few examples by which we shall satisfy your knowledge of this *Ens Spirituale* and conclude our discussion of it. To start in, you know well the wax figurines which are made because of a spiritual antagonism between two persons. If, then, these replicas are buried and weighed down with stones, the person against whom they are made is sorely troubled in those spots where the stones lie and does not get well until the replica is destroyed. Then the person, too, is relieved. Now, if a leg is broken in this replica, the same fracture will occur also to the person against whom it is made. In like manner with stabs, wounds and other injuries. The cause in these instances is this. You are acquainted with the powers of necromancers who can bring it about that by the art of necromancy an apparition may be made of a thing not in existence. But, necromancy cannot injure the body, except when the spirit of the other person is injured by this spirit. Thus, let a necromancer produce a tree and set it up. Whoever hews into it, will cut himself. The reason is that his spirit is cut through the spirit of the tree. This spirit has hands and feet like yourself, and where it is chopped into, there you are being cut. For you and your mind are one. However, understand that it is not your body that receives the wound, although it may be felt as in your body and be visible. Your mind causes that, who has the shape of your limbs and your body. Take care not to treat the body with medicines. For that would be in vain. However, treat the mind, and the body will get well. For, the spirit is sore, and not the body.

TRACT CONCERNING THE "ENS DEI"

Having written four separate treatises on pagan usage as advertised in the beginning of our books, we shall now abstain from these pagan customs in our *Parenthesis* and speak in our own manner in a Christian style, composing the fifth book on the *Ens Dei* so you will no longer accuse us of being pagan. For, any Christian who writes otherwise than in the faith he holds, writes like a pagan. Although we are going to write five books on medical practice after we have finished this *Parenthesis,* in order to round out this book we would like you to know that in the fifth book we shall conclude Christian style, while treating the four initial ones according to pagan conceptions.

This we may well do without detriment to our faith, because pagan medical practice follows nature and with it what is destined us by God. However, even though the diseases arise thus from nature and in accordance with the four powers that have been discussed, we ought to seek their cure in faith, and not in nature, as the fifth book on medical practice will demonstrate.

Therefore, we are addressing Christians so they will peruse this fifth *Parenthesis* and come to realize that they ought to make all their diseases dependent on one thing and search for this thing as follows. All health and sickness comes from God as you know, nothing comes from man. The diseases of mankind may be classified into two groups: Natural ones and inflictions. The natural ones are the first, second, third and fourth powers. Infliction is the fifth. Be well aware that God has instituted punishment, a sign to make known to us by our sicknesses that we should realize that all our affairs are nothing and that we are well grounded in nothing and are ignorant of the truth. Rather, in all things we are feeble and our debilities and knowledge are as nothing. But, touching the core of the matter and holding it up to you, be assured that God gives sickness and health as well as medical practice for our diseases. However, in medical practice everything has a certain purpose and is predestined. This certain thing is time. Hence one should bear in mind that all of our diseases should be healed at a certain hour and not according to our desire and will. By this we mean that no physician is to know when the time for health is at hand, for God has that in his power. Moreover, every disease is a purgatory. Hence no physician is able to heal, except the purgatory has been extinguished by God. Thus, the physician is he who works in harmony with the predestined purgatory.

You ought to know that at the time of Hippocrates, Rasis, Galen etc. it was a sheer pleasure to practice medicine. The reason: Purgatory was a small affair. But at present and henceforth, gradually less happiness may be found in medicine because evil is on the increase; for this reason there have never been so many bad physicians as there are now. Purgatory is so intense that no physician can stem it. Even if these great ones were here now, they would be groping in the dark. Because on top of it we have the plague. Hence, we demand in this *Tract* a Christian method to the effect that we require faith to recognize that all of our diseases are inflictions, examples and warnings that God may take them from us by virtue of our Christian faith, not by pagan medicine, but through Christ. For, the patient who puts his hope in medicine, is no Christian. But who puts it in God, he is a Christian. He will then let God take care of how he will be made well, be it wondrously by saints, by one's own art, by a physician or by old women. You, as Christians, should realize that God is the archphysician. For He is the highest no less who is greater and most powerful, without whom nothing happens. But the pagans, the unbelievers, they cry to man for help. You, however, ought to cry to God. He will assuredly send you the healer, be it a saint, or a physician, or himself.

God has created medicine and physician even though He Himself is the physician and operates through the physician and works nothing Himself without the physician. Let us explain why that should be. Our interpretation is that it is God's secret why He does not want the patient to know that He Himself is the physician, but that He promotes the medical art and practice so that man may experience His help not merely in miraculous workings performed by Himself as God, but also by His creatures who, in the person of the medical expert, provide succor at the time decreed.

Clerical Investigation into the Case of Benedetta Carlini (1619–1623)

Among the documents stored in the State Archives of Florence there is a collection labeled "Papers relating to a trial against Sister Benedetta Carlini of Vellano, abbess of the Theatine nuns of Pescia, who pretended to be a mystic, but who was discovered to be a woman of ill-repute." Here, in this brief heading, lies the sad career of Benedetta, who was discovered to be engaging in sexual relations with another nun, while claiming to be in a state of holy rapture. Sentenced to imprisonment for life, Benedetta lived out her remaining thirty-five years in a small cell within the Theatine convent whose affairs she had once directed. Benedetta's life began auspiciously enough: Born under "miraculous" circumstances, she was pledged by her parents to the order of the Theatines, which she joined at the age of nine. When she was twenty-three, Benedetta started having visions, and shortly after this began experiencing "travails"—episodes of excruciating pain over her entire body that eluded any medical diagnosis or treatment. Five years later, she received an uncontestable sign of her blessedness: the stigmata— wounds in her hands, feet, and side that resembled those of the crucified Christ. An even greater miracle followed: On the night of March 21, 1619, Christ appeared to her as a handsome youth and extracted her heart, replacing it three days later with his own, which he inserted into her chest with His own hands. Within a few months of these occurrences, Pescia's leading ecclesiastical official, Provost Stefano Cecchi, had arrived at the convent to begin his investigation of Benedetta's experiences, thoroughly examining her bodily wounds as well as her ecstatic visions. In reading the ambiguous text of her body, Cecchi had to decide whether its signs were true or forged, a legitimate or a counterfeit image of the Word made Flesh. What he was not prepared to find was a case of lesbian "fornication."

SELECTIONS FROM FIRST INVESTIGATION
On the twenty-seventh day of May, 1619

On the first visit, the provost saw on the hands, feet, and side of Benedetta signs of dry blood as large as a *crazia* [a small Tuscan coin]; and when they were washed with warm water, one could see a small cut from which blood ran out; in several places on the head one could see many signs of dry blood like the blood on the hands; and when they were washed with warm water, one could see in the places that had

From *Immodest Acts: The Life of a Lesbian Nun in Renaissance Italy,* by Judith C. Brown, Studies in the History of Sexuality (New York: Oxford University Press, 1986).

been washed, punctures from which blood poured out and which remained on the cloth with which she was dried.

Benedetta confesses that on the second Friday of Lent of the year 1619, while in bed between two and three hours of the night [7 to 8 P.M.] the thought came to her to suffer all the things suffered by Jesus Christ; and there appeared in front of her a crucified man as large as a good-sized man, and he was alive and asked her if she were willing to suffer for his love because he was Jesus Christ; and she protested that if this were an illusion of the Devil she did not want to consent and would tell her Spiritual Father [her confessor] and she made the sign of the cross. He assured her that he was God and that he wanted her to suffer for the duration of her life, that she should arrange herself in the form of a cross because he wanted to imprint his holy wounds in her body. When she did this, a flash burst forth from all of them, which she thought imprinted themselves on her hands. And on her head she saw many small rays that seemed to delineate her entire head and she felt great pains in it and in her hands. But afterwards a great contentment came into her heart. The large rays she saw were five, but those of the head were a great many more, but small ones; that she did not arrange her feet one on top of the other, but found them wounded and arranged without realizing it; and she felt pain there. On Sundays they seem to be numb; on Mondays and Tuesdays she feels little or no pain; on all other days great pain; on Fridays more than any other days and on that day there is more bleeding, except for this morning as you have seen.

On the first day of August, 1619

This visit begins with the testimony of the Abbess Felice and Sister Angelina and is followed by the testimony of Mea Crivelli excerpted below:

The above-mentioned Mea, under oath—She sleeps next to the superior, Felice; and last year next to Benedetta; and I began to sleep next to Felice when we came here last November, if I'm not mistaken. When we came up here I put myself near the large window and Benedetta was here below near the door, but because she was in pain at night, I went to stay down there with her so that I could get up and help her. And often I did not go to sleep at night until the eighth or ninth hour [1 or 2 A.M.] so that I could help her because she had those pains. She had those pains in her heart and often throughout her entire body, but the former were the strongest. And I know it because she had me put my hand on her heart because she seemed to feel less pain that way. And while I had my hand there it felt as if a dagger were hitting it, so strong was it. And with my hand in place she seemed to flail around less but when I didn't have my hand there, she would not stay in bed because of the great pains she experienced. And I would work so hard that I would sweat. The pains lasted two years, and during a period of four months they were continuous.

Sometimes she would call me twice a night because she was still mindful of the dead abbess. She would tell her, "hold me, help me," and as soon as I heard her I would put my hand on her heart and would quiet her. And she would tell me this because she could not hold still on account of her great pains. She never told me what caused them, but when I would say that Jesus wanted to test her, she would confirm it. And when she had these pains one could smell an awful sulphurous stink coming out of her mouth. At night I never saw anyone appear in front of her. But I heard her talk; I heard her say that she did not want to leave this place but that she would rather be ill for love of Jesus and she answered the same thing many times. And she wanted to persevere in this monastery. And when she touched her heart she never heard her say anything else, except when Jesus took out her heart. I went to her and I put my hand on the side of her heart. I seemed to feel a hole. Benedetta's heart was removed and I thought to myself that it was Jesus that did it. The night of the second day of Easter, her heart was removed after the same hour as her signs had appeared. Because I found myself present and heard her, she began to speak and said that she saw Jesus approaching, "but I don't know if it is the devil's work, pray to God for me." (Benedetta confessed this but these words were left.) "If it is the devil's work, I will make the sign of the cross on my heart and he will disappear." Shortly thereafter, she began to laugh and became all happy. And I heard her saying, "What would you do my Jesus! You came to take my heart but I don't want to do it without permission from my Spiritual Father." And then I heard her say, "You will see that he will have no objections. Do it." And I saw that she laid down on her back and said, "where will you take my heart from?" And I heard her say, "from the side." And I saw that she suffered a great deal of pain and I heard her say, "Oh my Jesus, show it to me. That is it. No wonder I felt such pain." And I heard her say, "I would like it as a sign of your love and in conformity with your will, but how can I live without a heart now that you have left me without one? How will I be able to love you?" And I saw all these things because I was there by the bed, secretly. But she didn't see me because when I realized that she was returning to her senses, I retreated behind the curtain so she wouldn't see me. I realized that she was not herself because she seemed like one who dreams and this was very obvious. And she would have sent me away and she wouldn't have spoken in this manner. And I touched her near the heart and one could feel an empty space and she remained there apparently out of her senses.

I did not say anything about this because I didn't see it, but knew that for God it is not impossible to live without a heart. She was without it for three days. I was present when he put it back in and I think it was the second hour of the night, when she had gone to bed. And she said, "Oh my bridegroom did you come to give me back my heart?" And she remained thus, a bit quiet. Then gaily she opened her arms as when people want to embrace each other, saying, "My Jesus, don't show it to me because I will lose my sight." And she turned her head in the other direction, saying that it was so beautiful that she couldn't watch it. And she asked him what those rays meant. "It is the capacity of your love. And that circle of gold is the conformity of your will. And it is just as I wanted it." And I heard her say: "Put it back in the same place that you took it from, but I don't want to disrobe here in the presence of so many people." And she retreated and she let go the cloths, uncovering her side, and I saw that the sign on her side was larger and redder than at other times. And I saw that she was very happy. And when He put it [the heart] inside her I began to see that the flesh rose up and she moved slowly, slowly with those rays in front; and all the ribs, which I could see, were lifted up. And when it arrived at the place where the heart belongs, it stopped. And she slowly turned with her forehead bent down

BATTISTA PIERGILIUS

The Life of Sister Chiara
of Montefalco (1663)

In his book *The Incorruptible Flesh, Bodily Mutation and Mortification in Religion and Folklore,* Piero Camporesi, professor of Italian Literature at the University of Bologna, cites Battista Piergilius's life of Sister Chiara of Montefalco (1268–1308), an Augustinian abbess who died amidst "the odor of sanctity," a condition in which the processes of bodily decomposition purportedly are forestalled. In his account of Chiara's life, Piergilius described an autopsy performed on her corpse by four nuns with the aim of finding and giving witness to signs of her saintliness. They were not disappointed. Discovering several anatomical wonders upon opening Chiara's body, the nuns of Montefalco proceeded to extract her organs and then to dissect her heart. Every year thereafter, on the eve of the feast of St. John the Baptist, the nuns removed the body from its coffin, dressed it anew, and displayed it for the populace on the altar of their church. Such practices, which entailed repeated and intimate handling of "sanctified" corpses—and at times contact with their viscera and effluvia—were not at all uncommon among the religious communities that thrived throughout the Middle Ages.

Having decided that the body of Sister Chiara of Montefalco, known as 'of the Cross,' who had died in an 'odour of sanctity' and had been declared blessed by all, should be opened and embalmed, the Augustinian nuns—whose abbess she had been—deemed that 'it was not proper for that virgin flesh to be touched by any man whatsoever,' and that 'her saintly body' which had been a 'living temple to the Holy Ghost,' should not be contaminated by the hands of a barber-surgeon. Therefore, one hot and still Saturday night in August 1308, while the convent slept, four of their number, tucking up their sleeves, embarked on a series of (for us) astonishing operations.

They went into the oratory and with the utmost respect undressed the saintly body. Sister Francesca, inexperienced though she was, opened it as best she could with a razor. They then began to remove the intestines. She noticed that the gall-bladder was white and when she touched it she felt inside it three hard objects like stones, which were round in shape and together formed a triangle. . . . As they continued removing the intestines, they reached the heart and all saw that it was inordinately large, larger than an infant's head. . . . The nuns decided that it was right and proper to put the heart to one side: this they

From *The Incorruptible Flesh: Bodily Mutation and Mortification in Religion and Folklore,* by Piero Camporesi, trans. Tania Croft-Murray, Latin texts trans. Helen Elsom, Cambridge Studies in Oral and Literate Culture (Cambridge: Cambridge University Press, 1988).

did, and placing all the other intestines in an earthenware jar, they buried them within the oratory itself where the saint had died, to one side of the altar where to this day they are thought to lie. Taking up the heart again, Sister Francesca said 'behold this heart, in which the Lord has worked so many wonders.' Placing it in a wooden bowl, they locked it up in a chest. This done, they dressed the body again and set it to rights.

After being told the results of the autopsy carried out by their four dissecting colleagues, the thought of this heart of extraordinary dimensions caused the nuns to lie awake at night. It began to be suspected that the matter 'was not without mystery.' Some of the nuns then recalled that Sister Chiara had been much given to contemplating Christ's Passion, and that during her final illness

she had more than once repeated these words: 'I bear the crucified Christ within my heart.' All the nuns were agreed that in this heart there lay Christ's cross. 'I am the more inclined to believe this,' added Sister Marina, 'since I remember our holy Mother Abbess saying to me seven years ago that Christ had appeared to her in the guise of a Pilgrim bearing a cross on his shoulder, and told her that He wanted to plant the cross in her heart'; the nuns finally decided that her heart should be opened for the purposes of embalming, whether a mystery were found or no.

And so one Sunday night, with this in mind, Sisters Lucia, Margarita, Caterina and Francesca betook themselves to a room where the heart lay locked away in its box; and taking it up they all four knelt. Sister Francesca opened it, uttering with great humility the following words: 'Lord, I believe that in this heart there lies your holy Cross, although I believe my sins to be so many that they make me unworthy to find it.' Thus saying, she took the heart in one hand and in the other a razor and, not knowing where to make her incision because the heart, consistent with the general condition of the body, was all covered in fat, she finally decided to start the incision at the top where the heart is broader, took it to the lower extremity, and thus opened the heart easily with one cut.

The excess of blood was such that they did not at first see what was contained therein; they knew well enough that the heart is concave and divided into two parts, being a whole only in its circumference; then Sister Francesca felt with her finger that in the middle of one section there ran a nerve; and when she drew it out, they saw to their amazement that it was a cross, formed of flesh, which had been ensconced in a cavity of the same shape as the cross. Upon seeing this, Sister Margarita began shouting, 'A miracle, a miracle.' . . .

It occurred to Sister Giovanna, after observing this phenomenon, that the heart might harbour other mysteries: so she told Sister Francesca to continue her inspection with greater attention. . . . And in so doing, she encountered another small nerve standing up in the heart, like the Cross; and studying it carefully, they realized that it represented the Whip, or Scourge, with which Christ was beaten at the Pillar.

The nuns were so astonished at the extraordinary nature of these mysteries, that they could do no less than praise the Lord, who worked such miracles.

The news spread like wildfire outside the bounds of the convent and an 'heretic of the sect of the Little Brothers' [Minorite Friars], feigning devout orthodoxy, and at the instigation of the Devil, hastened to the Bishop at Spoleto, Berengario Donadei, in order to denounce this 'credulousness born of gossip and the fantasies of women' and the probably bogus nature of the operation performed by 'meddlesome hands.' Having thanked the heretic, Berengario set off for Montefalco to 'bury the news which he already considered scandalous and foolhardy and severely to punish those nuns.'

Before a chosen gathering of theologians, judges, doctors and churchmen of every kind and persuasion, Berengario caused the heart to be brought to him. He took it and 'with a gesture of scorn and disdain he opened it.'

> Whereupon he observed both Cross and Scourge with great circumspection, as he did the whole heart. And behold an even greater miracle: both he and the others foregathered discovered, when they touched the heart and examined it carefully, that there were other mysteries of the Passion, to wit the Pillar, the Crown of Thorns, the three Nails, the Spear and the Pole with the Sponge, all so truly represented that Berengario on touching the point of the Spear and the thee Nails was pricked by them as though they had really been of iron. At this point everyone was awe-struck and filled with amazement. . . .

The same fate awaited the gall bladder which, when disinterred and taken from the jar together with the other intestines, and separated from the liver and dissected by Sister Francesca again with the same razor, yielded three globules or balls, linked together to form a triangle. These were washed in wine by Sister Tommasa, dissected and examined by the theologians, who decreed that 'the three globules were without doubt a symbol of the ineffable mystery of the Holy Trinity.' It was found that the heart and its mysteries remained miraculously intact

> since these were never kept in any preservative; indeed, for a period of some years at a time, the chaplain or some other priest exhibited them, and taking the heart he would open it, remove the Crucifix and the Scourge from its cavity; after showing these to the congregation, he would replace them. . . .

The blood which 'was collected from the heart of this saintly woman . . . is still today to be seen in a phial and it is red in colour just like a ruby.' At times this blood would boil, portentously and 'terribly,' especially in periods of mourning or catastrophe, war or epidemic.

The remainder of the body was placed in a coffin and lowered into a deep grave inside the church of Montefalco. It became necessary, nonetheless, to satisfy the 'devout importunings' of the populace which 'clamoured repeatedly to be allowed to see Chiara's saintly remains,' and the chaplain of Montefalco ordered 'that the body be disinterred and kept in a place where it might be seen by all.'

As in the case of the intestines hidden away in a jar which, when exhumed were found 'to have no unwholesome odour,'

> it being the fifth day since the death of this saintly woman: her body, despite its being plentifully covered in flesh and fat, and although it had not yet been embalmed, the day being hot too—for it was the twenty-first of August—not

only remained intact and unblemished in every way but with a countenance fresh, nay, almost resplendent, she exhaled a gentle odour, a heavenly fragrance.

The nuns had requested of the apothecary, Tomaso di Bartolone, the necessary ointments in order to embalm the body: It was God's will that the apothecary should bring the said ointments ten days after the death of the holy woman. He delivered them into the nuns's hands and showed them what to do. Accordingly, the nuns undressed the body and following the apothecary's instructions, removed the brain and embalmed the body in its entirety. They then wrapped it in the fine cloth which they sewed up, allowing face, hands and feet to show—just as they may be seen today.

PART 2

The Body Secularized

HIPPOCRATES (460–377 B.C.)

"The Nature of Man"

Owing to Plato, we are certain of at least two facts concerning Hippocrates: He was born on the Greek island of Cos, and being an Asklepiad, he belonged to the guild believed to have been founded by the legendary physician Aesculapius. Much of the rest of Hippocrates' life is shrouded in mystery, as is his work. A diverse and often self-contradictory collection of manuals, textbooks, lectures, and notes, the "Hippocratic corpus" could not possibly have been authored by one man. What these writings do have in common, however, is a new ethos: They systematized a medical outlook that had largely broken free of its magical and religious sources and had turned its attention to the study of the natural world through disciplined observation and experiment. Symptoms were delineated, disease pictures were described, clinical histories were recorded, and a theory of health and illness was formulated. This theory rested on the notion that the body was composed of four "humors," or fluids—blood, phlegm, yellow bile, and black bile—that needed to be kept in a state of equilibrium. An imbalance of the humors—a surfeit or deficit of one or the other substance—resulted in disease. Because of each individual's unique temperament, history, and habits, treatment was specifically tailored to restore the balance appropriate to any given patient by a daily regimen that relied almost entirely on the curative powers of nature. By prescribing the proper diet and type of exercise, by aiding the body's own efforts to rid itself of excess or corrupt humors, the physician acted mainly as nature's facilitator, dispensing drugs solely as a last resort. The doctrine of the four humors, then, encompassed not only an approach to medicine and disease but a theory of the natural world and of the body; and it is in the Hippocratic corpus that this doctrine, which was to prevail in Western civilization for over a millennium and a half, finds its first unified expression.

The human body contains blood, phlegm, yellow bile and black bile. These are the things that make up its constitution and cause its pains and health. Health is primarily that state in which these constituent substances are in the correct proportion to each other, both in strength and quantity, and are well mixed. Pain occurs when one of the substances presents either a deficiency or an excess, or is separated in the body and not mixed with the others. It is inevitable that when one of these is separated from the rest and stands by itself, not only the part from which it has come, but also that where it collects and is present in excess, should become diseased, and because it contains too much of the particular substance, cause pain and distress.

From *The Medical Works of Hippocrates,* trans. John Chadwick and W. N. Mann (Springfield, Ill.: Charles C. Thomas, 1950). Used by permission of Blackwell Scientific Publications Ltd.

Whenever there is more than slight discharge of one of these humours outside the body, then its loss is accompanied by pain. If, however, the loss, change or separation from the other humours is internal, then it inevitably causes twice as much pain, as I have said, for pain is produced both in the part whence it is derived and in the part where it accumulates.

Those who assert that the human body is a single substance seem to have reasoned along the following lines. Having observed that when men died from excessive purgation following the administration of drugs, some vomited bile and some phlegm, they concluded from this that whatever was the nature of the material voided at death, this was indeed the fundamental constituent of man. Those who insist that blood is the basic substance use a similar argument; because they see blood flowing from the body in the fatally wounded, they conclude that blood constitutes the soul. They all use similar arguments to support their theories. But, to begin with, no one ever yet died from excessive purgation and brought up only bile; taking medicine which causes the bringing up of bile, produces first the vomiting of bile, but subsequently, the vomiting of phlegm as well. This is followed by the vomiting of black bile in spite of themselves and they end up by vomiting pure blood and that is how they die. The same effects result from taking a drug which brings up phlegm; the vomiting of phlegm is followed by yellow bile, then black bile, then pure blood, and so death ensues. When a drug is ingested, it first causes the evacuation of whatever in the body is naturally suited to it, but afterwards, it causes the voiding of other substances too. It is similar in the case of plants and seeds; when these are put into the ground, they first absorb the things which naturally suit them; they may be acid, bitter, sweet, salty and so forth. But although at first the plant takes what is naturally suited to it, afterwards it absorbs other things as well. The action of drugs in the body is similar; those which cause the bringing up of bile at first bring it up undiluted, but later on it is voided mixed with other substances; the same is true of drugs which bring up phlegm. In the case of men who have been fatally wounded the blood at first runs very warm and red, but subsequently it becomes more like phlegm and bile.

Now the quantity of phlegm in the body increases in winter because it is that bodily substance most in keeping with the winter, seeing that it is the coldest. You can verify its coldness by touching phlegm, bile and blood; you will find that the phlegm is the coldest. It is however the most viscous and is brought up with greater force than any other substance with the exception of black bile. Although those things which are forcibly expelled become warmer owing to the force to which they are subjected, nevertheless phlegm remains the coldest substance, and obviously so, owing to its natural characteristics. The following signs show that winter fills the body with phlegm: people spit and blow from their noses the most phlegmatic mucus in winter; swellings become white especially at that season and other diseases show phlegmatic signs.

During the spring, although the phlegm remains strong in the body, the quantity of blood increases. Then, as the cold becomes less intense and the rainy season comes on, the wet and warm days increase further the quantity of blood. This part of the year is most in keeping with blood because it is wet and hot. That this is so, you can

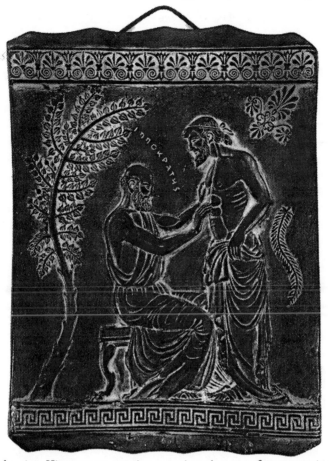

4. Relief showing Hippocrates treating a patient (anon., after an ancient source). Wellcome Institute Library, London. The Greek inscription at the top center of this plaque identifies the physician as "Hippocrates." One of the scene's notable features is that it depicts Hippocrates touching the patient, demonstrating that medicine, from its earliest days, had a privileged authority over the (naked) body.

judge by these signs: it is in spring and summer that people are particularly liable to dysentery and to epistaxis, and these are the seasons too at which people are warmest and their complexions are ruddiest.

During the summer, the blood is still strong but the bile gradually increases, and this change continues into the autumn when the blood decreases since the autumn is contrary to it. The bile rules the body during the summer and the autumn. As proof of this, it is during this season that people vomit bile spontaneously, or, if they take drugs, they void the most bilious sort of matter. It is plain too from the nature of fevers and from people's complexions in that season. During the summer, the phlegm is at its weakest since this season, on account of its dryness and heat, is most contrary to that substance.

The blood in the body reaches its lowest level in autumn, because this is a dry season and the body is already beginning to cool. Black bile is strongest and preponderates in the autumn. When winter sets in the bile is cooled and decreases while the phlegm increases again owing to the amount of rain and the length of the nights.

All these substances, then, are all always present in the body but vary in their relative quantities, each preponderating in turn according to its natural characteristics. The year has its share of all the elements; heat, cold, dryness and wetness. None of these could exist alone, while, on the other hand, were they missing, all would disappear, for they are all mutually interdependent. In the same way, if any of these primary bodily substances were absent, life would cease. And just as the year is governed at one time by winter, then by spring, then by summer and then by autumn; so at one time in the body phlegm preponderates, at another time blood, at another time yellow bile and this is followed by the preponderance of black bile. A very dear proof of this can be obtained by giving the same man the same emetic at four different times in the year; his vomit will be most phlegmatic in winter, most wet in spring, most bilious in summer and darkest in autumn.

In addition to these considerations, certain further points should be known. Diseases caused by over-eating are cured by fasting; those caused by starvation are cured by feeding up. Diseases caused by exertion are cured by rest; those caused by indolence are cured by exertion. To put it briefly; the physician should treat disease by the principle of opposition to the cause of the disease according to its form, its seasonal and age incidence, countering tenseness by relaxation and *vice versa*. This will bring the patient most relief and seems to me to be the principle of healing.

Some diseases are produced by the manner of life that is followed; others by the life-giving air we breathe. That there are these two types may be demonstrated in the following way. When a large number of people all catch the same disease at the same time, the cause must be ascribed to something common to all and which they all use; in other words to what they all breathe. In such a disease, it is obvious that individual bodily habits cannot be responsible because the malady attacks one after another, young and old, men and women alike, those who drink their wine neat and those who drink only water; those who eat barley-cake as well as those who live on bread, those who take a lot of exercise and those who take but little. The régime cannot therefore be responsible where people who live very different lives catch the same disease.

However, when many different diseases appear at the same time, it is plain that the regimen is responsible in individual cases. For, in such a case, it is obvious that all, most, or at least one of the factors in the regimen does not agree with the patient; such must be sought out and changed having regard to the constitution of the patient, his age and appearance, the season of the year and the nature of the disease. The treatment prescribed should vary accordingly by lessening this or increasing that, and the regimen and drugs should be appropriately adapted to the various factors already mentioned.

When an epidemic of one particular disease is established, it is evident that it is not the regimen but the air breathed which is responsible. Plainly, the air must be harmful because of some morbid secretion which it contains. Your advice to patients at such a time should be not to alter the regimen since this is not to blame, but they should gradually reduce the quantity of food and drink taken so that the body is as little loaded and as weak as possible. A sudden change of regimen involves the risk of starting a fresh complaint, so you should deal with the regimen in this way when it is clearly not the cause of the patient's illness. Care should be taken that the amount of air breathed should be a small as possible and as unfamiliar as possible. These points may be dealt with by making the body thin so that the patient will avoid large and frequent breaths, and, wherever practicable, by a change of station from the infected area.

Most fevers are caused by bile. Apart from those arising from local injury, they are of four types. These are called continued, quotidian, tertian and quartan.

Continued fever is produced by large quantities of the most concentrated bile and the crisis is reached in the shortest time; as the body enjoys no periods of coolness, the great heat it endures results in rapid wasting.

Quotidian fever is caused by a large quantity of bile, but less than that which causes continued fever. This is quicker than the others to depart although it lasts longer than a continued fever by as much as there is less bile causing it, and because the body has some respite from the fever whereas continued fever allows none.

Tertian fever lasts longer than quotidian fever and is caused by less bile. A tertian fever is longer in proportion to the longer respites from fever allowed to the body compared with quotidian fevers.

Quartans behave similarly to the tertians but last longer, as they arise from still less of the heat-producing bile and because they give the body longer respites in which to cool down. A secondary reason for their chronic character and difficult resolution is that they are caused by black bile; this is the most viscous of the humours in the body and remains the longest. As evidence of this note the association of quartan fevers with melancholy. Quartan fever has its highest incidence in the autumn and in those between the ages of twenty-five and forty-five. This is the time of life when the body is most subject to black bile, and the autumn is the corresponding season of the year. If a quartan fever occurs at any other time of the year, or at any other age, you may be sure that it will not be chronic unless some other malady be present.

PLATO (429–347 B.C.)

Timaeus

Born into an aristocratic Athenian family, Plato planned to follow a political career but became bitterly disillusioned with affairs of state after the execution of Socrates. In 385 B.C., Plato founded the Academy, a school of philosophy that remained an active center of teaching and research until its suppression by the Roman emperor Justinian in A.D. 529. The translation of "the good" into "the actual," of the moral ideal into the political reality, was a problem whose solution profoundly concerned Plato, particularly in his later years, during which he wrote the *Timaeus*. His only treatise on natural science, the *Timaeus* was meant to be the first in a trilogy of dialogues on the implementation of the ideal polis. Plato never completed the project, but its aims are implicit in the *Timaeus*'s premise that the "miniature cosmos" of the human being—the microcosm—corresponds in all its parts and relations to the macrocosm—the larger cosmos that contains it. Unlike Democritus, who conceived the universe to be the result of random collisions of eternal particles, Plato argued that the cosmos was governed by ineluctable laws and principles instituted by the Creator. This conviction rules the *Timaeus*, starting from its account of the making of the universe and the birth of mankind to its description of the human frame and the causes of its disorder and decline. A synthesis of Socratic philosophy, the *Timaeus* is also a compendium of the most recent scientific and medical theories of its day. It was one of the few works by Plato known to medieval Europe, and nowhere is its centrality in Renaissance thought and culture more vividly attested to than in Raphael's *School of Athens*. Here, alongside Aristotle, Plato strides forth into the midst of its pantheon of scholars with the *Timaeus* firmly grasped in his hand.

. . . [S]o long as a creature's constitution is still youthful, and the triangles of its constituents, so to say, fresh from the workshop, they are locked firmly together, though the mass as a whole is soft, since it has been but recently formed from marrow and fed upon milk. So, as the intruding foreign triangles contained in the system and supplied by its meat and drink are older and feebler than its own, which are fresh, it succeeds in cutting them up; the organism is sustained by an abundance of triangles like its own and waxes great. But when the root of the triangles is loosened by buffetings endured from many a storm for many a year, they can no longer cut up the triangles of the food as they enter the body into their own likeness, but are themselves easily divided by the intruders. So all creatures at this period fail and dwindle, and the condition is called age. Finally, when the bonds of the triangles of the marrow no longer hold out but break under the tempest, they, in their turn, relax the

---

From *Plato: Timaeus and Critias*, ed. and trans. A. E. Taylor (London: Methuen, 1929).

bonds of the soul; she comes to her natural release and takes her flight with pleasure. For while unnatural processes are always painful, the natural are always pleasant. Death itself, on this principle, is painful and contrary to nature when it follows on disease or wounds, but when it comes in age as the end of a natural process, it is the easiest of all deaths and is attended rather by pleasure than by pain.

As for diseases, their origin should, I take it, be obvious. Since the body is compacted of four ingredients, earth, fire, water and air, disorders and diseases arise from abnormal usurpation or deficiency of these ingredients, or from their moving from their own place to a foreign one, or, again,—since there are several varieties of fire and the rest—from the reception in the system of an inappropriate variety, and from similar causes. For when there is abnormality in the formation or location of any of these ingredients, parts which were formerly warmed are chilled, the dry become damp—(it is the same, of course, with the light and the heavy)—and all are exposed to all kinds of changes. My thesis, in fact, is this: only when same accedes to, or is withdrawn from, same by self-same, uniform, proportional rule—only then will a thing be left self-same, intact and sound; a false note struck by accession or withdrawal beyond these limits will occasion manifold degeneration, and endless diseases and corruptions.

Once more, since secondary formations exist in nature, there is a second class of diseases to be noted by all who would understand. Since, in fact, marrow, bone, flesh, sinew are all compacted of the substances already named, while blood, also, is formed of the same ingredients, though in a different fashion, though most disorders have the same causes as those already mentioned, the gravest maladies of all afflict us from another cause: the formations just specified suffer corruption when the order of formation is inverted. In the normal order, in fact, flesh and sinews are formed from blood, sinew from the fibrine, with which it is akin, flesh from the coagulation of the residue left when the fibrine is removed. The viscous and oily product given off by sinews and flesh, in its turn, not only glues the flesh to the bones, but feeds the growth of the bone enclosing the marrow; finally, that which percolates through the dense substance of the bones, smooth and oily in extreme degree, with triangles of superlative refinement, drops and trickles from the bones and waters the marrow. When this order is observed in the several processes, the regular result is health, but disease, if the order is inverted. Thus when the decomposing flesh infects the blood-vessels with the decomposition, against natural order, these vessels contain abundant blood mixed with air; this exhibits a great variety of colours and bitter tastes, to say nothing of acid and briny characters, and develops divers forms of bile, serum and phlegm. These perverse and corrupted secretions begin by poisoning the very blood, and are carried in the blood-vessels all over the body, no longer providing it with nutriment nor observing any orderly natural period, at strife among themselves, since they have no affinity for each other, and at open war with such elements of the body as support the constitution and abide at their posts, spreading destruction and decomposition. Now when the flesh which is decomposed is of very ancient formation, it resists concoction, and turns black under its long exposure to inflammation, and the bitterness due to its thorough corrosion makes it a grave danger to all such parts of the body as are still uncorrupted. Sometimes the black colour is attended by acidity rather than bitterness, when the bitterness has been somewhat diluted; in other cases, the bitterness is suffused with blood and acquires a reddish, or, with an interfusion of black, a greenish tint. Or a yellow colour may be conjoined with this bitterness when the flesh decomposed by the fire of the inflammation is of recent formation. The name common to all these varieties, *bile,* may have come from physicians, or possibly from one who was capable of contemplating a variety of phenomena and discerning in them all a single type deserving of a name. The other currently recognized forms of bile are defined by their specific colours. As to serum, that of blood is a gentle lymph, that of black and acid bile, when rendered saline by heat, a virulent lymph which is known as acid phlegm. But as for that which results from the decomposition of soft young flesh, in combination with air, (the said substances being understood to be inflated by wind and enveloped by liquid, and thus to form bubbles, individually too minute to be visible but collectively having a visible bulk and a white colour due to the production of froth),—all this decomposition of soft flesh combined with air we call *white phlegm.* The lymph of freshly forming phlegm itself is sweat, tears and other bodies of that kind which are daily exuded as purgations. All these materials naturally become instrumental to disease when the blood is not replenished in normal fashion from meat and drink, but augments its bulk from the contrary quarter against nature's usage.

. . . [W]e have to consider a third type of disease, which may originate in three different ways, from wind, from phlegm, or from bile. When the lung, the body's steward of winds, is blocked by rheums and presents no clear passage, the wind does not reach some parts at all, and enters others in more than due measure. The parts which get no ventilation then suffer decomposition; in other parts, the wind forces its way into the blood-vessels, contorts them, dissolves the body and is intercepted in its central region where the diaphragm is located. This causes a great number of painful disorders, often accompanied by copious sweating. Often again, when a cavity has been formed in the body, wind gets in, is unable to escape and occasions the same distress as if it had entered from outside the frame. The suffering is worst when the wind besets the sinews and the connected blood-vessels, swells the tendons and the sinews continuous with them and gives them a backward curvature. From this symptom of tension such disorders have naturally received the names *tetanus* and *opisthotonus.* A cure, too, is difficult; in fact, these troubles are most commonly brought to a solution by the supervening of a fever. White phlegm may be serious if intercepted within the body, but is milder if it finds passages for escape, though it disfigures us by producing blotches, scabs and similar complaints. But when it combines with black bile to overlay and confound the divine circles in the head, the visitation, though comparatively mild if it occurs during sleep, is more difficult to escape when it attacks the waking. As the disorder affects a holy substance it fully deserves its name of 'the sacred disease.' Acid and briny phlegm is the fount of all disorders involving discharge, though the names which have been given to them are as various as the parts towards which the defluxion is directed. But inflammations of the various parts, so called from the burning and heat which attend them, are one and all caused by *bile.* When this bile finds an outward vent it bubbles up in superficial abscesses, but if confined within the body, causes a variety of acutely inflammatory

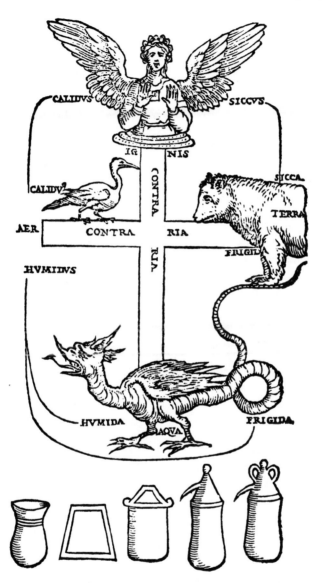

The labels in the woodcut include: CALIDVS, SICCVS, IGNIS, CALIDV², SICCA, AER, CONTRA, RIA, TERRA, CONTRARIA, FRIGID, HVMIDVS, HVMIDA, AQVA, FRIGIDA.

5. *Woodcut of the Four Humors for an alchemical book by Pietro Antonio Boni (fl.ca. 1494), from Giano Lacinio, ed.,* Pretiosa Margarita Novella de Thesauro Ac Pretiosissimo Philosophorum Lapide *(Venice: Apud Aldi Filios, 1546). The New York Academy of Medicine, New York. Part of a sixteenth-century treatise on alchemy, this woodcut is an allegorical representation of the four humors and elements. The angel, bear, dragon, and bird designate yellow bile (fire), black bile (earth), phlegm (water), and blood (air) along with their respective qualities. The temperaments associated with the humors are, in order, choleric, melancholic, phlegmatic, and sanguine.*

diseases. The gravest case is when it mingles with pure blood and disturbs its fibrine in its appointed function. That substance was dispersed through the blood to ensure a proper proportion in the matter of rarity and density, so that the blood should neither, from its fluidity, escape when heated through the pores of the body, nor yet, from overthickness, be sluggish and slow of circulation in the vessels. The right balance in this matter is preserved by the fibrine, when it is produced in the normal way; even in the case of blood from a corpse, which has lost its warmth, if the fibrine is collected, what is left of the blood liquefies, whereas if it is left in position, the blood is soon congealed by the fibrine and the cold environment acting together. Accordingly, since fibrine acts in the blood in this fashion, when bile, a product of old blood which is returned to the blood from decomposing flesh, begins to enter it, hot and liquid and in small quantity, it congeals under the action of the fibrine, and this congelation and unnatural loss of heat cause internal distress and shivering. When the influx of bile is more copious, its heat boils up, overpowers the fibrine and throws its action into disorder, and if powerful enough to retain the upper hand permanently, penetrates to the marrow, where it burns through the soul's mooring-cables and sets her at liberty. If there is less of it and the body resists dissolution, it is itself overpowered and either completely expelled from the whole body or forced through the blood-vessels into the stomach or abdomen, when it causes diarrhoeas, dysenteries and the like disorders, much like a factionary in process of expulsion from the community after a civil tumult.

So much, then, for the causation of disorders of body; disorders of soul are caused by bodily condition in the following way. We shall admit, of course, that disease of soul is the same thing as mindlessness, and of this there are two varieties, frantic madness and stupidity. Consequently, any condition which involves either is to be called disease, and we must pronounce that the gravest of all these diseases of soul are excessive pleasures and pains. Indeed, when a man is transported by delight, or its contrary, distress, in his haste to grasp the pleasure or escape the pain unseasonably he can neither see nor hear aright; for the time being, he is in a frenzy and all but incapable of reflection. And when the seed in a man's marrow is copious and turbid—a condition like that of a tree yielding far more than the due proportion of fruits—his appetites and their consequences bring with them many a specific pang of pain, but also many a thrill of pleasure; so he passes most of his life in a frenzy of passionate pleasure and pain, with a soul diseased and mindless by the fault of its body, and is commonly held not for a sick man but for one deliberately vicious. But in plain fact, sexual incontinence is, for the most part, a malady of soul caused by a turbid and over-moist condition of one of the constituents of the body, due to porosity of the bones. And so, speaking more generally, the charges of incontinence in pleasures which are brought against the vicious, as though their conduct were voluntary, are not really deserved. No man, in fact, is deliberately vicious; those who are vicious become so from some flaw in their physical constitution or in their education, both of them unwelcome conditions which come to a man against his will. So, too, on the other side, the soul contracts a great deal of vice in the matter of pains from the body. When acid and saline phlegmatic or bitter bilious humours roaming through a man's body can find no vent, but collect within and their commingled vapours interfere with the revolutions of the soul, they occasion a great variety of disorders of soul, more or less severe and extensive. As the vapours reach the three regions of the soul, according to the region they invade, they give rise to manifold types of irritable temper and low spirits, rashness and cowardice, or, finally, forgetfulness and slowness in learning. And when, on the top of all this, men with so vicious a composition live under bad forms of government where corrupt discourses are held in their societies by private or public persons, and where there is no course of study they can undertake at an early age to remedy their faults, one has the conditions in which all of us who are vicious acquire our vices, through two causes utterly independent of our own will. The blame must be laid on parents rather than on children, on those who bestow nurture rather than on those who receive it; still a man must do his utmost endeavour, alike by regimen, by daily practice and by study, to shun vice and embrace its opposite. But that belongs to another story.

ANDREAS VESALIUS (1514–1564)

The Fabric of the Human Body

Like many other Renaissance physicians and artists, Andreas Vesalius was driven by a desire to know the human body in all its parts and aspects. An irresistible urge to dissect had mastered him even as a child, periodically leaving in its wake a succession of dismembered neighborhood dogs, cats, mice, and moles that had succumbed to his curiosity. The son of a court apothecary, Vesalius was born in Brussels, and sent to Paris to study medicine. Once there, however, he was greatly disappointed to find that his anatomy teachers were content to expound on Galen while poking around in the bodies of dead dogs. Having reappeared at the beginning of the fourteenth century in Bologna, the practice of dissecting human bodies was spreading; more and more authorities began placing the corpses of executed criminals at the disposal of universities. Searching for more rigorous training in anatomy, Vesalius left Paris and returned to Brussels, where, risking imprisonment, he stole a body from the gallows to acquire a complete human skeleton. Next, Vesalius moved on to the University of Padua, where he received his medical degree in 1537 and was appointed professor of surgery and anatomy. Here, as elsewhere, anatomical demonstrations were highly ritualized events, with the professor seated above the corpse reading from a Galenic text, the surgeon dissecting, and the demonstrator pointing to the indicated parts of the body. Not content with this division of labor, Vesalius took scalpel in hand, with the result that he soon proved many of Galen's centuries-old observations to be false. Because it was still unthinkable to dispute Galen's claims, however, discrepancies between what was seen in the sixteenth-century corpse and what was written in the second-century text were ascribed to the "fact" that the human body had changed since antiquity. Vesalius offered another explanation: He was certain that Galen, in most cases, had dissected not human bodies but those of monkeys, goats, and pigs. Setting out to portray a true picture of the human anatomy, Vesalius published the results of his anatomical work in *De Humanis Corporis Fabrica, Libri Septem* (1543), one of the most important of the early generation of printed books. Containing 663 folio pages and more than three hundred illustrations by the painter Jan Stefan von Kalkar, the great treatise appeared in the same year that Copernicus redrew the anatomy of the heavens.

From *The Source Book of Medical History,* comp. Logan Clendening (New York: Dover, 1942).

To the Divine Charles the Fifth, Greatest and Most Invincible Emperor.
The preface of Andrew Vesalius to his books
On the Fabric of the Human Body

Whenever various obstacles stand seriously in the way of the study of the arts and sciences and keep them from being learned accurately and applied advantageously in practice, Charles, Most Clement Caesar, I think a great deal of damage is done. I think also that great harm is caused by too wide a separation of the disciplines which work toward the perfection of each individual art, . . .

Although once upon a time three schools of doctors existed, namely, the Logical, the Empirical and the Methodic, nevertheless the founders of these schools directed the aim of the art as a whole to the preservation of health and the elimination of diseases. In short, they referred to this end all the things which the individual men in their schools deemed necessary to their art, and they were accustomed to make use of three aids. Of these the first was a rational plan of diet; the second, all the uses of drugs; the third, surgery. The last shows with particular aptness that medicine consists in the supplying of deficiencies and the removal of superfluities; and it ever stands ready for the cure of affections. Time and use have shown that, as often as we engage in medical work, surgery is very helpful to the human race in its benefit to these affections.

This three-fold scheme of doctoring was equally familiar to the doctors of each sect. The doctors themselves accommodated their own hands to curing in accordance with the nature of the affections; and they expended no less energy in training their hands than in the business of arranging the diet or of knowing and compounding drugs. For instance, over and above his other books, the volumes which the divine Hippocrates wrote on the Rôle of the Doctor, on the Fractures of Bones, on the Dislocations of Joints, and evils of this type—the best written of all his works—show this clearly. Indeed, Galen, that prince of medicine after Hippocrates, in addition to boasting frequently that the care of the Pergamene gladiators had been entrusted to him alone, and to being unwilling, although his years were heavy upon him, that the apes which were to be dissected by himself should be skinned by the labor of his servants, frequently impresses upon [his readers] how much he delighted in the craft of the hand, and how zealously he and the other doctors of Asia practiced it.

But no one of the ancients seems to have handed down to posterity with equal care the curing which is wrought by the hand and that which is accomplished by diet and medicines. After the devastation of the Goths particularly, when all the sciences, which had previously been so flourishing and had been properly practiced, went to the dogs, the more elegant doctors at first in Italy in imitation of the ancient Romans began to be ashamed of working with their hands, and began to prescribe to their servants what operations they should perform upon the sick, and they merely stood alongside after the fashion of architects. When, soon, others also began to refuse the inconveniences of those practicing true medicine, meanwhile subtracting nothing from their profit and honor, they promptly fell away from the standards of the early doctors. They left the manner of cooking, and in fact the whole preparation, of the diet for the sick, to their attendants, and they left the composition of drugs to the vendors of medicines, and surgery to the barbers. And so in the course of time the technique of curing was so wretchedly torn apart that the doctors, prostituting themselves under the names of "Physicians," appropriated to themselves simply the prescription of drugs and diets for unusual affections; but the rest of medicine they relegated to those whom they call "Chirugians" and deem as if they were servants. They shamefully reject that which is the principal and the most ancient branch of medicine, the one which rests primarily upon the observation of nature (if indeed it is anything else!). Yet this branch of medicine even the kings in India practice to-day; and by the law of heredity in Persia they pass it all on to their children, as once the families of the Asclepiades did. The Thracians, along with many other peoples cultivate and venerate it. Although this art accomplishes absolutely nothing without the help of nature, but rather desires to aid her as she works to free herself from disease; when a part of the art, which the Romans in times past have proscribed from the state as if designed to deceive and destroy men, has been almost wholly neglected, the result is that the utility of the art as a whole is removed and destroyed. To this primarily we owe the fact that this most sacred art is ridiculed, although many censures are normally cast at doctors anyway, since that part of the art which those educated in the liberal arts have shamefully allowed to be torn away is the part which permanently illuminates medicine with its especial glory.

When Homer, the fount of talents, affirms that the medical man is more pre-eminent than many, and when he and the other Greek poets celebrate Podalirius and Machaon, these sons of the divine Aesculapius are not lauded because they did away with a little fever—which Nature alone cures more easily without the aid of a doctor than when the aid is applied—or because they humored the palate of men in peculiar and lamentable affections. They were celebrated because they were especially pre-eminent in the cure of haemorrhages, dislocations, fractures, contusions, wounds, and the other breaks in the continuity of the body. They freed the most noble soldiers of Agamemnon from arrow points, javelins, and other evils of this sort which are principally caused by wars and which demand the careful attention of the doctor.

But, Most August Caesar, Charles, I have in no manner proposed to exalt any one instrument of medicine above the others, since the aforesaid three-fold method of help absolutely can not be disjoined and taken apart. The whole method belongs to one workman. To effect this synthesis properly, all the parts of medicine should be constituted and prepared equally so that all the individual elements can be put to use more advantageously, and each element in turn unites all together more perfectly. Now and then an extremely rare disease does turn up which does not immediately require the three-fold instrument of the safeguards. And so a fitting plan of diet should be instituted, and finally something must be attempted by medicines and then by surgery. Therefore tyros in the art should be encouraged in all the methods, and, if it please the gods, scorning the whisperings of the "physicians," they should apply their hands likewise to curing in whatever manner the nature of the art and reason really demand, as the Greeks did. This they should do lest they turn mutilated medicine to the destruction of the common life of man. And they must be encouraged in this more diligently in proportion as we see today that the men who are more thoroughly grounded in the art abstain from surgery as from the plague. They are afraid that they will be traduced by the fanatics of the medical profession before the unlettered populace as "barbers." They also fear that afterwards they may not get half the profit, honor, or reputation in the eyes of either the unlearned mob or the leaders. This detestable opinion of many people in the first place keeps us from taking up the *whole* craft of healing; and we arrogate to ourselves only the cure of internal affections, we desire to be doctors only in a small way (to tell the truth for once!). The ensuing damage to mortals is great. Indeed, when all the compounding of drugs were relegated to the pharmacists, the doctors in turn soon lost completely the knowledge of the simple drugs that were necessary to them. The shops were filled with barbarous labels and crooked pharmacists.

Furthermore, this most perverse surrender of the instruments of healing to various artificers, has brought a much more execrable disaster and far more frightful calamity upon an outstanding part of natural philosophy. To anatomical study, Hippocrates and Plato gave a high rank, since it embraces the study of man and since it correctly must be considered the solidest foundation of the medical art and the beginning of the constitution. They did not doubt that it should be included in the first parts of medicine. When this subject used to be practiced exclusively by the doctors, they stretched every nerve to master it. But when they surrendered the surgical work to others and forgot their anatomical knowledge, it ultimately began to collapse.

As long as the doctors thought that only the curing of internal affections belonged to them, they considered that the mere knowledge of the viscera was abundantly sufficient. They neglected the fabric of bones, muscles, nerves, veins and of the arteries which creep through the bones and muscles, as being of no concern of theirs. When the whole business was committed to the barbers, not only did the true knowledge of the viscera disappear from among the doctors, but also their activity in dissecting straightway died. This went so far that the doctors did not even attempt cutting; but those barbers, to whom the craft of surgery was delegated, were too unlearned to understand the writings of the professors of dissection. It is far from the truth that this group of men preserved for us this most difficult art, transmitted manually to them; but it is true that this deplorable dispersion of the curative rôle brought a detestable procedure into our Gymnasiums, wherein some were accustomed to administer the cutting of the human body while others narrated the history of the parts. The latter, indeed, from a lofty chair arrogantly cackle like jackdaws about things which they never have tried, but which they commit to memory from the books of others or which they place in written form before their eyes. The former, however, are so unskilled in languages that they cannot explain the dissections to the spectators. They merely chop up the things which are to be shown on the instructions of the physician, who, having never put his hand to cutting, simply steers the boat from the commentary—and not without arrogance. And thus all things are taught wrongly, and days go by in silly disputations. Fewer facts are placed before the spectators in that tumult than a butcher could teach a doctor in his meat market. I shall not mention those schools where they hardly ever think of dissecting the structure of the human body, with the result that ancient medicine declined from its pristine glory years ago.

When at length in the great happiness of this age, which the gods have willed to be ruled by Your power, medicine had begun to revive along with all the studies, and had begun to lift up its head from the profoundest darkness so that it almost seems to have recovered its old splendor in some Academies; and since medicine now needs nothing more acutely than the dead knowledge of the parts of the human body, I decided to go to work on this book with whatever strength and brains I had, and with the encouragement of the example of so many distinguished men. For fear that I alone might go slack at a time when all men are, with great success, essaying something for the sake of the common studies, or even for fear that I might fall away from the standards set by my progenitors, who were by no means obscure doctors, I thought that this branch of natural philosophy should be called back from the depths, so that, even if it should not be more complete among us than among the early doctors of dissection, nevertheless it should some day reach a point where one would not be ashamed to state that our method of dissection compares favorably with the ancient. And one might say that nothing had been so broken down by time, and then so quickly restored, as anatomy.

But this ambition of mine would never have succeeded if, when I was studying medicine at Paris, I myself had not applied my hand to this business, and incidentally had the pleasure of being present at several public dissections put on by certain barbers for my colleagues and me when some viscera were superficially shown. At that time, when we first saw the prosperous re-birth of medicine, anatomy was given rather perfunctory treatment there. When some dissections of animals were being performed under the direction of that celebrated and most praiseworthy gentleman, Jacobus Sylvius, I was encouraged by colleagues and preceptors, although I had been trained only by my own efforts, to perform in public the third dissection at which I ever happened to be present—a dissection which dealt purely and simply with the viscera as was the custom there—and I did it more thoroughly than was usual. Moreover, when I next attacked a dissection, I attempted to show the muscles of the hand along with the more accurate dissection of the viscera. For, aside from the eight muscles of the abdomen, badly mangled and in the wrong order, no one had ever shown a muscle to me, nor any bone, much less the succession of nerves, veins, and arteries.

. . . [At Padua] and at Bologna I performed dissections rather more often, and, having exploded the ridiculous custom of the schools, I taught in such a way that in anatomy we might want nothing which has been handed down to us by the ancients.

But indeed it should be noted that the sluggishness of the doctors has taken too little care that the writings of Eudemus, Herophilus, Marinus, Andrew, Lycus and the other leaders in dissection be preserved for us; not even a fragment of any page survives from the many illustrious authors, more than twenty of whom Galen mentions in his second commentary on Hippocrates' book *De natura humana*. Why, hardly half of his own anatomical books have been saved from destruction! But those who have followed Galen, in which class I consider Oribasius, Theophilus, the Arabs, and all of our men however many I have chanced to read thus far (with your permission I would have written of these), if they handed down anything worth reading, they took it straight from Galen. And, by heaven, to the man who is diligently dissecting they seem to have done nothing less than the dissection of the human body! And so, with their teeth set, the principal followers of Galen put their trust in some kind of talking, and relying upon the inertia of others in dissecting, they shamelessly abridge Galen into elaborate compendia. They do not depart from him a hair's breadth while they are following his sense; but to the front of their books they add writings of their own, stitched together completely from the opinions of Galen—and all of theirs is from him. The whole lot of them have placed their faith in him, with the result that you can not find a doctor who has thought that even the slightest slip has ever been detected in the anatomical volumes of Galen, much less *could* be found (now).

Meanwhile (especially since Galen corrects himself frequently, and in later works written when he became better informed he points out his own slips perpetrated in certain books, and teaches the contrary) it now becomes obvious to us from the reborn art of dissection, from diligent reading of the books of Galen, and from impeccable restoration in numerous places of (the text of) these books, that he himself never dissected the body of a man who had recently died. Although the dried cadavers of men prepared, so to speak, for the inspections of the bones were available to him, he was misled by his apes, and he undeservedly censures the ancient doctors who had busied themselves with the dissection of men. Nay, you may even find a great many things in his writings which he has not followed correctly in the apes; not to mention the fact that in the manifold and infinite difference between the organs of the human body and the body of apes, Galen noticed almost none, except in the fingers and in the bending of the knee. This difference he doubtless would have omitted too, if it had not been obvious to him without the dissection of man.

But in the present work, I have in no wise set out to reprimand the false doctrines of Galen, easily the chief of the professors of dissection; and much less would I wish to be considered disloyal and too little respectful of authority toward that author of all good things right at the beginning of my work. For I am not unaware of how much disturbance the doctors—far less than the adherents of Aristotle—raise when they observe that Galen deviated more than two hundred times from the correct description of the harmony, use, and function of the parts of man in treatment of anatomy alone, as I now exhibit it in the schools, while they examine sharply the dissected particles with the greatest zeal in defending him. Although these men, led by the love of truth, gradually grow milder and put a little more trust in their rational faculties and their eyes—by no means ineffectual eyes and brains—than to the writings of Galen, they are now writing hither and thither to their friends about these truly paradoxical things which have neither been borrowed from the attempts of others or buttressed by congeries of authorities so sedulously and they have been urging their friends to learn some true anatomy so eagerly and amicably, that there is hope of its being fostered in all our Universities as it once was practiced at Alexandria.

In order that this may succeed under the happier auspices of the Muses, besides the works on this subject which I published elsewhere and which certain plagiarists, thinking me far absent from Germany, sent forth as their own; I have now prepared afresh, and to the best of my ability, the history of the parts of the human body in seven books, arranged in the order in which in this city, at Bologna, and at Pisa I have been accustomed to treat it in the assembly of learned men. I have done this with the specific idea that those who have attended the dissector [at work] will have commentaries of the demonstrated facts, and will show anatomy to others with lighter work; although the [commentaries] will not be entirely useless to those to whom direct observation is denied, since of each particle of the human body the site, form, substance, connection to other parts, use, function, and very many things of this sort which we have been accustomed to turn up during dissections in the nature of the parts, together with the technique of dissecting both dead and live men, are pursued at adequate length. The books contain pictures of all the parts inserted into the context of the narrative, so that the dissected body is placed, so to speak, before the eyes of those studying the works of nature.

Truly, there is no one who does not find out in geometry and in the other mathematical disciplines how much pictures help in the understanding of them, and place the matter before the eyes more clearly, even though the text itself is very explicit. But however that may be, in the whole of this work I have striven with the purpose that, in an exceedingly recondite and no less arduous business, I should help as many as possible and that I should treat as truly and completely as possible the history of the fabric of the human body, a fabric not built of ten or twelve parts, as it appears to the casual observer, but of several thousand diverse parts; and finally that I might bring to the candidates in medicine a grist not to be scorned for the understanding of the books of Galen in this field which, among his other monuments, require especially the help of a preceptor.

But in the meanwhile, it is perfectly clear to me that my attempt will have all too little authority because I have not yet passed the twenty-eighth year of my life; it is equally clear that, because of the numerous indications of the false dogmas of Galen, it will be exceedingly unsafe from the attacks of the conservatives, who, as with us in the Italian schools, have sedulously avoided anatomy, and who, being old men, will be consumed with envy because of the correct discoveries of the young, and will be ashamed of having been blind thus far, along with the other followers of Galen.

Andreas Vesalius' First Public Anatomy at Bologna, 1540: An Eyewitness Report

Born in Liegnitz, in Silesia, Baldasar Heseler came from a German family of public officials and businessmen. Before undertaking the study of medicine, Heseler completed a degree in theology under Martin Luther at the University of Wittenberg. From there, he went to the University of Leipzig and, like many of his fellow students, rounded out his medical education at the University of Bologna. After graduating in 1540, Heseler returned to Silesia, becoming a physician of high repute in the town of Breslau. Although thousands of students attended Vesalius's presentations, Heseler's account survives as the only set of notes actually taken during these demonstrations. Also included in Heseler's text are Matthaeus Curtius's commentaries on the *Anatomy* of Mundinus; these always preceded the demonstrations of Vesalius, who adroitly used the text of the body to disprove the text of Mundinus.

THE FIRST ANATOMICAL DEMONSTRATION, IN THE MORNING

The anatomy of our subject was arranged in the place where they use to elect the Rector medicorum; a table on which the subject was laid, was conveniently and well installed with four steps of benches in a circle, so that nearly 200 persons could see the anatomy. However, nobody was allowed to enter before the anatomists, and after them, those who had paid 20 sol. More than 150 students were present and D. Curtius, Erigius, and many other doctors, followers of Curtius. At last, D. Andreas Vesalius arrived, and many candles were lighted, so that we all should see, etc.

Then D. Vesalius began: Domini, you know how doctors, both ancient and modern, use to divide the human body. The Egyptians and the Arabs begin with the trunk and the extremities, but Galen, whom also Mundinus has followed, begins with the three venters. But leaving these questions (because Curtius requested him to demonstrate what [Curtius] had lectured) we shall proceed to our anatomy. And there was the body cut up and prepared beforehand, already shaved, washed and cleaned. He began with the outer skin, to which the inner one adhered, that is rightly called the skin, cutis, the outer one being better named hide. And, he said, these two cannot well be separated, because the inner one is too subtle and really spermatic, which when ruptured or cut cannot be healed. And he proved the difference between these

From *Andreas Vesalius' First Public Anatomy at Bologna, 1540: An Eyewitness Report*, ed. and trans. Ruben Eriksson (Uppsala and Stockholm: Almquist & Wiksells, 1959). Used by permission.

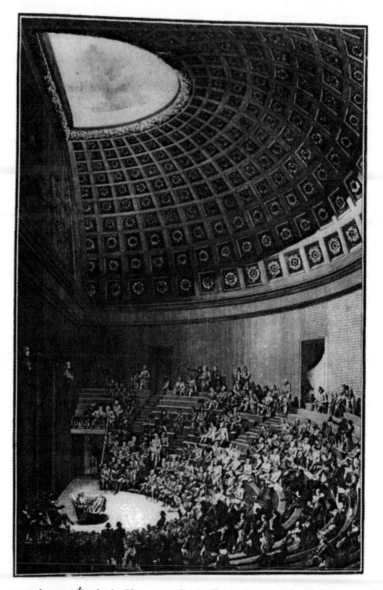

6. *Anatomy theater, École de Chirurgie, Paris. From Jacques Gondouin,* Description des Écoles de Chirurgie *(Paris: P. D. Pierres, 1780). Wellcome Institute Library, London. The glorification of the anatomy theater is apparent in the artist's use of classical models in designing it. Architectural elements from the Pantheon—the Roman temple dedicated to all the gods—as well as from the famous Greek theater at Epidaurus—the religious center devoted to the healing arts in classical antiquity— are invoked. Gondouin, however, literally throws a sinister light on the grandeur of the proceedings, transforming the midsection of observers into cadaverous spectators.*

two in the following way: with a candle he burnt the outer skin which is called corium, and showed us how it turned into blisters, while the inner skin, however, did not blister because it was more fleshy and fleshlike than the outer one. The inner skin was whitish, having the form of the sperma, out of which it has its origin. Because, he said, the complexion always takes the form and nature of the components, out of which they originate, as the skin, in otherwise the same conditions, in colour take and appropriate the nature of its humours. Then there was the fat adhering to the fleshy layer beneath the skin, that had been separated from it with a razor, and he declared that the fat which moistened the skin, coagulated because of the coldness of the skin. In this membrane or layer he demonstrated to us the black ends of the veins and the openings of the nerves, the veins for the nourishment of both kinds of skin and the nerves for the feeling of the inner skin. This he showed us in the left side. In the right side, again, he had not removed this layer. In this way, he said, the butchers strip the carcases. At last he came to the anatomy of the muscles, which, extremely skilled in dissecting as he was, he had dissected with the utmost diligence so that the substance, the size, the position, the beginning and the end of each one of them could be clearly seen.

THE SECOND DEMONSTRATION, IN THE AFTERNOON

He had stripped off the skin of the entire inner side of the arm to the tips of the nails of the hand. And before he demonstrated the dissection [of the muscles], their position etc., it is necessary, he said, for you beforehand to know the anatomy of the bones; for from the extremities of them all the muscles have their origin beginning at the head with a sinew and ending tied [to the bones] at their caudae with the tendons or cordae. Accordingly he demonstrated to us in the promised anatomy of the bones, how the muscles begin at the heads of the bones and how they end with their tendons at the hands and at each of the joints of each finger. Thereafter, he enumerated to us the muscles of the interior side of the arm, which tend towards our head, and he showed by dissection how the muscles with a thin sinew begin at the head of the bones of the arm and how after a long course they end in the hand and the joints of the fingers, how the muscles in double layers are situated one over the other, always four over four, and how the lower ones tend to the first joints, the upper ones to the second and third joints, and always pass through the first ones. Certainly this was very beautiful to see. And he showed us how these sinews at the same time were covered by a special membrane, and he separated them from each other and followed them to the joints of the fingers. About this he said: please, read Galen, *De usu partium,* I and II, *De anatomicis administrationibus,* I, and about the muscles of the organs. Tomorrow we shall see the anatomy of the muscles of the exterior part of the forearm or the cubitus.

THE ELEVENTH DEMONSTRATION
The Anatomy of the 'Didimi'

Mundinus goes on to the spermatic vessels of the female, to the uterus etc. but all that we shall pass, as we now have no female body. But we shall explain the anatomy of the spermatic vessels of the male and first the anatomy of the testicles. . . . Galen says that the organs of procreation are the same in the male and in the female, only that in the female all is reversed to the male, in whom that which is inside in the female is outside. And again in the male all is contrary to the female. For if you turn the scrotum, the testicles and the penis inside out you will also have all the genital organs of the female, like they are in the male. (Yet the penis of the male is more solid, the neck of the uterus of the female more excavated and concave and much more extendable in time of coitus and parturition.) Vice versa, if you turn inside out the genital organs of the female, you will have all the organs of the male. Thus, they differ only by being reversed. The reason of this reversion in the female is that they have all their genital organs inside, and that is, I maintain, owing to their lack of natural warmth. Therefore in women these organs have stayed inside. This results in three great advantages in woman. One is that their genital organs are inside in order to receive man's seed. The second reason is that women increase the superfluous blood and humidities, which they have attracted, and that thus they overflow with superfluous blood, namely for the production and nourishment of the foetus. This is why not-pregnant women menstruate naturally each month, but when they become pregnant, the fluids are retained for the said purpose, namely conserved for the nourishment of the foetus. The third reason is that they cannot conceive by their own seed without the intercourse of the male. For [the seed of the male] is required, because it is hotter and more perfect, but that of the female colder.

THE FOURTEENTH DEMONSTRATION, IN THE MORNING

Because our next subject was hanged this morning (there were two of them) during Curtius' lecture and they were still hanging, as I myself saw, the students in the meantime had killed a pregnant bitch, which was the fourth dog. Hence, this morning D. Vesalius demonstrated the anatomy of the uterus and of the embryos contained in it, the puppies. He showed how the arteries and the veins outside the uterus converging ran to the umbilicus of each foetus, and there was always an interval or an interspace between them at each foetus. And in this dog there were seven puppies. Thereafter he opened the substance of the uterus, which was membranous, sinewy, elastic and rather soft. Thereafter a second membrane appeared where the umbilical vein and artery ran together. Then there was another sack in which the sweat of the foetuses was received. The fourth and last was that in which the urine of the foetuses was contained. When we had seen this, he dissected two puppies showing us in them the composition of the umbilicus, namely how two veins ran to the liver conveying the nourishment, and two arteries to the heart conveying spirits and warmth. And there was one white duct that tended to the side of the bladder, and it was strongly connected to and entered the bladder, and through this duct the urine was transmitted into the fourth and last sack mentioned before. And thus the anatomy of the pregnant [dog] and the foetuses is completed.

THE TWENTY-SECOND DEMONSTRATION, IN THE EVENING

When the lecture of Curtius was finished, Vesalius, who had been present and heard the refutation of his arguments, asked Curtius to accompany him to the anatomy. For he wanted to show him that his theory was quite true. Therefore he brought Curtius to our two bodies. Now, he said, excellentissime Domine, here we have our bodies. We shall see whether I have made an error. Now we want to look at this and we should in the meantime leave Galen, for I acknowledge that I have said, if it is permissible to say so, that here Galen is in the wrong, because he did not know the position of the vein without pair in the human body, which is the same to-day just as it was in his time. Curtius answered smiling, for Vesalius, choleric as he was, was very excited: No, he said, Domine, we must not leave Galen, because he always well understood everything, and, consequently, we also follow him. Do you know how to interpret Hippocrates better than Galen did? Vesalius answered: I do not say so, but I show you here in these bodies the vein without pair, how it nourishes all the lower ribs, except the two upper ones, in which there is no pleurisy. For always here—he knocked with his hands against the middle of the chest—occurs inflammation and pleurisy, not at the two upper ribs. Consequently, as this vein also is distant from the heart, as you see, by three fingers' breadth, it will always in pleurisy and all morbus lateralis be better to bleed from this vein only; or it ought to be no difference from what part the bleeding is done, because the ribs are nourished exclusively by this vein. Curtius replied: I am no anatomista, but there can be also other veins nourishing the ribs and the muscles besides these. Where, please, Vesalius said, show them to me. Curtius said: Do you want to deny the ducts of Nature? Oh!, Vesalius said, you want to talk about things not visible and concealed. I, again, talk about what is visible. Curtius answered: Indeed, I always deal with what is most obvious. Domine, you do not well understand Hippocrates and Galen concerning this. Vesalius replied: It is quite true, because I am not so old a man as you are. Thus, with much quarrel and scoffing they attacked each other, and in the meantime they accomplished nothing. Vesalius said: D. Doctor, I beg Your Excellency not to think me so unskilled that I do not know and understand this. Smiling Curtius said: Domine, I did not say so, for I have said that you are excellent, but I have rejected the wrong explanation of Hippocrates implying that Galen should have erred in this. Vesalius replied: I acknowledge that I have said that Galen has erred in this, and this is evident here in these bodies, as also many other mistakes of his. When Curtius asked Vesalius not to be angry with him, Vesalius said: not at all, Domine. And thus Curtius left.

FELIX PLATTER (1536–1614)

Journal

In 1552, Felix Platter, following his father's wishes, set out from Basle to Montpellier to take up the study of medicine, keeping a journal of his adventures. His father, the head of a school and printing establishment, had chosen his son's profession and education shrewdly. By the sixteenth century, a career in medicine promised social prestige as well as financial security, and the medical school at Montpellier was one of Europe's best. Platter did not disappoint his father's hopes; after returning home from Montpellier, he became the chief physician of Basle, professor and rector of its university, and attendant to several of the great families of France and Switzerland. The study of mental illness became his speciality, and in his efforts to understand its nature and causes, he went so far as to live with the mad in the dungeons where they were confined. It was, no doubt, this same relentless spirit of inquiry that had urged him on as a medical student in 1554, during his nightmarish raids on the graveyards of Montpellier.

I had always desired to know everything concerning medicine, even those parts commonly neglected. I was mindful, too, of the multitude of physicians in Basle, among whom I could make my way only by superior knowledge. I could not expect to be assisted by my father, who was overwhelmed with debt, had only a small income, and was reduced to living on what revenue came from the boarders in his school. I could not have imagined then that he would remarry in his old age and have a large number of children. The desire to learn made me follow with attention not only the lectures and ordinary studies, but also the preparation of remedies in the pharmacy, a matter I found very useful later. Further, I collected plants, and arranged them properly on paper. But my principal study was anatomy. Not only did I never miss the dissections of men and animals that took place in the College, but I also took part in every secret autopsy of corpses, and I came to put my own hand to the scalpel, despite the repulsion I had felt at first. I joined with French students and exposed myself to danger to procure subjects. A bachelor of medicine named Gallotus, who had married a woman from Montpellier and was passing rich, would lend us his house. He invited me, with some others, to join him in nocturnal expeditions outside the town, to dig up bodies freshly buried in the cloister cemetery, and we carried them to his house for dissection. We had spies to tell us of burials and to lead us by night to the graves.

Our first excursion of this kind took place on the 11th of November 1554. As night fell Gallotus led us out of the town to the monastery of the Augustins, where we met a monk, called Brother Bernhard, a determined fellow, who had disguised him-

From *Beloved Son Felix: The Journal of Felix Platter, a Medical Student in Montpellier in the Sixteenth Century*, trans. Seán Jennett (London: Frederick Muller, 1961).

self in order to help us. When we came to the monastery we stayed to drink, quietly, until midnight. Then, in complete silence, and with swords in hand, we made our way to the cemetery of the monastery of Saint-Denis. There we dug up a corpse with our hands, the earth being still loose, because the burial had taken place only that day. As soon as we had uncovered it we pulled it out with ropes, wrapped it in a *flassada,* and carried it on two poles as far as the gates of the town. It must then have been about three o'clock in the morning. We put the corpse to one side and knocked on the postern that is opened for coming and going at night, and the old porter came in his shirt to open it for us. We asked him to bring us something to drink, under the pretext that we were dying of thirst, and while he went in search of wine three of us brought the cadaver in and carried it directly to Gallotus's house, which was not far away. The porter was not suspicious, and we rejoined our companions. On opening the winding sheet in which the body was sewn, we found a woman with a congenital deformity of the legs, the two feet turned inwards. We did an autopsy and found, among other curiosities, various veins *vasorum spermaticorum,* which were not deformed, but followed the curve of the legs towards the buttocks. She had a lead ring, and as I detest these it added to my disgust.

Encouraged by the success of this expedition, we tried again five days later. We had been informed that a student and a child had been buried in the same cemetery of Saint-Denis. When night came we left the town to go to the monastery of the Augustins. It was the 16th of December. In Brother Bernhard's cell we ate a chicken cooked with cabbage. We got the cabbage ourselves, from the garden, and seasoned it with wine supplied by the monk. Leaving the table, we went out with our weapons drawn, for the monks of Saint-Denis had discovered that we had exhumed the woman, and they had threatened us direly should we return. Myconius carried his naked sword, and the Frenchmen their rapiers. The two corpses were disinterred, wrapped in our cloaks, and carried on poles as before as far as the gates of the town. We did not dare to rouse the porter this time, so one of us crawled inside through a hole that we discovered under the gate—for they were very negligently maintained. We passed the cadavers through the same opening, and they were pulled through from the inside. We followed in turn, pulling ourselves through on our backs; I remember that I scratched my nose as I went through.

The two subjects were carried to Gallotus's house and their coverings were removed. One was a student whom we had known. The autopsy revealed serious lesions. The lungs were decomposed and stank horribly, despite the vinegar that we sprinkled on them; we found some small stones in them. The child was a little boy, and we made a skeleton of him.

When I returned to my lodging early in the morning, the shop boy who slept with me did not hear me ring, and he did not wake even when I threw stones against the shutters. I was obliged to go for some sleep to the house of one of the Frenchmen who had been with us. After this the monks of Saint-Denis guarded their graveyard, and if a student came near he was received with bolts from a crossbow.

WILLIAM HARVEY (1578–1657)

An Anatomical Study on the Motion of the Heart and the Blood in Animals

William Harvey received his B.A. from Cambridge, where he studied with John Caius, once a pupil of Vesalius. Like Caius before him, Harvey chose Padua for his medical education, and after completing his degree in 1602, he returned to England to set up a private practice. In 1609, Harvey was appointed physician at St. Bartholomew's Hospital and began to consider a problem that had as yet been barely formulated: How is it that blood moves through the body? An anatomist by training, Harvey focused his attention on the heart, dissecting hundreds of animals from nearly eighty different species. Although Galen had speculated that blood flows from the heart's right side to the left through pores in the septum, Harvey could not find them. In watching the heart, he noted that it contracted seventy-two times per minute, forcing blood into the arteries with every movement. Harvey's next question was inspired: How much blood does the heart pump every hour? Calculating that it ejects two fluid ounces per beat, seventy-two times per minute ($72 \times 60 \times 2$), he came up with the astounding figure of 8,640 ounces per hour. Finding it impossible to believe that the heart could make such a quantity of blood every hour, Harvey was forced to conclude that the heart does not continually produce new blood but rather circulates or "recycles" it. The path of return to the heart could only be the veins, and Harvey was able to demonstrate this by applying pressure to the veins of the forearm. Although most of Harvey's discoveries were in place by the time he was appointed physician to James I in 1618, he delayed publishing them until 1628, in anticipation of the storm of controversy that would follow his "reinvention" of the body. Few readers would fail to grasp the fact that De Motu Cordis had leveled the old qualitative model of form and function, and that in its place, Harvey had erected a new physiology based on measurement and mathematics, and on the ceaseless dynamic of ordered motion.

To The Most Illustrious and Indomitable Prince CHARLES, KING *of* GREAT BRITAIN, FRANCE *and* IRELAND, DEFENDER *of the* FAITH

Most Illustrious Prince!
The heart of animals is the foundation of their life, the sovereign of everything within them, the sun of their microcosm, that upon which all growth depends, from which

From *Exercitatio Anatomica De Motu Cordis et Sanguinis in Animalibus,* trans. Chauncey D. Leake, 4th ed. (Springfield, Ill.: Charles C. Thomas, 1958). Used by permission of Blackwell Scientific Publications Ltd.

all power proceeds. The King, in like manner, is the foundation of his kingdom, the sun of the world around him, the heart of the republic, the fountain whence all power, all grace doth flow. What I have here written of the motions of the heart I am the more emboldened to present to your Majesty, according to the custom of the present age, because almost all things human are done after human examples, and many things in a King are after the pattern of the heart. The knowledge of his heart, therefore, will not be useless to a Prince, as embracing a kind of Divine example of his functions,—and it has still been usual with men to compare small things with great. Here, at all events, best of Princes, placed as you are on the pinnacle of human affairs, you may at once contemplate the prime mover in the body of man, and the emblem of your own sovereign power. Accept, therefore, with your wonted clemency, I most humbly beseech you, illustrious Prince, this, my new Treatise on the Heart; you, who are yourself the new light of this age, and, indeed, its very heart; a Prince abounding in virtue and in grace, and to whom we gladly refer all the blessings which England enjoys, all the pleasure we have in our lives.

Your Majesty's most devoted servant,
WILLIAM HARVEY

(London. . . . 1628.)

To His Very Dear Friend
DOCTOR ARGENT
the excellent and accomplished PRESIDENT *of* THE ROYAL COLLEGE *of*
PHYSICIANS, *and* to other learned PHYSICIANS, his esteemed COLLEAGUES.

I have already and repeatedly presented you, my learned friends, with my new views of the motion and function of the heart, in my anatomical lectures; but having now for nine years and more confirmed these views by multiplied demonstrations in your presence, illustrated them by arguments, and freed them from the objections of the most learned and skilful anatomists, I at length yield to the requests, I might say entreaties, of many, and here present them for general consideration in this treatise.

Were not the work indeed presented through you, my learned friends, I should scarce hope that it could come out scatheless and complete; for you have in general been the faithful witnesses of almost all the instances from which I have either collected the truth or confuted error; you have seen my dissections, and at my demonstrations of all that I maintain to be objects of sense, you have been accustomed to stand by and bear me out with your testimony. And as this book alone declares the blood to course and revolve by a new route, very different from the ancient and beaten pathway trodden for so many ages, and illustrated by such a host of learned and distinguished men, I was greatly afraid lest I might be charged with presumption did I lay my work before the public at home, or send it beyond seas for impression, unless I had first proposed its subject to you, had confirmed its conclusions by ocular demonstrations in your presence, had replied to your doubts and objections, and secured the assent and support of our distinguished President. For I was most intimately persuaded, that if I could make good my proposition before you and our College, illustrious by its numerous body of learned individuals, I had less to fear from others;

I even ventured to hope that I should have the comfort of finding all that you had granted me in your sheer love of truth, conceded by others who were philosophers like yourselves. For true philosophers, who are only eager for truth and knowledge, never regard themselves as already so thoroughly informed, but that they welcome further information from whomsoever and from whencesoever it may come; nor are they so narrow-minded as to imagine any of the arts or sciences transmitted to us by the ancients, in such a state of forwardness or completeness, that nothing is left for the ingenuity and industry of others; very many, on the contrary, maintain that all we know is still infinitely less than all that still remains unknown; nor do philosophers pin their faith to others' precepts in such wise that they lose their liberty, and cease to give credence to the conclusions of their proper senses. Neither do they swear such fealty to their mistress Antiquity, that they openly, and in sight of all, deny and desert their friend Truth. But even as they see that the credulous and vain are disposed at the first blush to accept and to believe everything that is proposed to them, so do they observe that the dull and unintellectual are indisposed to see what lies before their eyes, and even to deny the light of the noonday sun. They teach us in our course of philosophy as sedulously to avoid the fables of the poets and the fancies of the vulgar, as the false conclusions of the sceptics. And then the studious, and good, and true, never suffer their minds to be warped by the passions of hatred and envy, which unfit men duly to weigh the arguments that are advanced in behalf of truth, or to appreciate the proposition that is even fairly demonstrated; neither do they think it unworthy of them to change their opinion if truth and undoubted demonstration require them so to do; nor do they esteem it discreditable to desert error, though sanctioned by the highest antiquity; for they know full well that to err, to be deceived, is human; that many things are discovered by accident, and that many may be learned indifferently from any quarter, by an old man from a youth, by a person of understanding from one of inferior capacity.

INTRODUCTION

In discussing the movements and functions of the heart and arteries, we should first consider what others have said on these matters, and what the common and traditional viewpoint is. Then by anatomical study, repeated experiment, and careful observation, we may confirm what is correctly stated, but what is false make right.

Nearly all anatomists, physicians, and philosophers up to now have thought with Galen that the pulse has the same function as respiration, differing only in one respect, the former arising from an animal, the latter a vital faculty, but from the standpoint of function or movement behaving alike. Thus one finds, as in the recent book on *Respiration* by Hieronymus Fabricius of Aquapendente, that since the pulsation of the heart and arteries is not sufficient for the aeration and cooling of the blood, Nature has placed the lungs around the heart. So it seems that whatever has been said prior to this about the systole and diastole of the heart and arteries has been proposed with special reference to the lungs.

Since the movements and structure of the heart differ from those of the lungs, as those of the arteries from those of the chest, separate functions or purposes are likely. The pulsings and uses of the heart as well as of the arteries are distinct from those of the chest and lungs. If the pulse and respiration have the same purpose, if the arteries in diastole draw air into their cavities (as commonly said) and in systole give off waste vapors by the same pores in flesh and skin, and if also in the time between systole and diastole they contain air, in fact containing at all times either air, spirits, or sooty vapors, what may be answered to Galen? He declared that the arteries by nature contain blood and blood alone, neither air nor spirits, as may easily be determined by experiments and explanations found in his report.

It is not to be supposed that the function of the pulse is the same as that of respiration because the respiration is made more frequent and powerful, as Galen says, by the same causes as running, bathing or any other heating agent. Not only is experience opposed to this (though Galen strives to get around it), when by immoderate gorging the pulse becomes great and the respiration less, but in children the pulse is rapid when respiration is slow. Likewise in fear, trouble, or worry, in many fevers, of course, the pulse is very fast, the respiration slower than usual.

If one repeats Galen's experiment of opening the trachea of a living dog, forcing air into the lungs by a bellows, and then firmly tying off the trachea, a great abundance of air even out to the pleurae will be found in the lungs on opening the chest. No air, however, will be found in the pulmonary vein or in the left ventricle of the heart. It certainly should be if the heart drew in air from the lungs, or if the lungs transmitted air to the heart, in the living dog. On inflating the lungs of a cadaver in an anatomical demonstration, who doubts the air could be seen going this way if such a passage exists? This function of the pulmonary vein, the transmission of air from the lungs to the heart, is considered so significant that Hieronymus Fabricius of Aquapendente insists the lungs were made for the sake of this vessel and that it is their most important structure.

Even less tolerable is the opinion which supposes two materials, air and blood, necessary for the formation of vital spirits. The blood is supposed to ooze through tiny pores in the septum of the heart from the right to the left ventricle, while the air is drawn from the lungs by the large pulmonary vein. According to this many little openings exist in the septum of the heart suited to the passage of blood. But, damn it, no such pores exist, nor can they be demonstrated!

The septum of the heart is of denser and more compact material than any part of the body except bones and tendons. Even so, supposing the pores are there, how could the left ventricle draw blood from the right when both ventricles contract and dilate at the same time? Why not rather believe that the right ventricle draws spirits through these pores from the left instead of the left ventricle drawing blood from the right? It is surely miraculous and incongruous that plenty of blood should be drawn through obscure invisible openings in the same time as air through wide open ones. Why require invisible pores and obscure uncertain channels to get the blood to the left ventricle when there is such a wide open passage through the pulmonary vein?

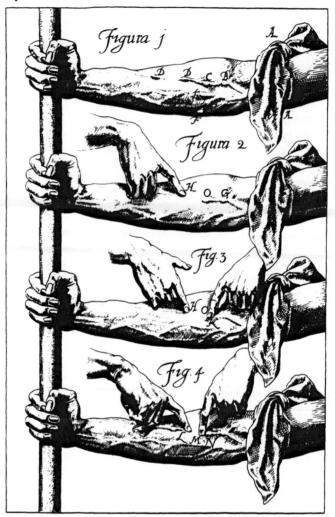

7. *Diagram illustrating William Harvey's experiments on the valves of the veins (1628);
after a drawing by S. Gooden for the Nonesuch edition of* De Motu Cordis *(London,
1928). Wellcome Institute Library, London. This diagram illustrates the simple exercise Harvey designed to demonstrate the fact that the veins carry blood back to the
heart. While his subject grasped a staff, Harvey pressed a finger on the veins of the
forearm and, through a sequence of movements, was able to show that the valves in
the veins are arranged in such a way that blood passing through them can flow only
toward the heart.*

THE AUTHOR'S REASONS FOR WRITING

When I first tried animal experimentation for the purpose of discovering the motions and functions of the heart by actual inspection and not by other people's books, I found it so truly difficult that I almost believed with Fracastorius, that the motion of the heart was to be understood by God alone. I could not really tell when systole or diastole took place, or when and where dilatation or constriction occurred, because of the quickness of the movement. In many animals this takes place in the twinkling of an eye, like a flash of lightning. Systole seemed at one time here, diastole there, then all reversed, varied and confused. So I could reach no decision, neither about what I might conclude myself nor believe from others.

Finally, using greater care every day, with very frequent experimentation, observing a variety of animals, and comparing many observations, I felt my way out of this labyrinth, and gained accurate information, which I desired, of the motions and functions of the heart and arteries. From that time I have not hesitated to declare my thoughts on this matter, not only in private to friends, but even publicly in my anatomical lectures, as in the ancient Academy.

CONCLUSION OF THE DEMONSTRATION OF THE CIRCULATION OF THE BLOOD

Briefly let me now sum up and propose generally my idea of the circulation of the blood.

It has been shown by reason and experiment that blood by the beat of the ventricles flows through the lungs and heart and is pumped to the whole body. There it passes through pores in the flesh into the veins through which it returns from the periphery everywhere to the center, from the smaller veins into the larger ones, finally coming to the vena cava and right auricle. This occurs in such an amount, with such an outflow through the arteries, and such a reflux through the veins, that it cannot be supplied by the food consumed. It is also much more than is needed for nutrition. It must therefore be concluded that the blood in the animal body moves around in a circle continuously, and that the action or function of the heart is to accomplish this by pumping. This is the only reason for the motion and beat of the heart.

THE CIRCULATION OF THE BLOOD IS CONFIRMED BY PLAUSIBLE METHODS

It will not be irrelevant here to point out further that even according to common ideas, the circulation is both convenient and necessary. In the first place, since death is a dissolution resulting from lack of heat, all living things being warm, all dying things cold *(Aristotle, De Respir., lib. 2 & 3, De Part. Animal., etc.),* there must be a place of origin for this heat. On this hearth, as it were, the original native fire, the warming power of nature, is preserved. From this heat and life may flow everywhere in the body, nourishment may come from it, and on it all vegetative energy may depend.

That the heart is this place and source of life, in the manner just described, I hope no one will deny.

The blood, then, must move, and in such a way that it is brought back to the heart, for otherwise it would become thick and immobile, as Aristotle says *(De Part. Animal., lib. 2)*, in the periphery of the body, far from its source.

Hence as long as the heart is uninjured, life and health can be restored to the body generally, but if it is exhausted or harmed by any severe affliction, the whole body must suffer and be injured. The heart alone is so situated and constructed as a reservoir and fountain that blood may be apportioned from it and distributed by its beat to all regions according to the size of the artery serving them.

Moreover, force and effort, such as given by the heart, is needed to distribute and move the blood this way. Blood easily concentrates toward the interior, as drops of water spilled on a table tend to run together, from such slight causes as cold, fear, or horror. It also tends to move from the tiny veins to the intermediate branches and then to the larger veins because of the movements of the extremities and the compression of muscles. So it is more inclined to move from the periphery toward the interior, even though valves offered no opposition to the contrary. Therefore, blood requires force and impulse to be moved from its origin against its inclination into more narrow and cooler channels. Only the heart can furnish this.

THE MOTION AND CIRCULATION OF THE BLOOD IS ESTABLISHED BY WHAT IS DISPLAYED IN THE HEART AND ELSEWHERE BY ANATOMICAL INVESTIGATION

I do not find the heart a separate and distinct organ in all animals. Some, called plant-animals, have no heart at all. These animals are colder, have little bulk, are softer, and of uniform structure, such as grubs, worms, and many which come from decayed material and do not preserve their species. These need no heart to impel nourishment to their extremities, for their bodies are uniform and they have no separate members. By the contraction and relaxation of the whole body they take up and move, expel and remove aliment. Oysters, mussels, sponges and the whole genus of zoophytes or plant-animals have no heart, for the whole body functions as a heart, and the animal itself is a heart.

The auricles exist as the initial motive power of the blood. Especially the right auricle, the first to live and the last to die, ... They are necessary in order to cast the blood conveniently into the ventricles. These, continually contracting, throw out more fully and forcibly the blood already in motion, just as a ball-player can send a ball harder and farther by striking it on a rebound than if he simply throws it.

It is noteworthy that the auricles are disproportionately large in the fetus, because they are present before the rest of the heart is made or can take up its function, so that ... they assume the duty of the whole heart.

While the fetus is still soft like a worm, or as is said, in the milk, there is a single bloody spot, or pulsating sac, as if a part of the umbilical vein were dilated at its base or origin. After a while when the fetus is outlined and the body begins to be more substantial, this vesicle becomes more fleshy and stronger, and its constitution changing, it turns into the auricles. From these the bulk of the heart begins to sprout, although as yet it has no function. When the fetus is really developed, with bones separated from fresh, when the body is perfected and has motion, then the heart actually beats and, as I said, pumps blood by both ventricles from the vena cava to the arteries.

Thus divine Nature making nothing in vain, neither gives a heart to an animal where it is not needed, nor makes one before it can be used. By the same steps in the development of every animal, passing through the structural stages, I might say, of egg, worm, and fetus, it obtains perfection in each. These points are confirmed elsewhere by many observations on the formation of the fetus.

. . . [The heart] is the first to exist, and contains in itself blood, vitality, sensation and motion before the brain or liver are formed, or can be clearly distinguished, or at least before they can assume any function. Being finished first, Nature wished the rest of the body to be made, nourished, preserved, and perfected by it, as its work and home. The heart is like the head of a state, holding supreme power, ruling everywhere. So in the animal body power is entirely dependent on and derived from this source and foundation.

PART 3

Anatomy and Destiny

ARISTOTLE (384–322 B.C.)

The Generation of Animals

If in Raphael's *School of Athens* Plato is pointing upward to the realm of Ideal Forms, Aristotle is gesturing downward toward the earth, indicating that the ideal can be grasped only by studying its manifestations in the natural world. A student in Plato's Academy, Aristotle went on in 355 to found the Lyceum, his own school of philosophy, where he and his students conducted research in a diversity of fields, including political science, music, ethics, zoology, botany, and biology. *The Generation of Animals,* which is the West's first systematic treatise on reproduction and embryology, represents a synthesis of Aristotle's thought; he believed that the processes of reproduction were the means by which humanity achieved the eternal, and as such, they involved not only the natural endowments of the individual but the collective forces of the cosmos. In these processes, the female—possessing sexual organs that are inverse and inferior analogues of the male's—plays an integral but secondary role. Within Aristotle's binary hierarchy, the male imparts Form to the fetus, while the female contributes Matter, a gendered dichotomy of spirit and flesh, mind and body, whose social and political ramifications are made explicit in the *Politics.* Here, Aristotle asserts that "the relation of male to female is naturally that of the superior to the inferior—of the ruling to the ruled."

. . . [T]he exhaustion consequent on the loss of even a very little of the semen is conspicuous because the body is deprived of the ultimate gain drawn from the nutriment.

. . . [W]e must distinguish of what sort of nutriment it is a secretion, and must discuss the catamenia which occur in certain of the vivipara. For thus we shall make it clear (1) whether the female also produces semen like the male and the foetus is a single mixture of two semens, or whether no semen is secreted by the female, and, (2) if not, whether she contributes nothing else either to generation but only provides a receptacle, or whether she does contribute something, and, if so, how and in what manner she does so.

We have previously stated that the final nutriment is the blood in the sanguinea and the analogous fluid in the other animals. Since the semen is also a secretion of the nutriment, and that in its final stage, it follows that it will be either (1) blood or that which is analogous to blood, or (2) something formed from this. But since it is from the blood, when concocted and somehow divided up, that each part of the body is made, and since the semen if properly concocted is quite of a different character from the blood when it is separated from it, but if not properly concocted has been

From *The Works of Aristotle,* ed. J. A. Smith and W. D. Ross, Vol. 5: *De Generatione Animalium,* trans. Arthur Platt (Oxford: Clarendon Press, 1912).

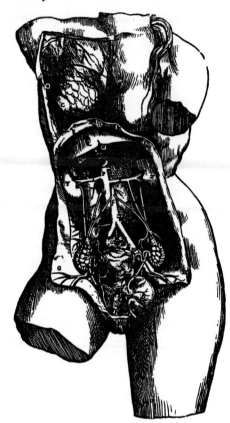

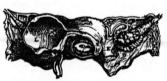

8. *Woodcut of female reproductive organs from Andreas Vesalius,* Suorum de Humani Corporis Fabrica Librorum Epitome *(Basle: Johannes Oporinus, 1543). From J. B. deC. M. Saunders and Charles D. O'Malley,* Illustrations from the Works of Andreas Vesalius of Brussels *(New York: Dover Publications, 1973).*

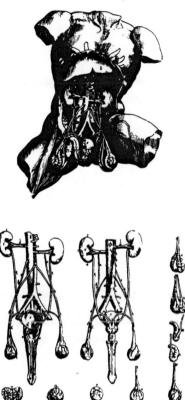

9. Woodcut of male reproductive organs from Andreas Vesalius, Suorum de Humani Corporis Fabrica Librorum Epitome *(Basle: Johannes Oporinus, 1543). From J. B. deC. M. Saunders and Charles D. O'Malley,* Illustrations from the Works of Andreas Vesalius of Brussels *(New York: Dover Publications, 1973). Vesalius's illustrations of human genitalia were guided by the centuries-old notion that the female reproductive organs were but the inverse of the male's. In keeping with Galen's remark that "the organs of procreation are the same in the male and the female," Vesalius aimed to demonstrate that "if you turn the scrotum, the testicles and the penis inside out, you will . . . have all the genitals of the female."*

known in some cases to issue in a bloody condition if one forces oneself too often to coition, therefore it is plain that semen will be a secretion of the nutriment when reduced to blood, being that which is finally distributed to the parts of the body. And this is the reason why it has so great power, for the loss of the pure and healthy blood is an exhausting thing; for this reason also it is natural that the offspring should resemble the parents, for that which goes to all the parts of the body resembles that which is left over. So that the semen which is to form the hand or the face or the whole animal is already the hand or face or whole animal undifferentiated, and what each of them is actually such is the semen potentially, either in virtue of its own mass or because it has a certain power in itself. I mention these alternatives here because we have not yet made it clear from the distinctions drawn hitherto whether it is the matter of the semen that is the cause of generation, or whether it has in it some faculty and efficient cause thereof, for the hand also or any other bodily part is not hand or other part in a true sense if it be without soul or some other power, but is only called by the same name as the living hand.

On this subject, then, so much may be laid down. But since it is necessary (1) that the weaker animal also should have a secretion greater in quantity and less concocted, and (2) that being of such a nature it should be a mass of sanguineous liquid, and (3) since that which Nature endows with a smaller portion of heat is weaker, and (4) since it has already been stated that such is the character of the female—putting all these considerations together we see that the sanguineous matter discharged by the female is also a secretion. And such is the discharge of the so-called catamenia.

It is plain, then, that the catamenia are a secretion, and that they are analogous in females to the semen in males. The circumstances connected with them are evidence that this view is correct. For the semen begins to appear in males and to be emitted at the same time of life that the catamenia begin to flow in females, and that they change their voice and their breasts begin to develop. So, too, in the decline of life the generative power fails in the one sex and the catamenia in the other.

Now since this is what corresponds in the female to the semen in the male, and since it is not possible that two such discharges should be found together, it is plain that the female does not contribute semen to the generation of the offspring. For if she had semen she would not have the catamenia; but, as it is, because she has the latter she has not the former.

And a proof that the female does not emit similar semen to the male, and that the offspring is not formed by a mixture of both, as some say, is that often the female conceives without the sensation of pleasure in intercourse, and if again the pleasure is experienced by her no less than by the male and the two sexes reach their goal together, yet often no conception takes place unless the liquid of the so-called catamenia is present in a right proportion. Hence the female does not produce young if the catamenia are absent altogether, nor often when, they being present, the efflux still continues; but she does so *after* the purgation. For in the one case she has not the nutriment or material from which the foetus can be framed by the power coming from the male and inherent in the semen, and in the other it is washed away with the catamenia because of their abundance. But when after their occurrence the greater part has been evacuated, the remainder is formed into a foetus.

It is clear then that the female contributes the material for generation, and that this is in the substance of the catamenia, and that they are a secretion.

Some think that the female contributes semen in coition because the pleasure she experiences is sometimes similar to that of the male, and also is attended by a liquid discharge. But this discharge is not seminal; it is merely proper to the part concerned in each case, for there is a discharge from the uterus which occurs in some women but not in others. The amount of this discharge, when it occurs, is sometimes on a different scale from the emission of semen and far exceeds it.

And as to the pleasure which accompanies coition it is due to emission not only of semen, but also of a spiritus, the coming together of which precedes the emission. This is plain in the case of boys who are not yet able to emit semen, but are near the proper age, and of men who are impotent, for all these are capable of pleasure by attrition. And those who have been injured in the generative organs sometimes suffer from diarrhoea because the secretion, which they are not able to concoct and turn into semen, is diverted into the intestine. Now a boy is like a woman in form, and the woman is as it were an impotent male, for it is through a certain incapacity that the female is female, being incapable of concocting the nutriment in its last stage into semen (and this is either blood or that which is analogous to it in animals which are bloodless owing to the coldness of their nature). As then diarrhoea is caused in the bowels by the insufficient concoction of the blood, so are caused in the blood-vessels all discharges of blood, including that of the catamenia, for this also is such a discharge, only it is natural whereas the others are morbid.

Thus it is clear that it is reasonable to suppose that generation comes from this. For the catamenia are semen not in a pure state but in need of working up, just as in the formation of fruits the nutriment is present, when it is not yet sifted thoroughly, but needs working up to purify it. Thus the catamenia cause generation by mixture with the semen, as this impure nutriment in plants is nutritious when mixed with pure nutriment.

. . . [W]hat the male contributes to generation is the form and the efficient cause, while the female contributes the material.

. . . [T]he female does not contribute semen to generation, but does contribute something, and that this is the matter of the catamenia, or that which is analogous to it in bloodless animals, is clear from what has been said, and also from a general and abstract survey of the question. For there must needs be that which generates and that from which it generates; even if these be one, still they must be distinct in form and their essence must be different; and in those animals that have these powers separate in two sexes the body and nature of the active and the passive sex must also differ. If, then, the male stands for the effective and active, and the female, considered as female, for the passive, it follows that what the female would contribute to the semen of the male would not be semen but material for the semen to work upon. This is just what we find to be the case, for the catamenia have in their nature an affinity to the primitive matter.

HEINRICH KRAMER (ca. 1430–1505)
AND JAMES SPRENGER (ca. 1436–1495)

Malleus Maleficarum

Members of the Dominican order, Heinrich Kramer and James Sprenger were designated as Inquisitors of Northern Germany by Pope Innocent III in 1484. Innocent's bull *Summis desideratus affectibus,* which decried the widespread power of witches and their leagues, was printed as a preface to *Malleus Maleficarum (The Witches' Hammer).* An encyclopedic collection of centuries of misogynistic beliefs, the book argued that women were far more likely to become witches than were men because of their inherently evil nature and voracious sexual appetite. Adopted by both Protestant and Catholic legislatures, the *Malleus* remained the bible of witch-hunters and prosecutors for nearly three centuries. Issued by the leading presses of Germany, France, and Italy, the treatise went through fourteen editions between 1487 and 1520, and at least sixteen more from 1574 to 1669. By the seventeenth century, it was reported to lie on the bench of every judge and on the desk of every magistrate in Europe.

WHY SUPERSTITION IS CHIEFLY FOUND
IN WOMEN

As for the first question, why a greater number of witches is found in the fragile feminine sex than among men; it is indeed a fact that it were idle to contradict, since it is accredited by actual experience, apart from the verbal testimony of credible witnesses. And without in any way detracting from a sex in which God has always taken great glory that His might should be spread abroad, let us say that various men have assigned various reasons for this fact, which nevertheless agree in principle. Wherefore it is good, for the admonition of women, to speak of this matter; and it has often been proved by experience that they are eager to hear of it, so long as it is set forth with discretion.

Now the wickedness of women is spoken of in *Ecclesiasticus* xxv: There is no head above the head of a serpent: and there is no wrath above the wrath of a woman. I had rather dwell with a lion and a dragon than to keep house with a wicked woman. And among much which in that place precedes and follows about a wicked woman, he concludes: All wickedness is but little to the wickedness of a woman. Wherefore S. John Chrysostom says on the text, It is not good to marry (*S. Matthew* xix): What else is woman but a foe to friendship, an unescapable punishment, a necessary evil, a natural temptation, a desirable calamity, a domestic danger, a delectable detriment, an evil of nature, painted with fair colours! Therefore if it be a sin to divorce her

From *Malleus Maleficarum,* ed. and trans. Montague Summers (1928; reprint, New York: Dover, 1971).

when she ought to be kept, it is indeed a necessary torture; for either we commit adultery by divorcing her, or we must endure daily strife. Cicero in his second book of *The Rhetorics* says: The many lusts of men lead them into one sin, but the one lust of women leads them into all sins; for the root of all woman's vices is avarice. And Seneca says in his *Tragedies*: A woman either loves or hates; there is no third grade. And the tears of a woman are a deception, for they may spring from true grief, or they may be a snare. When a woman thinks alone, she thinks evil.

Wherefore in many vituperations that we read against women, the word woman is used to mean the lust of the flesh. As it is said: I have found a woman more bitter than death, and a good woman subject to carnal lust.

Others again have propounded other reasons why there are more superstitious women found than men. And the first is, that they are more credulous; and since the chief aim of the devil is to corrupt faith, therefore he rather attacks them. See *Ecclesiasticus* xix: He that is quick to believe is light-minded, and shall be diminished. The second reason is, that women are naturally more impressionable, and more ready to receive the influence of a disembodied spirit; and that when they use this quality well they are very good, but when they use it ill they are very evil.

The third reason is that they have slippery tongues, and are unable to conceal from their fellow-women those things which by evil arts they know; and, since they are weak, they find an easy and secret manner of vindicating themselves by witchcraft. See *Ecclesiasticus* as quoted above: I had rather dwell with a lion and a dragon than to keep house with a wicked woman. All wickedness is but little to the wickedness of a woman. And to this may be added that, as they are very impressionable, they act accordingly.

But because in these times this perfidy is more often found in women than in men, as we learn by actual experience, if anyone is curious as to the reason, we may add to what has already been said the following: that since they are feebler both in mind and body, it is not surprising that they should come more under the spell of witchcraft.

For as regards intellect, or the understanding of spiritual things, they seem to be of a different nature from men; a fact which is vouched for by the logic of the authorities, backed by various examples from the Scriptures. Terence says: Women are intellectually like children.

But the natural reason is that she is more carnal than a man, as is clear from her many carnal abominations. And it should be noted that there was a defect in the formation of the first woman, since she was formed from a bent rib, that is, a rib of the breast, which is bent as it were in a contrary direction to a man. And since through this defect she is an imperfect animal, she always deceives. For Cato says: When a woman weeps she weaves snares. And again: When a woman weeps, she labours to deceive a man. And this is shown by Samson's wife, who coaxed him to tell her the riddle he had propounded to the Philistines, and told them the answer, and so deceived him. And it is clear in the case of the first woman that she had little faith; for when the serpent asked why they did not eat of every tree in Paradise, she answered: Of every tree, etc.—lest perchance we die. Thereby she showed that she doubted, and had little faith in the word of God. And all this is indicated by the etymology of the word; for *Femina* comes from *Fe* and *Minus,* since she is ever weaker to hold

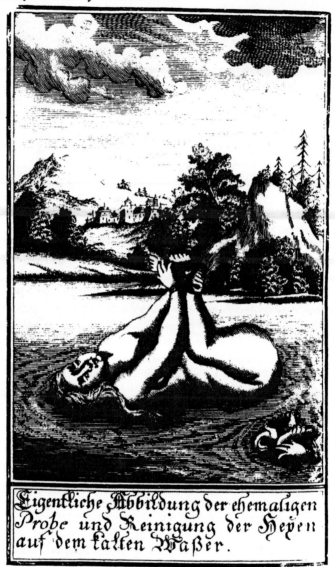

Eigentliche Abbildung der ehemaligen
Probe und Reinigung der Hexen
auf dem kalten Waßer.

10. A plate illustrating a witch from Bibliotheca sive Acta et Scripta Magica *(1745)
by Eberhard David Hauber. Henry Charles Lea Library, Department of Special Collections, Van Pelt-Dietrich Library, University of Pennsylvania. In keeping with the
common belief that witches would not sink in water, women accused of witchcraft
were frequently forced to undergo a trial-by-water. As the artist portrays her, the floating
witch is a seductive being whose body is sexualized through its suggestive pose. By
placing her against the backdrop of a village nestled in an idyllic mountain setting, he
indicates that she is a threat to communal stability and that her sorcery violates both
the civil and the natural order of things. The protruding hands and feet of an apparently innocent woman are visible to the right of the unsinkable one.*

and preserve the faith. And this as regards faith is of her very nature; although both by grace and nature faith never failed in the Blessed Virgin, even at the time of Christ's Passion, when it failed in all men.

Let us consider also her gait, posture, and habit, in which is vanity of vanities. There is no man in the world who studies so hard to please the good God as even an ordinary woman studies by her vanities to please men.

It is this which is lamented in *Ecclesiastes* vii, and which the Church even now laments on account of the great multitude of witches. And I have found a woman more bitter than death, who is the hunter's snare, and her heart is a net, and her hands are bands. He that pleaseth God shall escape from her; but he that is a sinner shall be caught by her. More bitter than death, that is, than the devil: *Apocalypse* vi, 8, His name was Death. For though the devil tempted Eve to sin, yet Eve seduced Adam. And as the sin of Eve would not have brought death to our soul and body unless the sin had afterwards passed on to Adam, to which he was tempted by Eve, not by the Devil, therefore she is more bitter than death.

More bitter than death, again, because that is natural and destroys only the body; but the sin which arose from woman destroys the soul by depriving it of grace, and delivers the body up to the punishment for sin.

More bitter than death, again, because bodily death is an open and terrible enemy, but woman is a wheedling and secret enemy.

And that she is more perilous than a snare does not speak of the snare of hunters, but of devils. For men are caught not only through their carnal desires, when they see and hear women: for S. Bernard says: Their face is a burning wind, and their voice the hissing of serpents: but they also cast wicked spells on countless men and animals. And when it is said that her heart is a net, it speaks of the inscrutable malice which reigns in their hearts. And her hands are as bands for binding; for when they place their hands on a creature to bewitch it, then with the help of the devil they perform their design.

To conclude. All witchcraft comes from carnal lust, which is in women insatiable. See *Proverbs* xxx: There are three things that are never satisfied, yea, a fourth thing which says not, It is enough; that is, the mouth of the womb. Wherefore for the sake of fulfilling their lusts they consort even with devils.

WHETHER WITCHES CAN HEBETATE THE POWERS OF GENERATION OR OBSTRUCT THE VENEREAL ACT

Now the fact that adulterous drabs and whores are chiefly given to witchcraft is substantiated by the spells which are cast by witches upon the act of generation. . . . [T]hey can take away the male organ, not indeed by actually despoiling the human body of it, but by concealing it with some glamour, . . . [I]t must in no way be believed that such members are really torn right away from the body, but that they are hidden by the devil through some prestidigitatory art so that they can be neither seen nor felt. And this is proved by the authorities and by argument; although it has been treated of before, where Alexander of Hales says that a Prestige, properly understood, is an illusion of the devil, which is not caused by any material change, but exists only in the perceptions of him who is deluded, either in his interior or exterior senses.

And what, then, is to be thought of those witches who in this way sometimes collect male organs in great numbers, as many as twenty or thirty members together, and put them in a bird's nest, or shut them up in a box, where they move themselves like living members, and eat oats and corn, as has been seen by many and is a matter of common report? It is to be said that it is all done by devil's work and illusion, for the senses of those who see them are deluded in the way we have said. For a certain man tells that, when he had lost his member, he approached a known witch to ask her to restore it to him. She told the afflicted man to climb a certain tree, and that he might take which he liked out of a nest in which there were several members. And when he tried to take a big one, the witch said: You must not take that one; adding, because it belonged to a parish priest.

All these things are caused by devils through an illusion or glamour, in the manner we have said, by confusing the organ of vision by transmuting the mental images in the imaginative faculty. And it must not be said that these members which are shown are devils in assumed members, just as they sometimes appear to witches and men in assumed aerial bodies, and converse with them. And the reason is that they effect this thing by an easier method, namely, by drawing out an inner mental image from the repository of the memory, and impressing it on the imagination.

"Remarks on Masturbation" (1835)

The early nineteenth century saw a steady proliferation of self-help guides for young men who aspired to reach an ideal of vigorous manhood and worldly success. Written by educators, ministers, and physicians, these guides invariably turned their readers' attention to the subject of masturbation—a habit that was believed to sap the vital juices necessary for a healthy mind and body, particularly during the critical developmental phase of adolescence. "W"'s remarks on masturbation were offered within this context of widespread anxiety about the debilitation of the American male. Beliefs regarding masturbation rested on a particular model of physiology which held that vital energy could be channeled into sexual activities only at the cost of draining it from mental ones, a model the historian G. J. Barker-Benfield has named "the spermatic economy." Despite the discovery of spermatozoa at the beginning of the nineteenth century, medical experts continued to believe that semen was the distilled essence of all the bodily fluids, and consequently, that its profligate expenditure enervated and depleted the entire body. Loss of stamina and concentration, lack of resolution and ambition, innumerable physical and mental disabilities—including insanity—were all part of the inevitable fate awaiting the chronic masturbator.

The pernicious and debasing practice of MASTURBATION is a more common and extensive evil with youth of both sexes, than is usually supposed. The influence of this habit upon both mind and body, severe as it has been considered, and greatly as it has been deprecated, is altogether more prejudicial than the public, and, as is believed, even the medical profession, are aware.

A great number of the evils which come upon the young at and after the age of puberty, arise from *masturbation,* persisted in, so as to waste the vital energies and enervate the physical and mental powers of man. Not less does it sap the foundation of moral principles, and blast the first budding of manly and honorable feelings which were exhibiting themselves in the opening character of the young.

Many of the weaknesses commonly attributed to growth and the changes in the habit by the important transformation from adolescence to manhood, are justly referable to this practice.

This change requires all the energy of the system, greatly increased as it is at this period of life, which if undisturbed will bring about a vigorous and healthy condition of both the mental and physical powers.

If masturbation be commenced at this period, it cannot fail to interrupt essentially this important process; and if continued, will inevitably impress imbecility on the

From *Boston Medical and Surgical Journal* 12 (6) (March 18, 1835).

constitution, not less apparent in the body than the mind, preventing, as it will not fail to do, the full development of the powers of both.

The individual becomes feeble, is unable to labor with accustomed vigor, or to apply his mind to study; his step is tardy and weak, he is dull, irresolute, engages in his sports with less energy than usual, and avoids social intercourse; when at rest he instinctively assumes a lolling or recumbent posture, and if at labor or at his games takes every opportunity to lie down or sit in a bent and curved position. The cause of these infirmities is *often* unknown to the subject of them, and *more generally* to the friends; and to labor, or study, or growth, is attributed all the evils which arise from the practice of this secret vice, which if persisted in will hardly fail to result in irremediable disease or hopeless idiocy. The natural consequence of indulgence in this, as in most other vices, is an increased propensity to them. This is particularly true of masturbation. In my intercourse with this unfortunate class of individuals, I have found a large proportion of them wholly ignorant of the causes of their complaints, and if not too far gone the abandonment of the habit has, after awhile, removed all the symptoms and resulted in confirmed health.

One young man, now under my care, was first arrested in his career by reading the chapters on the subject in the Young Man's Guide. For many months, he has totally abstained from the practice, and yet he is feeble, depressed, irresolute, and unable to fix his attention to any subject, or to pursue any active employment. But he is steadily convalescing, and will doubtless recover.

If the symptoms above enumerated do not lead in any way to a discontinuance of the habit, other symptoms more formidable, and more difficult of cure, will present themselves. The back becomes lame and weak, the limbs tremble, the digestion is disturbed, and costiveness or diarrhoea, or an alternation of them, take place. The head becomes painful—the heart palpitates—the respiration is easily hurried—the mind is depressed and gloomy—the temper becomes irritable—the sleep disturbed, and is attended by lascivious dreams, and not unfrequently nocturnal pollutions. With these symptoms the pulse becomes small, the extremities cold and damp; the countenance is downcast, the eye without natural lustre; shamefacedness is apparent, as if the unfortunate victim was conscious of his degraded condition.

The stomach often rejects food, and is affected with acidity, and loathing; the nervous system becomes highly irritable; neuralgia, tabes dorsalis, pulmonary consumption, or fatal marasmus, terminate the suffering, or else insanity and deplorable idiocy are the fatal result. Long before such an event, the mind is enfeebled, the memory impaired, and the power of fixing the attention wholly lost. These are symptoms which should awaken our attention to the danger of the case, and which should induce us to sound the alarm, and if possible arrest the victim from the inevitable consequences of persisting in the habit.

In females, leucorrhoea is often induced by masturbation, and I doubt not incontinence of urine, strangury, prolapsus uteri, disease of the clitoris, and many other diseases, both local and general, which have been attributed to other causes.

It is often difficult to obtain information on the subject of masturbation. Where it is suspected by the physician, the friends are wholly ignorant on the subject, and the individual, suffering, is not ready to acknowledge a practice which he is conscious is filthy in the extreme, although he may have had no suspicions of its deleterious influence upon his health.

It is not sufficient that we know the consequences of masturbation, for these are often irremediable disease; we ought to know the symptoms of its commencement, of the incipient stages of these diseases which result from it, as well as the influence which the moderate practice of it will have upon the physical and mental stamina of the man—for it is not too much to say that the practice cannot be followed by either sex, even in a moderate way, without injury, especially by the young.

Nature designs that this drain upon the system should be reserved to mature age, and even then that it be made but sparingly. Sturdy manhood, in all its vigor, loses its energy and bends under the too frequent expenditure of this important secretion; and no age or condition will protect a man from the danger of unlimited indulgence, legally and naturally exercised.

In the young, however, its influence is much more seriously felt; and even those who have indulged so cautiously as not to break down the health or the mind, cannot know how much their physical energy, mental vigor, or moral purity, have been affected by the indulgence.

Nothing short of total abstinence from the practice can save those who have become the victims of it. In this indulgence, no half way course will ever subdue the disease, or remove the effect of the habit from the system. Total abstinence is the only remedy. If the constitution is not fatally impaired—if organic disease has not taken place, this remedy will prove effectual, and must be adopted, especially in all cases in which the effects are visible, or the consequences cannot fail to be ultimately fatal.

This means of cure may be seconded by others, which may be found necessary to remove the effects upon the physical system. Suffice it to remark here, that total abstinence, in an aggravated form of masturbation, is not easily effected. Slight irritation will produce an expenditure of the secretion quite involuntary, and spontaneous emissions and nocturnal pollution may for a long time prolong the danger, and prevent that renovation of the powers which would otherwise be the result of the good resolution of the victim of the habit.

In a subsequent paper we may consider the influence of masturbation upon the mind, as a cause of insanity and idiocy, and suggest some remedies for the removal of its effects upon the health.

EDWARD HAMMOND CLARKE (1820–1877)

Sex in Education;
or,
A Fair Chance for Girls

The ninth son of a Massachusetts minister, Edward Hammond Clarke graduated Harvard College in 1841 and received his medical degree from the
University of Pennsylvania in 1846. Although a hemorrhage from his lungs
during his adolescence had left him in weak health, Clarke soon established
himself as one of Boston's most prominent physicians. In 1855, he became
professor of materia medica at Harvard, and in 1874, he published *Sex in
Education,* which argued that women's monthly "loss of blood" put their
health at grave risk; he warned that women who failed to take proper rest
or overtaxed their brains with study would develop atrophied uteruses. Published when pressure for coeducation at Harvard was at its height, Clarke's
book was enormously popular, going through seventeen editions in a few
years' time.

Woman, in the interest of the race, is dowered with a set of organs peculiar to herself, whose complexity, delicacy, sympathies, and force are among the marvels of
creation. If properly nurtured and cared for, they are a source of strength and power
to her. If neglected and mismanaged, they retaliate upon their possessor with weakness and disease, as well of the mind as of the body.

Ever since the time of Hippocrates, woman has been physiologically described as
enjoying, and has always recognized herself as enjoying, or at least as possessing, a
tri-partite life. The first period extends from birth to about the age of twelve or fifteen years; the second, from the end of the first period to about the age of forty-
five; and the third, from the last boundary to the final passage into the unknown.
The few years that are necessary for the voyage from the first to the second period,
and those from the second to the third, are justly called critical ones. Mothers are,
or should be, wisely anxious about the first passage for their daughters, and women
are often unduly apprehensive about the second passage for themselves. All this is
obvious and known; and yet, in our educational arrangements, little heed is paid to
the fact, that the first of these critical voyages is made during a girl's educational
life, and extends over a very considerable portion of it.

During the first of these critical periods, when the divergence of the sexes becomes
obvious to the most careless observer, the complicated apparatus peculiar to the female enters upon a condition of functional activity. "The ovaries, which constitute,"
says Dr. Dalton, "the 'essential parts' of this apparatus, and certain accessory or-

From *Sex in Education; or, A Fair Chance for Girls* (Boston, 1874).

gans, are now rapidly developed." No such extraordinary task, calling for such rapid expenditure of force, building up such a delicate and extensive mechanism within the organism,—a house within a house, an engine within an engine,—is imposed upon the male physique at the same epoch. The organization of the male grows steadily, gradually, and equally, from birth to maturity. The importance of having our methods of female education recognize this peculiar demand for growth, and of so adjusting themselves to it, as to allow a sufficient opportunity for the healthy development of the ovaries and their accessory organs, and for the establishment of their periodical functions, can not be overestimated. Moreover, unless the work is accomplished at that period, unless the reproductive mechanism is built and put in good working order at that time, it is never perfectly accomplished afterwards.

There have been instances, and I have seen such, of females in whom the special mechanism we are speaking of remained germinal,—undeveloped. It seemed to have been aborted. They graduated from school or college excellent scholars, but with undeveloped ovaries. Later they married, and were sterile.

The system never does two things well at the same time. The muscles and the brain cannot *functionate* in their best way at the same moment. One cannot meditate a poem and drive a saw simultaneously, without dividing his force. He may poetize fairly, and saw poorly; or he may saw fairly, and poetize poorly; or he may both saw and poetize indifferently. Brain-work and stomach-work interfere with each other if attempted together. The digestion of a dinner calls force to the stomach, and temporarily slows the brain. The experiment of trying to digest a hearty supper, and to sleep during the process, has sometimes cost the careless experimenter his life. The physiological principle of doing only one thing at a time, if you would do it well, holds as truly of the growth of the organization as it does of the performance of any of its special functions.

It is apparent, from these physiological considerations, that, in order to give girls a fair chance in education, four conditions at least must be observed: first, a sufficient supply of appropriate nutriment; secondly, a normal management of the catamenial functions, including the building of the reproductive apparatus; thirdly, mental and physical work so apportioned, that repair shall exceed waste, and a margin be left for general and sexual development; and fourthly, sufficient sleep. Evidence of the results brought about by a disregard of these conditions will next be given.

CLINICAL observation confirms the teachings of physiology. The sick chamber, not the schoolroom; the physician's private consultation, not the committee's public examination; the hospital, not the college, the workshop, or the parlor,—disclose the sad results which modern social customs, modern education, and modern ways of labor, have entailed on women.

. . . [I]n our factories, workshops, and homes,—may be found numberless pale, weak, neuralgic, dyspeptic, hysterical, menorraghic, dysmenorrhoeic girls and women, that are living illustrations of the truth of this brief monograph. It is not asserted here that improper methods of study, and a disregard of the reproductive apparatus and its functions, during the educational life of girls, are the sole causes of female diseases; neither is it asserted that all the female graduates of our schools and colleges are pathological specimens. But it is asserted that the number of these graduates who have been permanently disabled to a greater or less degree by these causes is so great, as to excite the gravest alarm, and to demand the serious attention of the community. If these causes should continue for the next half-century, and increase in the same ratio as they have for the last fifty years, it requires no prophet to foretell that the wives who are to be mothers in our republic must be drawn from trans-atlantic homes.

A woman, whether married or unmarried, whether called to the offices of maternity or relieved from them, who has been defrauded by her education or otherwise of such an essential part of her development, is not so much of a woman, intellectually and morally as well as physically, in consequence of this defect. Her nervous system and brain, her instincts and character, are on a lower plane, and incapable of their harmonious and best development, if she is possessed, on reaching adult age, of only a portion of a breast and an ovary, or none at all.

When arrested development of the reproductive system is nearly or quite complete, it produces a change in the character, and a loss of power, which it is easy to recognize, but difficult to describe. As this change is an occasional attendant or result of amenorrhoea, when the latter, brought about at an early age, is part of an early arrest, it should not be passed by without an allusion. In these cases, which are not of frequent occurrence at present, but which may be evolved by our methods of education more numerously in the future, the system tolerates the absence of the catamenia, and the consequent non-elimination of impurities from the blood. Acute or chronic disease, the ordinary result of this condition, is not set up, but, instead, there is a change in the character and development of the brain and nervous system. There are in individuals of this class less adipose and more muscular tissue than is commonly seen, a coarser skin, and, generally, a tougher and more angular makeup. There is a corresponding change in the intellectual and psychical condition,—a dropping out of maternal instincts, and an appearance of Amazonian coarseness and force. Such persons are analogous to the sexless class of termites. Naturalists tell us that these insects are divided into males and females, and a third class called workers and soldiers, who have no reproductive apparatus, and who, in their structure and instincts, are unlike the fertile individuals.

A closer analogy than this, however, exists between these human individuals and the eunuchs of Oriental civilization. When the school makes the same steady demand for force from girls who are approaching puberty, ignoring Nature's periodical demands, that it does from boys, who are not called upon for an equal effort, there must be failure somewhere. Generally either the reproductive system or the nervous system suffers. We have looked at several instances of the former sort of failure; let us now examine some of the latter.

Miss F—— was about twenty years old when she completed her technical education. She inherited a nervous diathesis as well as a large dower of intellectual and aesthetic graces. She was a good student, and conscientiously devoted all her time, with the exception of ordinary vacations, to the labor of her education. She made herself mistress of several languages, and accomplished in many ways. The catamenial function appeared normally, and with the exception of occasional slight attacks of menorrhagia, was normally performed during the whole period of her education.

She got on without any sort of serious illness. There were few belonging to my clientele who required less professional advice for the same period than she. With the ending of her school life, when she should have been in good trim and well equipped, physically as well as intellectually, for life's work, there commenced, without obvious cause, a long period of invalidism. It would be tedious to the reader, and useless for our present purpose, to detail the history and describe the protean shapes of her sufferings. With the exception of small breasts, the reproductive system was well developed. Repeated and careful examinations failed to detect any derangement of the uterine mechanism. Her symptoms all pointed to the nervous system as the *fons et origo mali.* First general debility, that concealed but ubiquitous leader of innumerable armies of weakness and ill, laid siege to her, and captured her. Then came insomnia, that worried her nights for month after month, and made her beg for opium, alcohol, chloral, bromides, any thing that would bring sleep. Neuralgia in every conceivable form tormented her, most frequently in her back, but often, also, in her head, sometimes in her sciatic nerves, sometimes setting up a tic douloureux, sometimes causing a fearful dysmenorrhoea and frequently making her head ache for days together. At other times hysteria got hold of her, and made her fancy herself the victim of strange diseases. Mental effort of the slightest character distressed her, and she could not bear physical exercise of any amount. This condition, or rather these varying conditions, continued for some years. She followed a careful and systematic regimen, and was rewarded by a slow and gradual return of health and strength, when a sudden accident killed her, and terminated her struggle with weakness and pain.

Words fail to convey the lesson of this case to others with any thing like the force that the observation of it conveyed its moral to those about Miss F——, and especially to the physician who watched her career through her educational life, and saw it lead to its logical conclusion of invalidism and thence towards recovery, till life ended.

GUIDED by the laws of development which we have found physiology to teach, and warned by the punishments, in the shape of weakness and disease, which we have shown their infringement to bring about, and of which our present methods of female education furnish innumerable examples, it is not difficult to discern certain physiological principles that limit and control the education, and, consequently, the co-education of our youth.

Before going farther, it is essential to acquire a definite notion of what is meant, or, at least, of what we mean in this discussion, by the term co-education. Following its etymology, *con-educare,* it signifies to draw out together, or to unite in education; and this union refers to the time and place, rather than to the methods and kinds of education.

Another signification of co-education, and, as we apprehend, the one in which it is commonly used, includes time, place, government, methods, studies, and regimen. This is identical co-education. This means, that boys and girls shall be taught the same things, at the same time, in the same place, by the same faculty, with the same methods, and under the same regimen. This admits age and proficiency, but not sex, as a factor in classification. It is against the co-education of the sexes, in this sense of identical co-education, that physiology protests; and it is this identity of education, the prominent characteristic of our American school-system, that has produced the evils described in the clinical part of this essay, and that threatens to push the degeneration of the female sex still farther on.

Identical education, or identical co-education, of the sexes defrauds one sex or the other, or perhaps both. It defies the Roman maxim, which physiology has fully justified, *mens sana in corpore sano.* The sustained regimen, regular recitation, erect posture, daily walk, persistent exercise, and unintermitted labor that toughens a boy, and makes a man of him, can only be partially applied to a girl. The regimen of intermittance, periodicity of exercise and rest, work three-fourths of each month, and remission, if not abstinence, the other fourth, physiological interchange of the erect and reclining posture, care of the reproductive system that is the cradle of the race, all this, that toughens a girl and makes a woman of her, will emasculate a lad. A combination of the two methods of education, a compromise between them, would probably yield an average result, excluding the best of both. It would give a fair chance neither to a boy nor a girl. Of all compromises, such a physiological one is the worst. It cultivates mediocrity, and cheats the future of its rightful legacy of lofty manhood and womanhood. It emasculates boys, stunts girls; makes semi-eunuchs of one sex, and agenes of the other.

MARY PUTNAM JACOBI (1842–1906)

"Do Women Require Mental and Bodily Rest during Menstruation?"

A physician and reformer, Mary Putnam Jacobi worked throughout her life to improve health care for the poor, enlarge opportunities for female physicians, and advance the cause of women's suffrage. The daughter of George Palmer Putnam, founder of the publishing firm G. P. Putnam's Sons, Jacobi began her studies at the Female Medical College of Philadelphia, and was the first woman to be admitted to Paris's École de Médecine, graduating in 1871 with high honors. After returning to the United States, Jacobi married Dr. Abraham Jacobi, one of the most distinguished pediatricians of the time, who shared her devotion to the welfare of impoverished families. From 1874 to 1879, Jacobi served as professor of materia medica at the Women's Medical College of New York; she also organized a pediatric dispensary at Mount Sinai Hospital, opened a children's ward at the New York Infirmary, and campaigned for a women's suffrage amendment to the New York State Constitution. In 1876, when Harvard announced that the topic for its Boylston Essay was the effects of menstruation on women, Jacobi rose to the occasion by writing "Do Women Require Mental and Bodily Rest during Menstruation?" Through a shrewd use of statistical information and analysis, she rebutted Clarke's and other physicians' claims that women's physiology rendered them unfit for higher education. To the dismay of many of her male colleagues, her essay was awarded the coveted prize.

An inquiry into the limits of human nature is always legitimate, and often exceedingly useful. When honestly made, it tends to increase real force while dissipating illusions concerning imaginary powers. Thus knowledge of the limits of muscular strength stimulates the invention of machines many times man power. Such indeed is the audacity of the human intellect, that the discovery of limits usually proves hopeless in only one case, namely, when they are perceived to apply to a different race, class, or sex, from that to which the investigator himself belongs. An inquiry into the limits to activity and attainments that may be imposed by sex, is very frequently carried on in the same spirit as that which hastens to ascribe to permanent differences in race all the peculiarities of a class, and this because the sex that is supposed to be limiting in its nature, is nearly always different from that of the person conducting the inquiry. It is true that men have inquired with great research into the influence exerted upon the general organization of man by the special character and working of his sexual organization, but it is rare that this influence has been regarded as "limiting" in its nature.

From *The Question of Rest for Women during Menstruation* (New York, 1886).

Physiologists and physicians again, while demonstrating the slavery that results from abuse of the sexual functions, have hinted of no danger consequent upon their normal exercise. On the contrary their stimulating effects upon the rest of the economy have been portrayed in brilliant colors by even sober pens. To the reproductive apparatus is generally ascribed a permanent influence upon the organism of whose maximum development it constitutes the most elaborate expression. The development and activity of this apparatus, by means of which the life of the individual is linked to that of the race, are said to be correlative with the development and activity of the organs of individual life, and not in inverse proportion to them. It may indeed be considered as quite a modern eccentricity to claim as an element of superiority in man, that, in the intervals of the voluntary exercise of sexual functions, "he is practically unsexed." Were the assertion true, which it is far from being, it would prove a marked inferiority on his part to organisms whose sexual characters are permanent, since both in plants and animals, sexual organisms rank higher than asexual; the development of sex marks a progress from the primitively neutral condition of young animals, and privation of the organs or sex is liable to seriously deteriorate some of the robust organs of individual life. All this is generally recognized in regard to the masculine sex. But as soon as there is question of the other, the fundamental conception of the subject seems to be changed. Not alone the accidents of sex or the abnormal exercise of its functions, but the sex itself seems to be regarded as a pathological fact, constantly detracting from the sum total of health, and of healthful activities. "Woman, in the interest of the race has been endowed with a set of organs peculiar to herself, whose complexity, delicacy, sympathies and force, are among the marvels of creation" (*Sex in Education*, p. 83). Comty (*Traité des maladies des femmes*, p. 274) enumerates the natural phenomena of menstruation, copulation, gestation, parturition, among the causes of the frequency of uterine disease. Dr. Guerin (*Movement medical* quoted by *Mundé Journal Obstetrics*, Aug., 1875) says, "There is no physiological condition so nearly resembling disease as that which produces every month in an adult woman a change so profound that it has been looked upon as the expression of a morbid condition." Tilt, who declares that diseases of menstruation have been the engrossing study of his life, defines this process to be a "sero sanguinolent secretion" propelled by an ovarian influence from all or different parts of the generative intestine, and principally from the womb. It is a natural function peculiar to women . . . who are subject to this *natural infirmity* for about seven out of the thirty years of reproductive life. Hutchins, in a prize essay accepted by a State Medical Association, says, "Woman has a sum total of nervous force equivalent to a man's, but this is distributed over a greater multiplicity of organs and directed to the development and support of special reproductive energies in addition to those of individual nutrition. The nervous force is therefore weakened in each organ,—and the period of resistance of each organ is weakened,—it is more sensitive, more liable to derangement." In another place the author quotes an experiment of Rabuteau, as a proof that during menstruation the general nutrition of the body is diminished. Hirt calls menstruation "a condition which, if not precisely morbid, is still often upon the limits of pathology; and under all circumstances determines a greater predisposition to different diseases." The author calculated that "every four weeks the uterus becomes hyperaemiated in such manner that almost the entire organism is involved in sympathetic suffering; and this during three to five days every month, or one to two months out of every year." Thus even for the non-pregnant woman, "a great portion of the time during the period of maturity is passed under the influence of the genital sphere." Storer, in his essay on criminal abortion, appends a note to the paragraph devoted to female physicians, considered as a special class of accomplices to this crime (p. 98), in which he remarks that, "granting that women in exceptional cases may have all the courage, tact, ability, pecuniary means, education, and patience necessary to fit persons for the cares and responsibilities of professional life, they still are and must be subject to the periodical *infirmity* of their sex; which for the time, and in every case, *however unattended by physical suffering,* unfits them for any responsible effort of mind, and in many cases of body also. It is not to women as physicians we would object; . . . but to their often *infirmity,* during which neither life nor limb submitted to them would be as safe as at other times. We could hardly allow to a female physician (?) convicted of criminal abortion, the plea that the act was committed during the *temporary insanity of her menstruation*; and yet at such times a woman is undoubtedly more prone than men to commit any unusual or outrageous act." In the same sense Dr. Tilt, in an address to the Obstetrical Society of London for 1874, congratulated the members upon their almost unanimous decision that women were not admissible,—"for the profession felt that the verdict really meant that women were not qualified by nature to make good midwifery practitioners; that they were unfit to bear the physical fatigues and mental anxieties of obstetrical practice, at *menstrual periods,* during pregnancy and puerperality; and that it was unfair to society to encourage women to suppose they could fit themselves to assume responsibilities in those formidable obstetric emergencies which too often completely paralyze even men of experience."

The plethoric theory of menstruation was based; first upon the general analogy of the menstrual flux with other evacuations; and second upon its relations to pregnancy, of which the most superficial observation showed it to be the substitute. The sense of discomfort or even experience of danger attendant on suppression of the evacuations of faeces or urine, offered a basis of sensation, upon which was easily built the theory, that all spontaneous evacuations implied the existence of some morbific material whose retention was extremely perilous to the economy. The menstrual "purgation" was included in the generalization. "The opinion, observes Kreiger, that the body was purified by the flux from the uterus, became permanent, and was asserted still more emphatically in the *Commentaries on Hippocrates* in the sixteenth and seventeenth centuries. So for instance, Bapt. Moretarus, de uterin affectionibus, p. 221." "The uterus is the sewer of all the excrements existing in the body; for all decrements flow to the uterus." On the other hand, the enormous amount of nutritive material required for the development of the foetus was supposed to be derived from some reserve habitually not utilized for individual nutrition; this reserve could be none other than the blood thrown away as superfluous during non-pregnant states, but retained as soon as the embryo began to develop. If women escaped annihilation during pregnancy, it could only be in virtue of a plethora existing in all other conditions.

It may therefore be confidently asserted that, previous to the discoveries which associated menstruation with the dehiscence of ova, this peculiar phenomena was almost universally regarded as a proof of an excess of nutritive force in the sex upon whom devolved the greatest cost of reproduction. From Hippocrates to Burdach, . . . this presumed excess or nutritive force in women is constantly contrasted with their deficiency of muscular force as compared with that of man, and with the arrest of the growth which is continuous in children. Menstruation in women, muscular force in man, growth in children, were held to be more or less exact equivalents to one another. But in 1845, with the establishment of the fact of spontaneous ovulation, the conditions of general nutrition upon which menstruation could be supposed to depend began to be lost sight of in comparison with the remarkable local phenomena with which they were asserted to be exclusively associated. The congestion of the ovary, ripening of the ovule, effusion of the serum and blood into the Graafian follicle; its rupture; the escape of the reproductive cell; its seizure by the fimbriae of the Fallopian tube; its journey along the oviduct and descent into the uterus; the hyperannia of the latter, the turgesence of its mucous membrane, the rupture of its blood vessels, and local hemorrhage; this entire succession of processes seemed the more surprising because more recently demonstrated, and to cause a greater perturbation of the economy, because occurring at intervals. For the first time the periodicity of menstruation began to be considered as a morbid circumstance. Although physiologists pointed out that the periodicity of menstruation belonged to the general law of vital phenomena, as earlier rude observations had associated it with the periodicity of cosmic phenomena, clinicians came gradually to look upon it as a fact which isolated menstruation from all other physiological processes, which rendered its ordinary course dangerous, its derangements fatal, and itself was sufficient to make any utero-ovarian disease baffle the skill of the physician.

Thus one of the most essential apparent peculiarities of the menstrual process, its periodicity, that formerly was supposed to indicate a periodical increase in the vital forces of the female organism, has come to be considered as a mark of constantly recurring debility, a means of constantly recurring exhaustion demanding rest as decidedly as a fracture or a paralysis. Although not yet proved, it is conceivable that all women should require an extra rest on account of it, as all children have been shown to require extra sleep on account of their immaturity. It is not impossible that the organization of the industrial world without reference to this physiological requirement, has been at least as great a hardship to women, as inattention to requirements of ventilation and drainage have proved to be to all laborers.

But if these hypotheses be true, the practical consequences are at once so important and so inconvenient, that they should only be accepted after the strictest scrutiny. It is well to glance for a moment at the statistics of the work performed by women in various parts of the world, without any attempt to secure for themselves rest during the menstrual period. Leroy Beaulieu, in his prize essay, has shown by a few well selected examples, that at no time and in no country have domestic occupations absorbed the existence of the woman in the working classes; that this ideal society where the man might suffice for the necessities of the family, and the woman only be obliged to look after the house and the education of the children, has never existed in the past; that whenever a branch of remunerative employment has been open to women, they have precipitated themselves upon it with avidity, and that in the absence of industrial pursuits, they have fallen back upon occupations coarser and less productive.

"The workshop existed in Europe long before the tenth century, under the name of gynecee, sometimes attached to the house of the lord of the manor and under the direction of his wife, sometimes belonging to abbeys, and controlled by a superintendent. In convents the nuns manufactured everything needed for their own use, then for sale in the world. Spinning and dyeing of wool occupied a large part of their days. In the Registers of trades and merchandises of Depping is proof that the trades corporations, contrary to a prevalent opinion, were arranged to include women. We find mentioned, workwomen in silk cloths, silk spinners, weavers of kerchiefs, embroideresses, combers of wool, silk hatters, and many other trades, where the women were not only admitted as aids, but might become mistresses, or even be eligible for the dignities of the corporation. The history of female labor in epochs nearer to us would be the history of industry itself. The more civilization is developed and refined, the more women participate in production, and this participation, constantly greater and more active, is regarded by women themselves as an advantage." In 1640, a decree of the parliament of Toulouse, on the pretext that lace manufacture carried off too many women from domestic occupations, forbade this work throughout the limits of its jurisdiction. Thousands of workwomen were thus deprived of their bread until the decree was reversed. Although the occupations of women under the old regime were much more numerous than is generally believed, they were nevertheless too little for the necessities of the women. In 1789 appeared the petition of the women of the Third Estate to the king, in which they claimed for their sex the right of working without (reglementary) hindrance, and even demanded that all trades for sewing, spinning, or knitting should be handed over exclusively to them. Thus before the new world about to open, the first cry of the women was, not to repudiate, but to invoke labor, not to decline and repulse the name of workwomen, but to claim it and make of it a title of honor. This in 1789. "In 1851 Paris alone contained 112,189 workingwomen, of whom 60,000 were employed in various kinds of needle-work. In 1873 it may be calculated that about 400,000 or 450,000 women are employed in France in manufactories of cotton, wool, linen, or silk. In 1861, in Great Britain, the textile industries occupied 467,261 women and 808,273 men, or about three women for every two men." In 1864—we continue to quote Leroy Beaulieu—"in 1864 a total of 747,261 women were engaged in the industrial establishments of Great Britain." Lord Brougham, in a speech before the Social Science Association in 1862, affirmed that "three-quarters of adult unmarried women, two-thirds of the widows, and a seventh of married women, are occupied in Great Britain on independent or isolated labors, without counting the multitude of wives, daughters, and sisters, who share in the work of their relatives at the counter, in the dairy, or by the needle."

In Germany, Hirt enumerates female laborers in manufactories for bronzes, (Nuremberg) pins, gold leaf, glass and porcelain, wool, flax, tobacco, paper, straw hats, india rubber, paints, looking-glasses, toys, phosphorus matches, sugar refineries, colors, etc., etc. In the United States, the census for 1870 shows that out of 9,750,000 females above ten years old, 1,594,783 are represented on tables of occupations taking part in the paid industry of the country. This is one-sixth of the entire female population.

. . . [T]o estimate the influence of steady occupation upon female existence, we must add to those engaged at any given time, a large proportion of the classes who do not then appear on the tables, but are registered as married or keeping house. Since marriage and domestic service constitute the only natural equivalent for the paid industry of women, everything which delays marriage tends to increase the extent to which they will engage in non-domestic professional or industrial occupations, and the regulation or their labor becomes therefore of more importance.

In Europe very much more than in America, and on the continent more than in Great Britain, marriage among the laboring classes does not interrupt industrial life, since the earnings of the woman are needed for the support of the family.

From this brief glance at the actual condition of modern society, it is evident that its existing regulations are little prepared to "yield to nature her inexorable demand for rest during one week out of every four" in the adult life of women. If the answer to the question asked by the committee be in the affirmative, a revolution in industrial customs should be required at least as radical as those enforced by the English Factory Laws of 1842. This question though apparently simple, is in reality difficult even to ask with precision. Each term is susceptible of various shades of meaning. If it be said, "It *is* necessary that women rest during menstruation," we must ask necessary for what purpose? The preservation of life? Evidently not, since the most superficial observation shows thousands of women of all races and ages engaged in work of various degrees of severity without attempting to secure repose at the menstrual epoch.

"The Dissolution of the Oedipus Complex"

An Austrian neurologist and the founder of psychoanalysis, Sigmund Freud was born in Moravia, and at the age of five moved to Vienna, where his father, a wool merchant, settled the family in the Jewish quarter of Leopoldstadt. A gifted student in literature and the classical languages, Freud also excelled in the sciences; by the time he received his medical degree from the University of Vienna in 1881, he had made several important discoveries about the structure and function of nerve cells. Being without the financial means to pursue a career in anatomical research, however, Freud soon turned to clinical work with the aim of readying himself for a practice in neurology. In 1883, he joined Theodor Meynert's Psychiatric Clinic in Vienna's General Hospital, and then the Department of Nervous Diseases. After having conducted seminal research in brain anatomy, the organic diseases of the nervous system, and the anesthetic properties of cocaine, he was appointed lecturer in neuropathology in 1885. This same year, he was awarded a traveling fellowship to study with Charcot at the Salpêtrière in Paris. Enthralled by Charcot's lectures and demonstrations on hysteria, Freud decided to investigate the illness, embarking on a journey that eventually led him to the study of sexuality as an etiological factor in the neuroses and, from there, to his discovery of infantile sexuality and the Oedipus complex. In treating patients with hysteria who reported they had been molested in childhood by their parents or other relatives, Freud began to suspect that their memories of such events were not always accurate, a finding that led him to the realization that a fantasied seduction could have as traumatic an effect on psychic life as an actual one. Freud meant none of this as a denial that some patients had in fact been molested; his intention was rather to emphasize the decisive role that infantile wishes and fantasies play in the emergence of neurosis, as well as in the construction of sexual identity and the development of personality and character. Although Freud initially believed that the psychosexual development of girls was "precisely analogous" to that of boys—an idea he elaborated in his "Three Essays on the Theory of Sexuality" (1905)—"The Dissolution of the Oedipus Complex" (1924) signals a decisive reversal of his opinion on the subject.

To an ever-increasing extent the Oedipus complex reveals its importance as the central phenomenon of the sexual period of early childhood. After that, its dissolution

From *The Standard Edition of the Complete Psychological Works of Sigmund Freud*, ed. and trans. James Strachey, Vol. 19: *The Ego and the Id and Other Works* (London: The Hogarth Press, 1961).

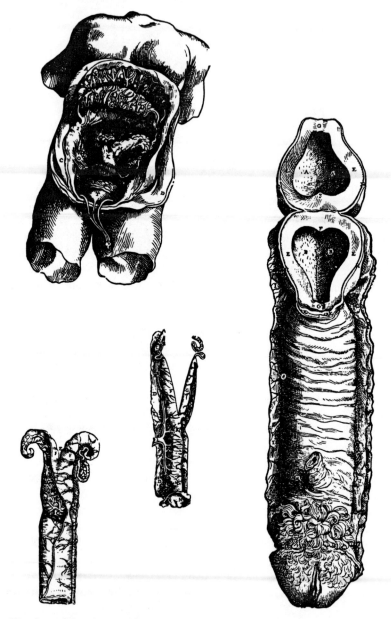

11. Woodcut of female reproductive organs from Andreas Vesalius, Suorum de Humani
Corporis Fabrica Librorum Epitome *(Basle: Johannes Oporinus, 1543). From
J. B. deC. M. Saunders and Charles D. O'Malley,* Illustrations from the Works of
Andreas Vesalius of Brussels *(New York: Dover Publications, 1973). The universal
fantasy that there is really only one sex—a fantasy that Freud claimed was central to
the psychological life of the pre-oedipal child—is vividly attested to by Vesalius's representation of the female genitalia as male, of the vagina and uterus as penis.*

takes place; it succumbs to repression, as we say, and is followed by the latency period. It has not yet become clear, however, what it is that brings about its destruction. Analyses seem to show that it is the experience of painful disappointments. The little girl likes to regard herself as what her father loves above all else; but the time comes when she has to endure a harsh punishment from him and she is cast out of her fool's paradise. The boy regards his mother as his own property; but he finds one day that she has transferred her love and solicitude to a new arrival. Reflection must deepen our sense of the importance of those influences, for it will emphasize the fact that distressing experiences of this sort, which act in opposition to the content of the complex, are inevitable. Even when no special events occur, like those we have mentioned as examples, the absence of the satisfaction hoped for, the continued denial of the desired baby, must in the end lead the small lover to turn away from his hopeless longing. In this way the Oedipus complex would go to its destruction from its lack of success, from the effects of its internal impossibility.

Another view is that the Oedipus complex must collapse because the time has come for its disintegration, just as the milk-teeth fall out when the permanent ones begin to grow. Although the majority of human beings go through the Oedipus complex as an individual experience, it is nevertheless a phenomenon which is determined and laid down by heredity and which is bound to pass away according to programme when the next pre-ordained phase of development sets in. This being so, it is of no great importance what the occasions are which allow this to happen, or, indeed, whether any such occasions can be discovered at all.

The justice of both these views cannot be disputed. Moreover, they are compatible. There is room for the ontogenetic view side by side with the more far-reaching phylogenetic one. It is also true that even at birth the whole individual is destined to die, and perhaps his organic disposition may already contain the indication of what he is to die from. Nevertheless, it remains of interest to follow out how this innate programme is carried out and in what way accidental noxae exploit his disposition.

We have lately been made more clearly aware than before that a child's sexual development advances to a certain phase at which the genital organ has already taken over the leading role. But this genital is the male one only, or, more correctly, the penis; the female genital has remained undiscovered. This phallic phase, which is contemporaneous with the Oedipus complex, does not develop further to the definitive genital organization, but is submerged, and is succeeded by the latency period. Its termination, however, takes place in a typical manner and in conjunction with events that are of regular recurrence.

When the (male) child's interest turns to his genitals he betrays the fact by manipulating them frequently; and he then finds that the adults do not approve of this behaviour. More or less plainly, more or less brutally, a threat is pronounced that this part of him which he values so highly will be taken away from him. Usually it is from women that the threat emanates; very often they seek to strengthen their authority by a reference to the father or the doctor, who, so they say, will carry out the punishment. In a number of cases the women will themselves mitigate the threat in a symbolic manner by telling the child that what is to be removed is not his genital, which actually plays a passive part, but his hand, which is the active culprit. It happens particularly often that the little boy is threatened with castration, not because he plays with his penis with his hand, but because he wets his bed every night and cannot be got to be clean. Those in charge of him behave as if this nocturnal incontinence was the result and the proof of his being unduly concerned with his penis, and they are probably right. In any case, long-continued bed-wetting is to be equated with the emissions of adults. It is an expression of the same excitation of the genitals which has impelled the child to masturbate at this period.

Now it is my view that what brings about the destruction of the child's phallic genital organization is this threat of castration. Not immediately, it is true, and not without other influences being brought to bear as well. For to begin with the boy does not believe in the threat or obey it in the least. Psycho-analysis has recently attached importance to two experiences which all children go through and which, it is suggested, prepare them for the loss of highly valued parts of the body. These experiences are the withdrawal of the mother's breast—at first intermittently and later for good—and the daily demand on them to give up the contents of the bowel. But there is no evidence to show that, when the threat of castration takes place, those experiences have any effect. It is not until a *fresh* experience comes his way that the child begins to reckon with the possibility of being castrated, and then only hesitatingly and unwillingly, and not without making efforts to depreciate the significance of something he has himself observed.

The observation which finally breaks down his unbelief is the sight of the female genitals. Sooner or later the child, who is so proud of his possession of a penis, has a view of the genital region of a little girl, and cannot help being convinced of the absence of a penis in a creature who is so like himself. With this, the loss of his own penis becomes imaginable, and the threat of castration takes its deferred effect.

We should not be as short-sighted as the person in charge of the child who threatens him with castration, and we must not overlook the fact that at this time masturbation by no means represents the whole of his sexual life. As can be clearly shown, he stands in the Oedipus attitude to his parents; his masturbation is only a genital discharge of the sexual excitation belonging to the complex, and throughout his later years will owe its importance to that relationship. The Oedipus complex offered the child two possibilities of satisfaction, an active and a passive one. He could put himself in his father's place in a masculine fashion and have intercourse with his mother as his father did, in which case he would soon have felt the latter as a hindrance; or he might want to take the place of his mother and be loved by his father, in which case his mother would become superfluous. The child may have had only very vague notions as to what constitutes a satisfying erotic intercourse; but certainly the penis must play a part in it, for the sensations in his own organ were evidence of that. So far he had had no occasion to doubt that women possessed a penis. But now his acceptance of the possibility of castration, his recognition that women were castrated, made an end of both possible ways of obtaining satisfaction from the Oedipus complex. For both of them entailed the loss of his penis—the masculine one as a resulting punishment and the feminine one as a precondition. If the satisfaction of love in the field of the Oedipus complex is to cost the child his penis, a conflict is bound to arise between his narcissistic interest in that part of his body and the libidinal cathexis of his parental objects. In this conflict the first of these forces normally triumphs: the child's ego turns away from the Oedipus complex.

I have described elsewhere how this turning away takes place. The object-cathexes are given up and replaced by identifications. The authority of the father or the parents is introjected into the ego, and there it forms the nucleus of the super-ego, which takes over the severity of the father and perpetuates his prohibition against incest, and so secures the ego from the return of the libidinal object-cathexis. The libidinal trends belonging to the Oedipus complex are in part desexualized and sublimated (a thing which probably happens with every transformation into an identification) and in part inhibited in their aim and changed into impulses of affection. The whole process has, on the one hand, preserved the genital organ—has averted the danger of its loss—and, on the other, has paralysed it—has removed its function. This process ushers in the latency period, which now interrupts the child's sexual development.

I see no reason for denying the name of a 'repression' to the ego's turning away from the Oedipus complex, although later repressions come about for the most part with the participation of the super-ego, which in this case is only just being formed. But the process we have described is more than a repression. It is equivalent, if it is ideally carried out, to a destruction and an abolition of the complex. We may plausibly assume that we have here come upon the borderline—never a very sharply drawn one—between the normal and the pathological. If the ego has in fact not achieved much more than a *repression* of the complex, the latter persists in an unconscious state in the id and will later manifest its pathogenic effect.

Analytic observation enables us to recognize or guess these connections between the phallic organization, the Oedipus complex, the threat of castration, the formation of the super-ego and the latency period. These connections justify the statement that the destruction of the Oedipus complex is brought about by the threat of castration. But this does not dispose of the problem; there is room for a theoretical speculation which may upset the results we have come to or put them in a new light. Before we start along this new path, however, we must turn to a question which has arisen in the course of this discussion and has so far been left on one side. The process which has been described refers, as has been expressly said, to male children only. How does the corresponding development take place in little girls?

At this point our material—for some incomprehensible reason—becomes far more obscure and full of gaps. The female sex, too, develops an Oedipus complex, a super-ego and a latency period. May we also attribute a phallic organization and a castration complex to it? The answer is in the affirmative; but these things cannot be the same as they are in boys. Here the feminist demand for equal rights for the sexes does not take us far, for the morphological distinction is bound to find expression in differences of psychical development. 'Anatomy is Destiny,' to vary a saying of Napoleon's. The little girl's clitoris behaves just like a penis to begin with; but, when she makes a comparison with a playfellow of the other sex, she perceives that she has 'come off badly' and she feels this as a wrong done to her and as a ground for inferiority. For a while still she consoles herself with the expectation that later on, when she grows older, she will acquire just as big an appendage as the boy's. Here the masculinity complex of women branches off. A female child, however, does not understand her lack of a penis as being a sex character; she explains it by assuming that at some earlier date she had possessed an equally large organ and had then lost it by castration. She seems not to extend this inference from herself to other, adult females, but, entirely on the lines of the phallic phase, to regard them as possessing large and complete—that is to say, male—genitals. The essential difference thus comes about that the girl accepts castration as an accomplished fact, whereas the boy fears the possibility of its occurrence.

The fear of castration being thus excluded in the little girl, a powerful motive also drops out for the setting-up of a super-ego and for the breaking-off of the infantile genital organization. In her, far more than in the boy, these changes seem to be the result of upbringing and of intimidation from outside which threatens her with a loss of love. The girl's Oedipus complex is much simpler than that of the small bearer of the penis; in my experience, it seldom goes beyond the taking of her mother's place and the adopting of a feminine attitude towards her father. Renunciation of the penis is not tolerated by the girl without some attempt at compensation. She slips—along the line of a symbolic equation, one might say—from the penis to a baby. Her Oedipus complex culminates in a desire, which is long retained, to receive a baby from her father as a gift—to bear him a child. One has an impression that the Oedipus complex is then gradually given up because this wish is never fulfilled. The two wishes—to possess a penis and a child—remain strongly cathected in the unconscious and help to prepare the female creature for her later sexual role. The comparatively lesser strength of the sadistic contribution to her sexual instinct, which we may no doubt connect with the stunted growth of her penis, makes it easier in her case for the direct sexual trends to be transformed into aim-inhibited trends of an affectionate kind. It must be admitted, however, that in general our insight into these developmental processes in girls is unsatisfactory, incomplete and vague.

I have no doubt that the chronological and causal relations described here between the Oedipus complex, sexual intimidation (the threat of castration), the formation of the super-ego and the beginning of the latency period are of a typical kind; but I do not wish to assert that this type is the only possible one. Variations in the chronological order and in the linking-up of these events are bound to have a very important bearing on the development of the individual.

Since the publication of Otto Rank's interesting study, *The Trauma of Birth* [1924], even the conclusion arrived at by this modest investigation, to the effect that the boy's Oedipus complex is destroyed by the fear of castration, cannot be accepted without further discussion. Nevertheless, it seems to me premature to enter into such a discussion at the present time, and perhaps inadvisable to begin a criticism or an appreciation of Rank's view at this juncture.

ALFRED C. KINSEY, WARDELL B. POMEROY, AND CLYDE E. MARTIN

Sexual Behavior in the Human Male

Born in Hoboken, New Jersey, Alfred Charles Kinsey (1894–1956) developed an intense interest in biology as a child but was steered toward engineering by his father, an instructor in mechanical arts at the Stevens Institute of Technology. After two unproductive years at Stevens, Kinsey completed his B.S. at Bowdoin College and entered the Bussey Institute at Harvard to study entomology, specializing in the gall wasp. In 1919, he undertook a year of fieldwork in the American South and West, covering some 18,000 miles and gathering over 300,000 gall wasp specimens. In 1920, upon receiving his Sc.D., Kinsey was appointed assistant professor at Indiana University, where he was to remain as a teacher and researcher for the rest of his career. The turning point in Kinsey's work came in 1938, when he was asked to deliver several lectures for a course on marriage at Indiana University. Surprised by the lack of scientific information on human sexual behavior, Kinsey decided to research the subject in full anticipation of the fact that the problems likely to arise in such a study "promised to be greater than those involved in studying insects." Starting with a handful of college students, Kinsey and his collaborators, Pomeroy and Martin, began recording what they called the "sexual histories" of as many subjects as they could recruit, a sample population that grew to twelve thousand in the course of a nine-year study. Covering various age and racial groups and all social levels, the project sought to investigate "all kinds of persons and all aspects of human sexual behavior" without any moral or social interpretation of the facts or any preconceptions about what was normal or abnormal.

In 1947, the Institute for Sex Research was founded to house the project and its vast archives. Its first book, *Sexual Behavior in the Human Male* (1948), based on 5,300 interviews, was followed seven years later with *Sexual Behavior in the Human Female*. Throughout the project, Kinsey and his investigators faced formidable opponents, including psychiatrists who claimed that interviewers were "practicing medicine without a license," scientists who argued that his work was methodologically unsound, religious leaders who branded it immoral, and members of the House of Representatives, who pronounced it "unscientific and un-American."

From *Sexual Behavior in the Human Male* (Philadelphia: W. B. Saunders, 1948). Reprinted by permission of the Kinsey Institute for Research in Sex, Gender, and Reproduction, Inc.

HOMOSEXUAL OUTLET

In the total male population, single and married, between adolescence and old age, 24 per cent of the total outlet is derived from solitary sources (masturbation and nocturnal emissions), 69.4 per cent is derived from heterosexual sources (petting and coitus), and 6.3 per cent of the total number of orgasms is derived from homosexual contacts. It is not more than 0.3 per cent of the outlet which is derived from relations with animals of other species.

Homosexual contacts account, therefore, for a rather small but still significant portion of the total outlet of the human male. The significance of the homosexual is, furthermore, much greater than the frequencies of outlet may indicate, because a considerable portion of the population, perhaps the major portion of the male population, has at least some homosexual experience between adolescence and old age. In addition, about 60 per cent of the pre-adolescent boys engage in homosexual activities, . . . and there is an additional group of adult males who avoid overt contacts but who are quite aware of their potentialities for reacting to other males.

Until the extent of any type of human behavior is adequately known, it is difficult to assess its significance, either to the individuals who are involved or to society as a whole; and until the extent of the homosexual is known, it is practically impossible to understand its biologic or social origins. It is one thing if we are dealing with a type of activity that is unusual, without precedent among other animals, and restricted to peculiar types of individuals within the human population. It is another thing if the phenomenon proves to be a fundamental part, not only of human sexuality, but of mammalian patterns as a whole. The present chapter is, therefore, wholly confined to an analysis of the data which we now have on the incidence and the frequencies of homosexual activity in the white male population in this country.

Definition

For nearly a century the term homosexual in connection with human behavior has been applied to sexual relations, either overt or psychic, between individuals of the same sex. Derived from the Greek root *homo* rather than from the Latin word for man, the term emphasizes the *sameness* of the two individuals who are involved in a sexual relation.

It is unfortunate that the students of animal behavior have applied the term homosexual to a totally different sort of phenomenon among the lower mammals. In most of the literature on animal behavior it is applied on the basis of the general conspectus of the behavior pattern of the animal, its aggressiveness in seeking the sexual contact, its postures during coitus, its position relative to the other animal in the sex relation, and the conformance or disconformance of that behavior to the usual positions and activities of the animal during heterosexual coitus. . . .

In most mammals the behavior of the female in a heterosexual performance usually involves the acceptance of the male which is trying to make intromission. The female at such a moment is less aggressive than the male, even passive in her acceptance of the male's approaches, and subordinate in position to him during actual coitus. This means that the female usually lies beneath the male or in front of him during copulation, either submitting from the very beginning of the sexual relation or (as in the cats, ferret, mink, and some other animals) being forced into submission by the assault of the male. In the case of the rat, the female which is in heat as the result of the hormones which her ovaries secrete near the time of ovulation, is more readily induced to crouch on the floor, arch her back (in lordosis) so her body is raised posteriorly, and pass into a nervous state which is characterized by a general rigidity of most of the body, but by a constant and rapid trembling of the ears and by peculiar hopping movements. This is the behavior which is characteristic of the female in a heterosexual contact, and this is what the students of animals describe as typically feminine behavior.

Throughout the mammals it is the male which more often (but not always) pursues the female for a sexual contact. In species where there is a struggle before the female submits to coitus, the male must be physically dominant and capable of controlling the female. In the ultimate act it is the male which more often mounts in back of the female and makes the active pelvic thrusts which effect intromission. This is the behavior that students of the lower mammals commonly refer to as typically masculine behavior.

But among many species of mammals and, indeed, probably among all of them, it not infrequently happens that males and females assume other than their usual positions in a sexual contact. This may be dependent upon individual differences in the physiology or anatomy of certain individuals, on differences in hormones, on environmental circumstances, or on some previous experience which has conditioned the animal in its behavior.

In a certain number of cases the assumption of the attitudes and positions of the opposite sex, among these lower mammals, seems to depend upon nothing more than the accident of the position in which the individual finds itself. The same male rat that has mounted a female in typical heterosexual coitus only a few moments before, may crouch on the floor, arch its back, and rear its posterior when it is approached by another rat from the rear. The same female which rises from the floor where she has been crouching in front of a copulating male may bump into another rat as she runs around the cage, rear on her haunches in front of the decumbent partner, and go through all of the motions that a male ordinarily goes through in heterosexual copulation. She may move her pelvis in thrusts which are quite like those of the male. She may strike her genital area against the genital area of the rat in front, quite as she would if she had a penis to effect entrance. And, what is most astounding, she may double up her body as she pulls back from the genital thrusts and manipulate her own genitalia with her mouth . . . exactly as the male rat ordinarily manipulates his penis between the thrusts that he makes when he is engaged in the masculine role in the usual type of heterosexual relation.

The assumption by a male animal of a female position in a sexual relation, or the assumption by a female of a position which is more typical of the male in a heterosexual relation, is what the students of animal behavior have referred to as homosexuality. This, of course, has nothing whatsoever to do with the use of the term among the students of human behavior, and one must be exceedingly careful how one transfers the conclusions based on these animal studies.

In studies of human behavior, the term inversion is applied to sexual situations in which males play female roles and females play male roles in sex relations. Most of the data on "homosexuality" in the animal studies actually refer to inversion. Inversion, of course, may occur in either heterosexual or homosexual relations, although there has been a widespread opinion, even among students of human psychology, and among some persons whose experience has been largely homosexual, that inversion is an invariable accompaniment of homosexuality. However, this generalization is not warranted. A more elaborate presentation of our data would show that there are a great many males who remain as masculine, and a great many females who remain as feminine, in their attitudes and their approaches in homosexual relations, as the males or females who have nothing but heterosexual relations. Inversion and homosexuality are two distinct and not always correlated types of behavior.

If the term homosexual is restricted as it should be, the homosexuality or heterosexuality of any activity becomes apparent by determining the sexes of the two individuals involved in the relationship. And although one may hear of a male "who has sex relations with his wife in a homosexual way," there is no logic in such a use of the term. . . .

On the other hand, the homosexuality of certain relationships between individuals of the same sex may be denied by some persons, because the situation does not fulfill other criteria that they think should be attached to the definition. Mutual masturbation between two males may be dismissed, even by certain clinicians, as not homosexual, because oral or anal relations or particular levels of psychic response are required, according to their concept of homosexuality. There are persons who insist that the active male in an anal relation is essentially heterosexual in his behavior, and that the passive male in the same relation is the only one who is homosexual. These, however, are misapplications of terms, which are often unfortunate because they obscure the interpretations of the situation which the clinician is supposed to help by his analysis.

These misinterpretations are often encouraged by the very persons who are having homosexual experience. Some males who are being regularly fellated by other males without, however, ever performing fellation themselves, may insist that they are exclusively heterosexual and that they have never been involved in a truly homosexual relation. Their consciences are cleared and they may avoid trouble with society and with the police by perpetrating the additional fiction that they are incapable of responding to a relation with a male unless they fantasy themselves in contact with a female. Even clinicians have allowed themselves to be diverted by such pretensions. The actual histories, however, show few if any cases of sexual relations between males which could be considered anything but homosexual.

Many individuals who have had considerable homosexual experience, construct a hierarchy on the basis of which they insist that anyone who has not had as much homosexual experience as they have had, or who is less exclusively aroused by homosexual stimuli, is "not really homosexual." It is amazing to observe how many psychologists and psychiatrists have accepted this sort of propaganda, and have come to believe that homosexual males and females are discretely different from persons who merely have homosexual experience, or who react sometimes to homosexual stimuli. Sometimes such an interpretation allows for only two kinds of males and two kinds of females, namely those who are heterosexual and those who are homosexual. But as subsequent data in this chapter will show, there is only about half of the male population whose sexual behavior is exclusively heterosexual, and there are only a few per cent who are exclusively homosexual. Any restriction of the term homosexuality to individuals who are exclusively so demands, logically, that the term heterosexual be applied only to those individuals who are exclusively heterosexual; and this makes no allowance for the nearly half of the population which has had sexual contacts with, or reacted psychically to, individuals of their own as well as of the opposite sex. Actually, of course, one must learn to recognize every combination of heterosexuality and homosexuality in the histories of various individuals.

It would encourage clearer thinking on these matters if persons were not characterized as heterosexual or homosexual, but as individuals who have had certain amounts of heterosexual experience and certain amounts of homosexual experience. Instead of using these terms as substantives which stand for persons, or even as adjectives to describe persons, they may better be used to describe the nature of the overt sexual relations, or of the stimuli to which an individual erotically responds.

Previous Estimates of Incidence

Many persons have recognized the importance of securing specific information on the incidence of the homosexual. The clinician needs to know how far the experience of his patient departs from norms for the remainder of the population. Counselors, teachers, clergymen, personnel officers, the administrators of institutions, social workers, law enforcement officers, and still others who are concerned with the direction of human behavior, may completely misinterpret the meaning of the homosexual experience in an individual's history, unless they understand the incidence and frequency of such activity in the population as a whole.

Satisfactory incidence figures on the homosexual cannot be obtained by any technique short of a carefully planned population survey. The data should cover every segment of the total population.

Unfortunately, no previous attempts to assess the incidence of the homosexual have begun to satisfy these demands for statistical adequacy. The incidence figures which are most often quoted are derived from the 2 to 5 per cent estimate which Havelock Ellis made for England . . . and from the more elaborate calculations made by Hirschfeld, chiefly for Germany. . . . The professional literature, if it does not cite these studies, rarely quotes any other sources except "the best informed students of the subject" . . . and through devious channels these data have become general property among people who have no idea of their origin.

Incidence Data in Present Study

The statistics given throughout this volume on the incidence of homosexual activity, and the statistics to be given in the present section of this chapter, are based on those persons who have had physical contacts with other males, and who were brought to orgasm as a result of such contacts. By any strict definition such contacts are homosexual, irrespective of the extent of the pychic stimulation involved, of the techniques employed, or of the relative importance of the homosexual and the heterosexual in the history of such an individual. These are not data on the number of persons who are "homosexual," but on the number of persons who have had at least some homosexual experience. . . .

In these terms (of physical contact to the point of orgasm), the data in the present study indicate that at least 37 per cent of the male population has some homosexual experience between the beginning of adolescence and old age. This is more than one male in three of the persons that one may meet as he passes along a city street. Among the males who remain unmarried until the age of 35, almost exactly 50 per cent have homosexual experience between the beginning of adolescence and that age. Some of these persons have but a single experience, and some of them have much more or even a lifetime of experience; but all of them have at least some experience to the point of orgasm.

Frequencies

Since the incidence of the homosexual is high, and since it accounts for only 8 to 16 per cent of the total orgasms of the unmarried males . . . and for a rather insignificant portion of the outlet of the married males . . . , it is obvious that the mean frequencies must be low in the population as a whole. Even when the calculations are confined to those males who are having actual experience, the average frequencies are never high.

These low rates are in striking discord with the fact that homosexual contacts could in actuality be had more abundantly than heterosexual contacts, if there were no social restraints or personal conflicts involved. The sexual possibilities of the average male in his teens or twenties are probably more often assayed by males than by females, and younger males who are attractive physically or who have attractive personalities may be approached for homosexual relations more often than they themselves would ever approach females for heterosexual relations. A homosexually experienced male could undoubtedly find a larger number of sexual partners among males than a heterosexually experienced male could find among females.

The heterosexual male finds a regular outlet if he locates a single female who is acceptable as a wife in marriage. The homosexual male is more often concerned with finding a succession of partners, no one of whom will provide more than a few contacts, or perhaps not more than a single contact. Some promiscuous males with homosexual histories become so interested in the thrill of conquest, and in the variety of partners and in the variety of genital experiences that may be had, that they deliberately turn down opportunities for repetitions of contacts with any one person. This necessity for finding new partners may result in their going for some days or weeks without sexual relations.

There are some males who are primarily or even exclusively homosexual in their psychic responses, but who may completely abstain from overt relations for moral reasons or for fear of social difficulties. Left without any socio-sexual contacts, some of these persons have essentially no outlet, and some of them are, therefore, very badly upset.

For these several reasons, average frequencies among males with homosexual histories are usually low, and there are very few high frequencies. In any particular age group, in any segment of the population, it is never more than about 5.5 per cent of the males who are having homosexual relations that average more than once every other day (3.5 per week). Calculating only for the males who actually have homosexual experience, there are never more than 5.2 per cent that have frequencies averaging more than 6.0 per week during their most active years. Considering that it is 25 per cent of the entire population which has total sexual outlets which average more than 3.5 per week, and considering that 24 per cent of the married males have outlets that average more than 6.0 per week in their most active period, it is apparent that outlets from the homosexual are definitely low.

Scientific and Social Implications

In view of the data which we now have on the incidence and frequency of the homosexual, and in particular on its co-existence with the heterosexual in the lives of a considerable portion of the male population, it is difficult to maintain the view that psychosexual reactions between individuals of the same sex are rare and therefore abnormal or unnatural, or that they constitute within themselves evidence of neuroses or even psychoses.

If homosexual activity persists on as large a scale as it does, in the face of the very considerable public sentiment against it and in spite of the severity of the penalties that our Anglo-American culture has placed upon it through the centuries, there seems some reason for believing that such activity would appear in the histories of a much larger portion of the population if there were no social restraints. The very general occurrence of the homosexual in ancient Greece . . . , and its wide occurrence today in some cultures in which such activity is not as taboo as it is in our own, suggests that the capacity of an individual to respond erotically to any sort of stimulus, whether it is provided by another person of the same or of the opposite sex, is basic in the species. That patterns of heterosexuality and patterns of homosexuality represent learned behavior which depends, to a considerable degree, upon the mores of the particular culture in which the individual is raised, is a possibility that must be thoroughly considered before there can be any acceptance of the idea that homosexuality is inherited, and that the pattern for each individual is so innately fixed that no modification of it may be expected within his lifetime.

The opinion that homosexual activity in itself provides evidence of a psychopathic personality is materially challenged by these incidence and frequency data. Of the 40 or 50 per cent of the male population which has homosexual experience, certainly a high proportion would not be considered psychopathic personalities on the basis of anything else in their histories. It is argued that an individual who is so obtuse to social reactions as to continue his homosexual activity and make it any material portion of his life, therein evidences some social incapacity; but psychiatrists and clinicians in general might very well re-examine their justification for demanding that all persons conform to particular patterns of behavior. As a matter of fact, there is an increasing proportion of the most skilled psychiatrists who make no attempt to re-direct behavior, but who devote their attention to helping an individual accept himself, and to conduct himself in such a manner that he does not come into open conflict with society.

There are, of course, some persons with homosexual histories who are neurotic and in constant difficulty with themselves and not infrequently with society. That is also true of some persons with heterosexual histories. Some homosexual individuals are so upset that they have difficulty in the accomplishment of their business or professional obligations and reach the point where they find it difficult to make the simplest sort of social contact without friction. It is, however, a considerable question whether these persons have homosexual histories because they are neurotic, or whether their neurotic disturbances are the product of their homosexual activities and of society's reaction to them. These are matters that must be investigated in more detail in a later volume; but they are questions that become more significant when one realizes the actual extent of homosexual behavior.

SIMONE DE BEAUVOIR (1908–1986)

The Second Sex

Novelist, essayist, and political activist Simone de Beauvoir was an advocate of women's rights and an acute analyst of the social meanings and roles
relegated to women. Born in Paris, Beauvoir studied philosophy with Jean-
Paul Sartre at the Sorbonne, where she became a professor in 1941. Much
of Beauvoir's writing is autobiographical in nature: *The Mandarins* (1954),
a novel for which she won the Prix Goncourt, portrays the leading existentialist figures of her day; *Memoirs of a Dutiful Daughter* (1958) describes
her oppressive upbringing; and *Adieux* (1984) chronicles the last ten years
of her life with Sartre. When it was first published in France in 1949, *The
Second Sex* was violently attacked by the Church and drew fire from both
the political left and right. Justly called "the feminist bible," the book
launched the women's liberation movement in the 1960s and has been translated into dozens of languages. Ranging over philosophy, sociology, literature, and biology, the book is a devastating critique of the discourses that
define women as the feminine "other"—the inferior or second sex. In the
weeks that followed the book's publication, Beauvoir received a barrage of
letters from "some very active members of the First Sex," who variously
accused her of being frigid, priapic, a nymphomaniac, a lesbian, and "even
an unwed mother."

For a long time I have hesitated to write a book on woman. The subject is irritating,
especially to women; and it is not new. Enough ink has been spilled in the quarreling over feminism, now practically over, and perhaps we should say no more about
it. It is still talked about, however, for the voluminous nonsense uttered during the
last century seems to have done little to illuminate the problem. After all, is there a
problem? And if so, what is it? Are there women, really? Most assuredly the theory
of the eternal feminine still has its adherents who will whisper in your ear: "Even in
Russia women still are *women*"; and other erudite persons—sometimes the very
same—say with a sigh: "Woman is losing her way, woman is lost." One wonders if
women still exist, if they will always exist, whether or not it is desirable that they
should, what place they occupy in this world, what their place should be. "What has
become of women?" was asked recently in an ephemeral magazine.

But first we must ask: what is a woman? "*Tota mulier in utero*," says one, "woman
is a womb." But in speaking of certain women, connoisseurs declare that they are
not women, although they are equipped with a uterus like the rest. All agree in recognizing the fact that females exist in the human species; today as always they make

up about one half of humanity. And yet we are told that femininity is in danger; we are exhorted to be women, remain women, become women. It would appear, then, that every female human being is not necessarily a woman; to be so considered she must share in that mysterious and threatened reality known as femininity. Is this attribute something secreted by the ovaries? Or is it a Platonic essence, a product of the philosophic imagination? Is a rustling petticoat enough to bring it down to earth? Although some women try zealously to incarnate this essence, it is hardly patentable. It is frequently described in vague and dazzling terms that seem to have been borrowed from the vocabulary of the seers, and indeed in the times of St. Thomas it was considered an essence as certainly defined as the somniferous virtue of the poppy.

If her functioning as a female is not enough to define woman, if we decline also to explain her through "the eternal feminine," and if nevertheless we admit, provisionally, that women do exist, then we must face the question: what is a woman?

To state the question is, to me, to suggest, at once, a preliminary answer. The fact that I ask it is in itself significant. A man would never get the notion of writing a book on the peculiar situation of the human male. But if I wish to define myself, I must first of all say: "I am a woman"; on this truth must be based all further discussion. A man never begins by presenting himself as an individual of a certain sex; it goes without saying that he is a man. The terms *masculine* and *feminine* are used symmetrically only as a matter of form, as on legal papers. In actuality the relation of the two sexes is not quite like that of two electrical poles, for man represents both the positive and the neutral, as is indicated by the common use of *man* to designate human beings in general; whereas woman represents only the negative, defined by limiting criteria, without reciprocity. In the midst of an abstract discussion it is vexing to hear a man say: "You think thus and so because you are a woman"; but I know that my only defense is to reply: "I think thus and so because it is true," thereby removing my subjective self from the argument. It would be out of the question to reply: "And you think the contrary because you are a man," for it is understood that the fact of being a man is no peculiarity. A man is in the right in being a man; it is the woman who is in the wrong. It amounts to this: just as for the ancients there was an absolute vertical with reference to which the oblique was defined, so there is an absolute human type, the masculine. Woman has ovaries, a uterus; these peculiarities imprison her in her subjectivity, circumscribe her within the limits of her own nature. It is often said that she thinks with her glands. Man superbly ignores the fact that his anatomy also includes glands, such as the testicles, and that they secrete hormones. He thinks of his body as a direct and normal connection with the world, which he believes he apprehends objectively, whereas he regards the body of woman as a hindrance, a prison, weighed down by everything peculiar to it. "The female is a female by virtue of a certain *lack* of qualities," said Aristotle; "we should regard the female nature as afflicted with a natural defectiveness." And St. Thomas for his part pronounced woman to be an "imperfect man," an "incidental" being. This is symbolized in Genesis where Eve is depicted as made from what Bossuet called "a supernumerary bone" of Adam.

Thus humanity is male and man defines woman not in herself but as relative to him; she is not regarded as an autonomous being. Michelet writes: "Woman, the relative being. . . . " And Benda is most positive in his *Rapport d'Uriel*: "The body of man makes sense in itself quite apart from that of woman, whereas the latter seems wanting in significance by itself. . . . Man can think of himself without woman. She cannot think of herself without man." And she is simply what man decrees; thus she is called "the sex," by which is meant that she appears essentially to the male as a sexual being. For him she is sex—absolute sex, no less. She is defined and differentiated with reference to man and not he with reference to her; she is the incidental, the inessential as opposed to the essential. He is the Subject, he is the Absolute—she is the Other.

The category of the *Other* is as primordial as consciousness itself. In the most primitive societies, in the most ancient mythologies, one finds the expression of a duality—that of the Self and the Other. This duality was not originally attached to the division of the sexes; it was not dependent upon any empirical facts. It is revealed in such works as that of Granet on Chinese thought and those of Dumézil on the East Indies and Rome. The feminine element was at first no more involved in such pairs as Varuna-Mitra, Uranus-Zeus, Sun-Moon, and Day-Night than it was in the contrasts between Good and Evil, lucky and unlucky auspices, right and left, God and Lucifer. Otherness is a fundamental category of human thought.

Thus it is that no group ever sets itself up as the One without at once setting up the Other over against itself. If three travelers chance to occupy the same compartment, that is enough to make vaguely hostile "others" out of all the rest of the passengers on the train. In small-town eyes all persons not belonging to the village are "strangers" and suspect; to the native of a country all who inhabit other countries are "foreigners"; Jews are "different" for the anti-Semite, Negroes are "inferior" for American racists, aborigines are "natives" for colonists, proletarians are the "lower class" for the privileged.

But the other consciousness, the other ego, sets up a reciprocal claim. The native traveling abroad is shocked to find himself in turn regarded as a "stranger" by the natives of neighboring countries. As a matter of fact, wars, festivals, trading, treaties, and contests among tribes, nations, and classes tend to deprive the concept *Other* of its absolute sense and to make manifest its relativity; willy-nilly, individuals and groups are forced to realize the reciprocity of their relations. How is it, then, that this reciprocity has not been recognized between the sexes, that one of the contrasting terms is set up as the sole essential, denying any relativity in regard to its correlative and defining the latter as pure otherness? Why is it that women do not dispute male sovereignty? No subject will readily volunteer to become the object, the inessential; it is not the Other who, in defining himself as the Other, establishes the One. The Other is posed as such by the One in defining himself as the One. But if the Other is not to regain the status of being the One, he must be submissive enough to accept this alien point of view. Whence comes this submission in the case of woman?

There are, to be sure, other cases in which a certain category has been able to dominate another completely for a time. Very often this privilege depends upon inequality of numbers—the majority imposes its rule upon the minority or persecutes it. But women are not a minority, like the American Negroes or the Jews; there are as many women as men on earth. Again, the two groups concerned have often been

originally independent; they may have been formerly unaware of each other's existence, or perhaps they recognized each other's autonomy. But a historical event has
resulted in the subjugation of the weaker by the stronger. The scattering of the Jews,
the introduction of slavery into America, the conquests of imperialism are examples
in point. In these cases the oppressed retained at least the memory of former days;
they possessed in common a past, a tradition, sometimes a religion or a culture.

The parallel drawn by Bebel between women and the proletariat is valid in that
neither ever formed a minority or a separate collective unit of mankind. And instead
of a single historical event it is in both cases a historical development that explains
their status as a class and accounts for the membership of *particular individuals* in
that class. But proletarians have not always existed, whereas there have always been
women. They are women in virtue of their anatomy and physiology. Throughout history they have always been subordinated to men, and hence their dependency is not
the result of a historical event or a social change—it was not something that *occurred*. The reason why otherness in this case seems to be an absolute is in part that
it lacks the contingent or incidental nature of historical facts. A condition brought
about at a certain time can be abolished at some other time, as the Negroes of Haiti
and others have proved; but it might seem that a natural condition is beyond the possibility of change. In truth, however, the nature of things is no more immutably given,
once for all, than is historical reality. If woman seems to be the inessential which
never becomes the essential, it is because she herself fails to bring about this change.
Proletarians say "We"; Negroes also. Regarding themselves as subjects, they transform the bourgeois, the whites, into "others." But women do not say "We," except
at some congress of feminists or similar formal demonstration; men say "women,"
and women use the same word in referring to themselves. They do not authentically
assume a subjective attitude. The proletarians have accomplished the revolution in
Russia, the Negroes in Haiti, the Indo-Chinese are battling for it in Indo-China; but
the women's effort has never been anything more than a symbolic agitation. They
have gained only what men have been willing to grant; they have taken nothing, they
have only received.

The reason for this is that women lack concrete means for organizing themselves
into a unit which can stand face to face with the correlative unit. They have no past,
no history, no religion of their own; and they have no such solidarity of work and
interest as that of the proletariat. They are not even promiscuously herded together
in the way that creates community feeling among the American Negroes, the ghetto
Jews, the workers of Saint-Denis, or the factory hands of Renault. They live dispersed among the males, attached through residence, housework, economic condition, and social standing to certain men—fathers or husbands—more firmly than
they are to other women. If they belong to the bourgeoisie, they feel solidarity with
men of that class, not with proletarian women; if they are white, their allegiance is
to white men, not to Negro women. The proletariat can propose to massacre the ruling class, and a sufficiently fanatical Jew or Negro might dream of getting sole possession of the atomic bomb and making humanity wholly Jewish or black; but woman
cannot even dream of exterminating the males. The bond that unites her to her oppressors is not comparable to any other. The division of the sexes is a biological fact,

not an event in human history. Male and female stand opposed within a primordial *Mitsein,* and woman has not broken it. The couple is a fundamental unity with its two halves riveted together, and the cleavage of society along the line of sex is impossible. Here is to be found the basic trait of woman: she is the Other in a totality of which the two components are necessary to one anther.

Now, woman has always been man's dependent, if not his slave; the two sexes have never shared the world in equality. And even today woman is heavily handicapped, though her situation is beginning to change. Almost nowhere is her legal status the same as man's, and frequently it is much to her disadvantage. Even when her rights are legally recognized in the abstract, long-standing custom prevents their full expression in the mores. In the economic sphere men and women can almost be said to make up two castes; other things being equal, the former hold the better jobs, get higher wages, and have more opportunity for success than their new competitors. In industry and politics men have a great many more positions and they monopolize the most important posts. In addition to all this, they enjoy a traditional prestige that the education of children tends in every way to support, for the present enshrines the past—and in the past all history has been made by men. At the present time, when women are beginning to take part in the affairs of the world, it is still a world that belongs to men—they have no doubt of it at all and women have scarcely any. To decline to be the Other, to refuse to be a party to the deal—this would be for women to renounce all the advantages conferred upon them by their alliance with the superior caste. Man-the-sovereign will provide woman-the-liege with material protection and will undertake the moral justification of her existence; thus she can evade at once both economic risk and the metaphysical risk of a liberty in which ends and aims must be contrived without assistance. Indeed, along with the ethical urge of each individual to affirm his subjective existence, there is also the temptation to forgo liberty and become a thing. This is an inauspicious road, for he who takes it—passive, lost, ruined—becomes henceforth the creature of another's will, frustrated in his transcendence and deprived of every value. But it is an easy road; on it one avoids the strain involved in undertaking an authentic existence. When man makes of woman the *Other,* he may, then, expect her to manifest deep-seated tendencies toward complicity. Thus, woman may fail to lay claim to the status of subject because she lacks definite resources, because she feels the necessary bond that ties her to man regardless of reciprocity, and because she is often very well pleased with her role as the *Other.*

But it will be asked at once: how did all this begin? It is easy to see that the duality of the sexes, like any duality, gives rise to conflict. And doubtless the winner will assume the status of absolute. But why should man have won from the start? It seems possible that women could have won the victory; or that the outcome of the conflict might never have been decided. How is it that this world has always belonged to the men and that things have begun to change only recently? Is this change a good thing? Will it bring about an equal sharing of the world between men and women?

These questions are not new, and they have often been answered. But the very fact that woman *is the Other* tends to cast suspicion upon all the justifications that men have ever been able to provide for it. These have all too evidently been dictated by men's interest. A little-known feminist of the seventeenth century, Poulain de la Barre, put it this way: "All that has been written about women by men should be suspect, for the men are at once judge and party to the lawsuit." Everywhere, at all times, the males have displayed their satisfaction in feeling that they are the lords of creation. "Blessed be God . . . that He did not make me a woman," say the Jews in their morning prayers, while their wives pray on a note of resignation: "Blessed be the Lord, who created me according to His will." The first among the blessings for which Plato thanked the gods was that he had been created free, not enslaved; the second, a man, not a woman. But the males could not enjoy this privilege fully unless they believed it to be founded on the absolute and the eternal; they sought to make the fact of their supremacy into a right. "Being men, those who have made and compiled the laws have favored their own sex, and jurists have elevated these laws into principles," to quote Poulain de la Barre once more.

Legislators, priests, philosophers, writers, and scientists have striven to show that the subordinate position of woman is willed in heaven and advantageous on earth.

It was only later, in the eighteenth century, that genuinely democratic men began to view the matter objectively. Diderot, among others, strove to show that woman is, like man, a human being. Later John Stuart Mill came fervently to her defense. But these philosophers displayed unusual impartiality. In the nineteenth century the feminist quarrel became again a quarrel of partisans. One of the consequences of the industrial revolution was the entrance of women into productive labor, and it was just here that the claims of the feminists emerged from the realm of theory and acquired an economic basis, while their opponents became the more aggressive. Although landed property lost power to some extent, the bourgeoisie clung to the old morality that found the guarantee of private property in the solidity of the family. Woman was ordered back into the home the more harshly as her emancipation became a real menace. Even within the working class the men endeavored to restrain woman's liberation, because they began to see the women as dangerous competitors —the more so because they were accustomed to work for lower wages.

In proving woman's inferiority, the antifeminists then began to draw not only upon religion, philosophy, and theology, as before, but also upon science—biology, experimental psychology, etc. At most they were willing to grant "equality in difference" to the *other* sex. That profitable formula is most significant; it is precisely like the "equal but separate" formula of the Jim Crow laws aimed at the North American Negroes. As is well known, this so-called equalitarian segregation has resulted only in the most extreme discrimination. The similarity just noted is in no way due to chance, for whether it is a race, a caste, a class, or a sex that is reduced to a position of inferiority, the methods of justification are the same. "The eternal feminine" corresponds to "the black soul" and to "the Jewish character." True, the Jewish problem is on the whole very different from the other two—to the anti-Semite the Jew is not so much an inferior as he is an enemy for whom there is to be granted no place on earth, for whom annihilation is the fate desired. But there are deep similarities between the situation of woman and that of the Negro. Both are being emancipated today from a like paternalism, and the former master class wishes to "keep them in their place"—that is, the place chosen for them. In both cases the former masters lavish more or less sincere eulogies, either on the virtues of "the good Negro" with his dormant, childish, merry soul—the submissive Negro—or on the merits of the woman who is "truly feminine"—that is, frivolous, infantile, irresponsible—the submissive woman. In both cases the dominant class bases its argument on a state of affairs that it has itself created. As George Bernard Shaw puts it, in substance, "The American white relegates the black to the rank of shoeshine boy; and he concludes from this that the black is good for nothing but shining shoes."

The question is: should that state of affairs continue? Many men hope that it will continue; not all have given up the battle. The conservative bourgeoisie still see in the emancipation of women a menace to their morality and their interests. Some men dread feminine competition. Recently a male student wrote in the *Hebdo-Latin:* "Every woman student who goes into medicine or law robs us of a job." He never questioned his rights in this world. And economic interests are not the only ones concerned. One of the benefits that oppression confers upon the oppressors is that the most humble among them is made to *feel* superior; thus, a "poor white" in the South can console himself with the thought that he is not a "dirty nigger"—and the more prosperous whites cleverly exploit this pride.

I have lingered on this example because the masculine attitude is here displayed with disarming ingenuousness. But men profit in many more subtle ways from the otherness, the alterity of woman. Here is miraculous balm for those afflicted with an inferiority complex, and indeed no one is more arrogant toward women, more aggressive or scornful, than the man who is anxious about his virility. Those who are not fear-ridden in the presence of their fellow men are much more disposed to recognize a fellow creature in woman; but even to these the myth of Woman, the Other, is precious for many reasons. They cannot be blamed for not cheerfully relinquishing all the benefits they derive from the myth, for they realize what they would lose in relinquishing woman as they fancy her to be, while they fail to realize what they have to gain from the woman of tomorrow. Refusal to pose oneself as the Subject, unique and absolute, requires great self-denial. Furthermore, the vast majority of men make no such claim explicitly. They do not *postulate* woman as inferior, for today they are too thoroughly imbued with the ideal of democracy not to recognize all human beings as equals.

So it is that many men will affirm as if in good faith that women *are* the equals of man and that they have nothing to clamor for, while *at the same time* they will say that women can never be the equals of man and that their demands are in vain. It is, in point of fact, a difficult matter for man to realize the extreme importance of social discriminations which seem outwardly insignificant but which produce in woman moral and intellectual effects so profound that they appear to spring from her original nature. The most sympathetic of men never fully comprehend woman's concrete situation. And there is no reason to put much trust in the men when they rush to the defense of privileges whose full extent they can hardly measure. We shall not, then, permit ourselves to be intimidated by the number and violence of the attacks launched against women, nor to be entrapped by the self-seeking eulogies bestowed on the "true woman," nor to profit by the enthusiasm for woman's destiny manifested by men who would not for the world have any part of it.

We should consider the arguments of the feminists with no less suspicion, however, for very often their controversial aim deprives them of all real value. If the "woman question" seems trivial, it is because masculine arrogance has made of it a "quarrel"; and when quarreling one no longer reasons well. People have tirelessly sought to prove that woman is superior, inferior, or equal to man. Some say that, having been created after Adam, she is evidently a secondary being; others say on the contrary that Adam was only a rough draft and that God succeeded in producing the human being in perfection when he created Eve. Woman's brain is smaller; yes, but it is relatively larger. Christ was made a man; yes, but perhaps for his greater humility. Each argument at once suggests its opposite, and both are often fallacious. If we are to gain understanding, we must get out of these ruts; we must discard the vague notions of superiority, inferiority, equality which have hitherto corrupted every discussion of the subject and start afresh.

In particular those who are condemned to stagnation are often pronounced happy on the pretext that happiness consists in being at rest. This notion we reject, for our perspective is that of existentialist ethics. Every subject plays his part as such specifically through exploits or projects that serve as a mode of transcendence; he achieves liberty only through a continual reaching out toward other liberties. There is no justification for present existence other than its expansion into an indefinitely open future. Every time transcendence falls back into immanence, stagnation, there is a degradation of existence into the "*en-soi*"—the brutish life of subjection to given conditions—and of liberty into constraint and contingence. This downfall represents a moral fault if the subject consents to it; if it is inflicted upon him, it spells frustration and oppression. In both cases it is an absolute evil. Every individual concerned to justify his existence feels that his existence involves an undefined need to transcend himself, to engage in freely chosen projects.

Now, what peculiarly signalizes the situation of woman is that she—a free and autonomous being like all human creatures—nevertheless finds herself living in a world where men compel her to assume the status of the Other. They propose to stabilize her as object and to doom her to immanence since her transcendence is to be overshadowed and forever transcended by another ego (*conscience*) which is essential and sovereign. The drama of woman lies in this conflict between the fundamental aspirations of every subject (ego)—who always regards the self as the essential—and the compulsions of a situation in which she is the inessential. How can a human being in woman's situation attain fulfillment? What roads are open to her? Which are blocked? How can independence be recovered in a state of dependency? What circumstances limit woman's liberty and how can they be overcome? These are the fundamental questions on which I would fain throw some light.

WILLIAM H. MASTERS (1915–   )
AND VIRGINIA E. JOHNSON (1925–   )

Human Sexual Response

A physician and educator, William H. Masters received his M.D. from the University of Rochester in 1943 and interned in obstetrics and gynecology at the St. Louis Maternity Hospital. Four years later, he joined the faculty of the Washington University School of Medicine, where he became professor in 1969 and served as director of the Reproductive Biology Research Foundation from 1964 to 1973. In 1973, the Foundation was renamed the Masters and Johnson Institute, which Masters codirected for seven years with Virginia Johnson, the psychologist he had married in 1971. Johnson received an honorary doctorate from the University of Louisville in 1978. Before her work with Masters, she had done research in reproductive biology at the Washington University School of Medicine and the Reproductive Biology Research Foundation. In 1966, Masters and Johnson coauthored *Human Sexual Response,* the result of an investigation into sexual anatomy and physiology they had begun in 1954. By directly observing and measuring the physical changes accompanying each phase of response, Masters and Johnson sought to understand the mechanisms of sexual arousal in men and women. In the initial stages of the project, the histories of 118 female and 27 male prostitutes were elicited. Out of this group, eight women and three men were selected for anatomical and physiological observation during sexual activity. These initial subjects, however, were not included in the final study, which was based on a sample of 382 women and 312 men "weighted purposely toward higher than average intelligence levels and socioeconomic backgrounds." During the course of the project, Masters and Johnson and their team of researchers observed and recorded more than ten thousand complete cycles of sexual response.

The functioning role of the penis is as well established as that of any other organ in the body. Ironically, there is no organ about which more misinformation has been perpetrated. The penis constantly has been viewed but rarely seen. The organ has been venerated, reviled, and misrepresented with intent in art, literature, and legend through the centuries. These intentional misrepresentations have varied in magnitude with the culture. Our culture has been influenced by and has contributed to manifold misconceptions of the functional role of the penis. These "phallic fallacies" have colored our arts and, possibly of even more import to our culture, influenced our behavioral and biologic sciences.

From *Human Sexual Response* (Boston: Little, Brown, 1966). Used by permission of the Masters and Johnson Institute.

The twofold functioning role of the penis providing for both urinary release and seminal-fluid deposition has been accepted throughout recorded history. Why, with the functioning role unquestionably established, should the functional role of the penis have been shrouded so successfully by "phallic fallacy" concepts? This, indeed, is one of the great mysteries of biologic science.

The functional role of the penis is that of providing an organic means for physiologic and psychologic increment and release of both male and female sexual tensions. The penis as an organ of male sensual focus can be related to the functional role of the clitoris in the total of female sexual response. The gross difference between these two organs is that the clitoris serves only in a functional role, and the penis has both a functioning and a functional capacity.

Objective material relating to the functional role of the penis has been accumulated from over 2,500 directly observed sexual response cycles experienced by 312 male study subjects whose ages range from 21 to 89 years. Subjective material has been returned from team interrogation of 654 men screened as study-subject applicants before the 312 active participants were selected.

Thirty-five of the 312 male members of the study-subject population were uncircumcised. Although approximately one-quarter of the male study subjects were beyond 40 years of age, more than half (19) of the uncircumcised males were found in this age grouping. The fact that only 16 out of a total of 231 male members of the study-subject population between the ages of 21 and 40 years were uncircumcised is representative of the medical trend toward urging routine circumcision of the newborn male infant. More than 95 percent of all deliveries in this country now are hospital deliveries, and circumcision is recommended as a routine neonatal procedure. The uncircumcised male, particularly one born in an urban area, indeed, is becoming a rarity in our society.

The phallic fallacy that the uncircumcised male can establish ejaculatory control more effectively than his circumcised counterpart was accepted almost universally as biologic fact by both circumcised and uncircumcised male study subjects. This concept was founded upon the widespread misconception that the circumcised penile glans is more sensitive to the exteroceptive stimuli of coition or masturbation than is the glans protected by a residual foreskin. Therefore, the circumcised male has been presumed to have more difficulty with ejaculatory control and (as many study subjects believed) a greater tendency toward impotence.

A limited number of the male study-subject population was exposed to a brief clinical experiment designed to disprove the false premise of excessive sensitivity of the circumcised glans. The 35 uncircumcised males were matched at random with circumcised study subjects of similar ages. Routine neurologic testing for both exteroceptive and light tactile discrimination were conducted on the ventral and dorsal surfaces of the penile body, with particular attention directed toward the glans. No clinically significant difference could be established between the circumcised and the uncircumcised glans during these examinations.

Another widely accepted "phallic fallacy" is the concept that the larger the penis the more effective the male as a partner in coital connection. The size of the male organ both in flaccid and erect state has been presumed by many cultures to reflect directly the sexual prowess of the individual male. Dickinson was one of the first to record dimensions of the penis with some degree of objectivity. He supported Loeb's report that the normal range of penile length varies from 8.5 to 10.5 cm. in the flaccid state, with the general average in the 9.5 cm. range. The range of normalcy suggested by these measurements also has been supported by measurements returned from examinations of individual members of the male study-subject population.

The delusion that penile size is related to sexual adequacy has been founded in turn upon yet another phallic misconception. It has been presumed that full erection of the larger penis provides a significantly greater penile size increase than does erection of the smaller penis. This premise has been refuted by a small group of men selected from the study-subject population for clinical evaluation. Forty men whose penises measured 7.5–9 cm. in length in the flaccid state were compared to a similar number of study subjects whose penises in the flaccid state measured 10–11.5 cm. Measurement was crudely clinical at best and can only be presumed suggestive and certainly not specific in character. The length of the smaller penises increased by an average of 7.5–8 cm. at full (pleateau-phase) erection. This full erection essentially doubled the smaller organs in length over flaccid-size standards. In contrast, in the men whose organs were significantly larger in a flaccid state (10–11.5 cm.), penile length increased by an average of 7–7.5 cm. in the fully erect (plateau-phase) state.

These measurements of full penile erection are so crudely clinical that they have been adjusted arbitrarily to the nearest 0.5 cm. to facilitate presentation. In each instance, measurement was taken from the anterior border of the symphysis at the base of the penis along the dorsal surface to the distal tip of the glans. All 80 penises were measured on three different occasions both in flaccid and erect states by the same individual. Only one investigator conducted this clinical measurement so that any idiosyncrasy of measurement technique would be common to all results. One of the measurements of penile erection was taken during automanipulation, and two measurements were initiated immediately upon withdrawal of the plateau-phase penis from active coition. Measurement of an erect penis was not attempted until the final engorgement of late plateau phase had been accomplished. Since full penile engorgement is a short-term process before ejaculation intervenes, measurement frequently was rushed and, therefore, additionally unreliable. While the information returned obviously is not definitive, there certainly is no statistical support for the "phallic fallacy" that the larger penis increases in size with full erection to a significantly greater degree than does the smaller penis. The difference in average erective size increase between the smaller flaccid penis and the larger flaccid penis is not significant.

As Piersol has stated, the size of the penis has less constant relation to general physical development than that of any other organ of the body. This statement has been made in recognition of yet another "phallic fallacy." It has been presumed by many cultures that the bigger the man in skeletal and muscular development, the bigger the penis, not only in a flaccid but also in an erect state. Detailed examination of the study-subject population of 312 men aged 21 to 89 years supported Piersol's contention that there is no relation between man's skeletal framework and the size of his external genitalia. The largest penis in the study-subject population, measuring approximately 14 cm. long in the flaccid state, was in a man 5 feet, 7 inches tall weighing 152 pounds. The smallest penis, measuring just over 6 cm. in the flaccid state, was in a man 5 feet, 11 inches tall weighing 178 pounds.

Although there is little to support the concept that erective size is proportionally greater for the larger than the smaller penis, there remains the theoretical concern of the man with the small penis as to his potential coital effectiveness. Even with erective ability of the smaller penis (less than 9 cm.) presumed equal to that of the larger penis (more than 10 cm.), the smaller penis in the flaccid state usually remains somewhat smaller in an erect state. The factor that constantly is overlooked in theoretical discussions of penile coital effectiveness is the involuntary accommodative reactions of the vagina in its functional role under coital stimulation as a seminal receptacle.

"Phallic fallacies" relating to the functional role of the penis frequently devolve from the culturally conceived role for the male partner in human coition—that of actively satisfying the female partner.

The "fear of performance" developing from cultural demand for partner satisfaction has been in the past uniquely the burden of the responding male. Inevitably fear provides a breeding-ground for misconception. Among the male members of the study-subject population and males interrogated as applicants, phallic fallacies of subjective orientation were related to decades of life experience more than to any other single factor.

For the men forty years or younger, fears of performance centered about questions of excessive ejaculatory experience and concerns for premature ejaculation. The problem of too frequent ejaculation was associated in the minds of many study subjects with possible loss of physical strength and not infrequently was presumed to be a basis for emotional instability if not severe neurosis. These misconceptions have grown from the culturally centered fear that frequent or excessive masturbation may lead to mental illness. No study subject could provide a secure personal concept of what constituted frequent or excessive levels of masturbation, nor could anyone describe an instance known to them, even by report, of mental illness resulting from masturbation. The superstition that physical or mental deterioration results from excessive masturbation is firmly entrenched in our culture, if returns from the team questioning of the total male group of study-subject applicants are any criterion.

Reported masturbatory frequency in the male study-subject group ranged from once a month to two or three times a day. Every male questioned expressed a theoretical concern for the supposed mental effects of excessive masturbation, and in every case "excessive levels" of masturbation, although not defined specifically, were considered to consist of a higher frequency than did the reported personal pattern. One man with a once-a-month masturbatory history felt once or twice a week to be excessive, with mental illness quite possible as a complication of such a frequency maintained for a year or more. The study subject with the masturbatory history of two or three times a day wondered whether five or six times a day wasn't excessive and might lead to a "case of nerves." No study subject among the 312 questioned in depth expressed the slightest fear that his particular masturbatory pattern was excessive regardless of stated frequency.

There is no established medical evidence that masturbation, regardless of frequency, leads to mental illness. Certainly there is no accepted medical standard defining excessive masturbation. It is true, of course, that many severely neurotic or acutely psychotic men masturbate frequently. If a high-frequency pattern of masturbatory activity exists, it may be but one of a number of symptoms of underlying mental illness rather than in any sense the cause of the individual distress. The vague concept of excessive masturbatory activity is a phallic fallacy widely accepted in our culture, relating specifically to the functional role of the penis in male sexuality.

Problems of premature ejaculation also disturbed the younger members of the study-subject population. These fears of performance were not associated with problems of erection; rather, they were directed toward the culturally imposed fear of inability to control the ejaculatory process to a degree sufficient to satisfy the female partner. These expressed fears of performance were confined primarily to those study subjects who had attained college or postgraduate levels of formal education. Only 7 of the total of 51 men whose formal education did not include college matriculation expressed the slightest concern with responsibility for coital-partner satisfaction. These men felt that it was the female's privilege to achieve satisfaction during active coition if she could, but certainly it was not the responsibility and really not the concern of the male partner to concentrate on satisfying the woman's sexual demands. Out of a total of 261 study subjects with college matriculation, 214 men expressed concern with coital-partner satisfaction. With these men ejaculatory control sufficient to accomplish partner satisfaction was considered a coital technique that must be acquired before the personal security of coital effectiveness could be established.

The fear of performance reflecting cultural stigmas directed toward erective inadequacy was that associated with problems of secondary impotence. These fears were expressed, under interrogation, by every male study subject beyond forty years of age, irrespective of reported levels of formal education.

Regardless of whether the individual male study subject had ever experienced an instance of erective difficulty, the probability that secondary impotence was associated directly with the aging process was vocalized constantly. The fallacy that secondary impotence is to be expected as the male ages is probably more firmly entrenched in our culture than any other misapprehension. While it is true that the aging process, with associated physical involution, can reduce penile erective adequacy, it is also true that secondary impotence is in no sense the inevitable result of the aging process.

The functional role of the penis in male sexuality has not been established with the security of the organ's functioning role. It has been severely obscured by "phallic fallacies" of cultural origin. Further definitive research in the physiology of male sexual response will make the greatest contribution toward identifying and reversing these misconceptions. It is inevitably true that the psychology of human sexual response can best be appreciated when the physiology has been established.

MARY JANE SHERFEY (1933–1983)

The Nature and Evolution
of Female Sexuality

An American psychiatrist and writer on female sexuality, Mary Jane Sherfey received her medical degree from Indiana University, where she attended lectures on marriage and sexuality given by Alfred Kinsey. Sherfey had a private practice in New York City and was on the staff of the Payne Whitney Clinic of the New York Hospital–Cornell Medical Center. In 1961, Sherfey's interest in female biology was intensified when she came upon the inductor theory, which demonstrated that the human embryo is female until hormonally "induced" to become male. Determined to popularize a fact that had lain in neglect since its discovery in the 1950s, Sherfey began researching the subject and familiarizing herself with a variety of disciplines, including embryology, anatomy, primatology, and anthropology. Many of her findings appear in *The Nature and Evolution of Female Sexuality,* which initially took form as an article contesting the existence of vaginal orgasm, published in the *Journal of the American Psychoanalytic Association* in 1966.

PSYCHOANALYTIC THEORY AND THE
NATURE OF THE ORGASM

One of Freud's most useful, accepted, and enduring concepts is his theory of female psychosexual growth with its basic assumption that the female is endowed with two independent erotogenic centers; during development she must transfer the infantile erotogenic zone of the clitoris to the mature erotogenic zone of the vagina.

The clitorial-vaginal transfer theory has been held essentially unchanged by psychoanalysts and psychiatrists in spite of many doubts and objections. The objections are based mainly on four observations: the infrequency of vaginal orgasms in apparently normal women; the lack of sensory nerve endings in the main body of the vagina; the ease with which women can confuse a vaginal orgasm with a clitoral one; and the *seeming* absence of the vaginal orgasm in all subhuman animals. These are certainly cogent reasons but do not necessarily disprove the possibility of the vaginal orgasm.

In fact, we seem to be in a strange dilemma of having a developmental theory that explains so much so well and conforms to so many women's life histories and felt experiences, yet one that has shown surprisingly little therapeutic effectiveness and has had only a questionable basis in biology.

The question must be put and answered within the profession: Could the lack of psychiatric interest in the sociopsychological crisis of women today, the absence of deeper levels of understanding of the feminine personality, its functions and dysfunctions, and our serious therapeutic limitations and tragic failures stem, in part, from erroneous assumptions of vaginal and clitoral responsivity which form the basis of the clitoral-vaginal transfer theory? Could many of the sexual neuroses which seem to be almost endemic to women today be, in part, induced by doctors attempting to treat them?

If so, we have before us impressive proof of the extraordinary reach and depth of Freud's thinking, touching the minds of almost everyone. If so, we also have before us the formidable obstacle of a large block of professional and public opinion which exists because people *want* the vaginal orgasm to exist. If so, to dispel these erroneous concepts, we must first dispel them from the minds of psychoanalysts and psychiatrists. To accomplish this requires *indisputable* proof that *the vaginal orgasm as distinct from the clitoral orgasm* does not exist and that whatever does exist instead is compatible with the many observations on female psychosexuality we know to be true. If such proof is forthcoming, the psychoanalytic theory may not necessarily be refuted but will require amendations.

The question of the existence or nonexistence of the vaginal orgasm is a biological problem and must be answered by biology. This initial study attempts to marshal the biological evidence available at present for psychiatric consideration. We must turn our minds from the psyche to the soma long enough to make the biological data now to be presented a part of our felt knowledge—to accept knowledge without feeling its truth is not to know at all.

EMBRYOLOGY AND THE NATURE OF BISEXUALITY

For Freud, the woman's entire personality is colored and complicated by the dual nature of her sexuality with its fundamental struggle in childhood and early adolescence to relinquish the active, aggressive, masculine sexual pleasure emanating from infantile clitoral activity, which in turn is the result of the innately bisexual nature of the embryo, i.e., clitoral erotism is the remaining functional, masculine component after differentiation of the female has occurred and must undergo still further regression to practically a vestigial state before the fullest maturity can be reached.

From here, it is hardly another step to regard all the female external genitalia as more or less miniature structures derived from male anlagen, the primordial structures from which the adult male genitalia grow. (That the reverse could be true, i.e., the penis is an exaggerated clitoris, the phallus is "pleasure-physiologically clitoral," the scrotum is derived from the primordial cells of the labia majora, etc., has, until recently, never been given the least consideration.) Bonaparte carried this line of thinking to its logical conclusion, postulating that since the female retains a rudimentary masculine clitoris, relinquished with such difficulty, the basic libido of the external genitalia is innately masculine. All women are burdened with the extremely difficult task of shifting not only from the clitoris to the vagina, but also from an innately masculine sexual drive to an acquired passive and, in many ways, masochistic feminine sexual drive. This whole line of thought essentially states that normal feminine sexuality is derived from an innately masculine sexuality. Thus it is that psychoanalytic theory has led us through a series of perfectly logical steps to a position which is, in essence, anachronistic: a scientific restatement of the Eve-out-of-Adam myth.

The Inductor Theory of Primary Sexual Differentiation

The most important contribution from modern comparative embryology to psychiatry is the elucidation of the process of primary sexual differentiation and its relationship to the evolution of the bearing of live young. While many psychiatrists may be familiar with this theory, others no doubt are not; and its fundamental facts have not been integrated into psychiatric theory. To begin this integration, the inductor theory is now presented in sufficient detail to support its conclusions and to advance certain theoretical possibilities related to psychosexual development. Strictly speaking, we can no longer refer to the "undifferentiated" or "bisexual" phase of initial embryonic existence. The early embryo is not undifferentiated: "it" is a female. In the beginning, we were all created females; and if this were not so, we would not be here at all.

Genetic sex is established at fertilization; but the influence of the sex genes is not brought to bear until the fifth to sixth week of fetal life (in humans). During those first weeks, all embryos are morphologically females. If the fetal gonads are removed before differentiation occurs the embryo will develop into a normal female, lacking only ovaries, regardless of the genetic sex.

If the genetic sex is male, the primordial germ cells arising in the endoderm of the yolk sac and hindgut migrate to the gonadal medulla (future testes) during the fifth week of embryonic life. Once there, they stimulate the production of a "testicular inductor substance" which stimulates medullary growth and the elaboration of fetal androgen which suppresses the growth of the Mullerian ducts (oviducts) and the gonadal cortex (ovaries); subsequently fetal androgen induces the rest of the internal and external genital tract into the male growth pattern. Externally this becomes barely evident by the seventh week or a little later. From the seventh to the twelfth week, the full transformation of the male structures is slowly accomplished. After the twelfth week, the masculine nature of the reproductive tract is fully established; sex reversals of these tissues are then no longer possible. (Suppression of growth and function can take place, of course, throughout life.) The time limits during which reversals can occur vary considerably in the different species relative to the life spans. Within each species, the critical period of sexual differentiation is remarkably constant in its time limits and remarkably sensitive to the exact quantity of the heterologous hormone required to effect reversal.

If the genetic sex is female, the germ cells arrive at the gonadal cortex (ovaries) and eventually stimulate the production of the primordial nest of cells and fetal estrogens. However, these estrogens are not necessary for the continued feminization of the reproductive tract. If the gonads are removed before the seventh week so that no estrogen is produced, the embryo will still develop normal female anatomy. No ovarian inductor substance or estrogens are elaborated because none are needed. Female differentiation results from the innate, genetically determined female morphology of all mammalian embryos.

That the circulating maternal estrogens do not cause female differentiation has been demonstrated by ingenious experiments in which embryonic reproductive tracts are entirely removed, kept alive *in vitro* sufficiently long for the critical period to be completed. The growth pattern in all embryos remains female. However, just as androgen is needed for the fullest elaboration of the male pattern, so estrogens are required for the full development of the female pattern. It is not known to what extent the circulating maternal estrogens are involved in this task of secondarily "exploiting" the female pattern. Fetal ovaries could well play an insignificant role, and maternal estrogens an important one, at least for some organs. For example, both male and female human neonates have enlarged breasts which subside to the infantile level by the second postnatal week—in both sexes, the breasts may even secrete a few drops of milk, i.e., "witch's milk." It would seem that the material estrogens strongly affect male and female embryos to fairly equal degrees.

Therefore only the male embryo is required to undergo a differentiating transformation of the sexual anatomy; and only one hormone, androgen, is necessary for the masculinization of the originally female genital tract. Female development is autonomous.

The original mammalian femaleness came about as a biological necessity and carries all the biological appropriateness so regularly seen in adaptive changes. Evolution is only "concerned" that a necessary and sufficient degree of sexual differentiation and distinction exists in each species to insure species survival. Which sex differentiates from which is immaterial.

With this understanding of evolutionary and embryological development, one conclusion must force itself upon psychiatric theory: *to reduce clitoral erotism to the level of psychopathology because the clitoris is an innately masculine organ or the original libido is masculine in nature must now be considered a travesty of the facts.*

W. D. SNODGRASS (1926–   )

"An Envoi, Post-TURP"

A poet, translator, and teacher, William Dewitt Snodgrass was born in Wilkinsburg, Pennsylvania, and was educated at Geneva College and the University of Iowa, where he received his Master of Fine Arts degree in 1953. His first book of poetry, *Heart's Needle* (1959), which explored the grief and guilt surrounding severed family ties, won the Pulitzer Prize. Since then, Snodgrass has established himself as one of the most important and versatile poets of his generation, publishing more than twenty collections of poetry, critical essays, and translations of works ranging from gallows ballads to troubadour poems. Among Snodgrass's influences were the works not only of poets—most importantly his teachers, Randall Jarrell and Robert Lowell—but also those of painters, especially Matisse, Vuillard, and van Gogh. Snodgrass's early experiences as a ward aide in a veterans' hospital brought him in close contact with the vulnerabilities of the male body, a subject he appraises with wit and stoic irony in "An Envoi, Post-TURP."

(After Trans-Urethral Resectioning of the Prostate,
men experience retrograde ejaculation,
the semen being passed later during urination.)

Farewell, children of my right hand and bliss.
You'll come no more but in bright streams of piss,
Never more turn my bedroom towels stiff,
Whitewash the walls or glisten on the quiff;
Never more swim like salmon or rough Norse
Invaders swarming upstream to the source.
Once, ovaries were ovaries; sperms, sperms.
In nine short months you brought us all to terms
When captive loins were sentenced by your court
To long years, lawyers' fees, and child support.
You cared for just one thing—aye, that's the rub:
Each of you, at your Health and Country Club
Timed training laps, did pushups by the pool
Shunning each voice that cried, "Back, back you fools,
We'll all be killed—it's a blow job!" You hurled
Yourselves, bluff hardy semen, on the world

Like Noah's load that crested with the Flood
To populate the land and stand at stud.
Ink of my pen, you words spent ἐν ἀρχῆ,
This writer, knowing all he's cast away,
Knowing your creamy genes and DNA
Encodes our texts, pirates, and then reprints us, says,
"Good night, bad cess to you, sweet prince and princesses."

PART 4

Psyche and Soma

"The Sacred Disease"

Although little clinical evidence was available in ancient times to link the brain with mental activity, fifth-century-B.C. Greek philosophers and physicians already had begun to regard the brain as the seat of thought, sensation, and emotion—a view that would soon come into conflict with the Aristotelian notion that the heart was the site of such processes. Holding to a secular model, Hippocrates argued that the disruption of motor activity and consciousness brought on by epilepsy was the result of some disturbance in the brain, rather than the effect of supernatural intervention. Corrupted humors, not vengeful gods, were the agencies responsible for the so-called "sacred" disease. Like all diseases, Hippocrates asserted, epilepsy has a particular *physis*, or nature, and as such it falls within the province of the physician, not the priest or magician. In all of the Hippocratic corpus, "The Sacred Disease" is the most thorough exposition of the abnormal as well as normal functioning of the brain as it was understood in the classical era. At the same time, it is also one of the first salvos in a series of boundary disputes embroiling diverse groups of practitioners eager to stake their claims in the coveted terra incognita of the brain.

AN ATTACK ON THE POPULAR SUPERSTITIONS ABOUT EPILEPSY, FOLLOWED BY AN ACCOUNT OF THE NATURAL HISTORY OF THE DISEASE

I do not believe that the 'Sacred Disease' is any more divine or sacred than any other disease but, on the contrary, has specific characteristics and a definite cause. Nevertheless, because it is completely different from other diseases, it has been regarded as a divine visitation by those who, being only human, view it with ignorance and astonishment. This theory of divine origin, though supported by the difficulty of understanding the malady, is weakened by the simplicity of the cure consisting merely of ritual purification and incantation. If remarkable features in a malady were evidence of divine visitation, then there would be many 'sacred diseases.' Quotidian, tertian and quartan fevers are among other diseases no less remarkable and portentous and yet no one regards them as having a divine origin. I do not believe that these diseases have any less claim to be caused by a god than the so-called 'sacred' disease but they are not the objects of popular wonder. Again, no less remarkably, I have seen men go mad and become delirious for no obvious reason and do many strange things. I have seen many cases of people groaning and shouting in their sleep, some who choke; others jump from their bed and run outside and remain out of their mind till they wake, when they are as healthy and sane as they were before, although

From *The Medical Works of Hippocrates,* trans. John Chadwick and W. N. Mann (Springfield, Ill.: Charles C. Thomas, 1950). Used by permission of Blackwell Scientific Publications Ltd.

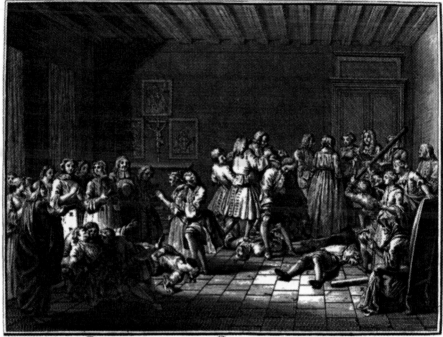

Différentes AGITATIONS *des* CONVULSIONAIRES.

12. Engraving of epileptics at the cemetery of Saint Medard, Paris, from Bernard Picart, Cérémonies Religieuses de tous les Peuples *(Paris: Rollins, 1741). Wellcome Institute Library, London. Despite attempts to secularize "the sacred disease," epilepsy continued to be understood as a species of demonic possession and madness. Picart's engraving shows patients being "treated" according to the therapeutic regimen of the day. Passive and prostrate, they are beaten and trampled under the supervision of religious authorities. The scene takes place at the cemetery of Saint Medard, Paris, where miraculous cures allegedly occurred by the tomb of François de Paris, propagator of the Jansenist doctrine. The two figures lying on the floor in the center and to the right (B and D) demonstrate the* arc de cercle *convulsion, while the man collapsing (figure A) on the left illustrates the first stages of an "attack."*

perhaps rather pale and weak. These things are not isolated events but frequent occurrences. There are many other remarkable afflictions of various sorts, but it would take too long to describe them in detail.

It is my opinion that those who first called this disease 'sacred' were the sort of people we now call witch-doctors, faith-healers, quacks and charlatans. These are exactly the people who pretend to be very pious and to be particularly wise. By invoking a divine element they were able to screen their own failure to give suitable treatment and so called this a 'sacred' malady to conceal their ignorance of its nature. By picking their phrases carefully, prescribing purifications and incantations along with abstinence from baths and from many foods unsuitable for the sick, they ensured that their therapeutic measures were safe for themselves.

It seems, then, that those who attempt to cure disease by this sort of treatment do not really consider the maladies thus treated of sacred or of divine origin. If the disease can be cured by purification and similar treatment then what is to prevent its being brought on by like devices? The man who can get rid of a disease by his magic could equally well bring it on; again there is nothing divine about this but a human element is involved. By such claims and trickery, these practitioners pretend a deeper knowledge than is given to others; with their prescriptions of 'sanctifications' and 'purifications,' their patter about divine visitation and possession by devils, they seek to deceive. And yet I believe that all these professions of piety are really more like impiety and a denial of the existence of the gods, and all their religion and talk of divine visitation is an impious fraud which I shall proceed to expose.

If these people claim to know how to draw down the moon, cause an eclipse of the sun, make storms and fine weather, rain and drought, to make the sea too rough for sailing or the land infertile, and all the rest of their nonsense, then, whether they claim to be able to do it by magic or by some other method, they seem to be impious rogues. Either they do not believe in the existence of the gods or they believe that the gods are powerless or would not refrain from the most dastardly acts. Surely conduct such as this must render them hateful to the gods. If a man were to draw down the moon or cause an eclipse of the sun, or make storms or fine weather by magic and sacrifices, I should not call any of these things a divine visitation but a human one, because the divine power had been overcome and forced into subjection by the human will. But perhaps these claims are not true and it is men in search of a living who invent all these fancy tales about this particular disease and all the others too. They make a different god responsible for each of the different forms of the complaint.

If the sufferer acts like a goat, and if he roars, or has convulsions involving the right side, they say the Mother of the Gods is responsible. If he utters a higher-pitched and louder cry, they say he is like a horse and blame Poseidon. If the sufferer should be incontinent of faeces, as sometimes happens under the stress of an attack, Enodia is the name. If the stools are more frequent and thin like those of kids, it is Apollo Nomius; if he foam at the mouth and kick out with his feet, Ares is to blame. If he suffers at night from fears and panic, from attacks of insanity, or if he jumps out of bed and runs outside, they talk of attacks of Hecate and the assaults of the heroes. In using purifications and spells they perform what I consider a most irreligious and impious act, for, in treating sufferers from this disease by purification with blood and like things, they behave as if the sufferers were ritually unclean, the victims of divine vengeance or of human magic or had done something sacrilegious. It would have been better if they had done the opposite and taken the sick into the temples, there, by sacrifice and prayer, to make supplication to the gods; instead they simply purify them and do none of these things. Charms are buried in the ground, thrown into the sea or carried off into the mountains where no one may touch them or tread on them. If a god really be responsible, surely these things should be taken into the temples as offerings.

Personally I believe that human bodies cannot be polluted by a god; the basest object by the most pure. But if the human body is polluted by some other agency or is harmed in some way, then the presence of a god would be more likely to purify and sanctify it than pollute it. It is the deity who purifies, sanctifies and cleanses us from the greatest and most unholy of our sins. We ourselves mark out the precincts of the temples of the gods so that no one should enter without purifying himself; as we go in, we sprinkle ourselves with holy water, not because we are thereby polluted, but to rid ourselves of any stain we may have contracted previously. This then is my opinion of the purifications.

I believe that this disease is not in the least more divine than any other but has the same nature as other diseases and a similar cause. Moreover, it can be cured no less than other diseases so long as it has not become inveterate and too powerful for the drugs which are given.

[T]he brain is the seat of this disease, as it is of other very violent diseases. I shall explain clearly the manner in which it comes about and the reason for it. It is through [the] blood-vessels that we respire, for they allow the body to breathe by absorbing air, and it is distributed throughout the body by means of the minor vessels. The air is cooled in the blood-vessels and then released. Air cannot remain still but must move; if it remains still and is left behind in some part of the body, then that part becomes powerless. A proof of this is that if we compress some of the smaller blood-vessels when we are lying or sitting down, so that air cannot pass through the vessels, then numbness occurs at once. Such, then, is the nature of blood-vessels.

Now this disease attacks the phlegmatic but not the bilious. Its inception is even while the child is still within its mother's womb, for the brain is rid of undesirable matter and brought to full development, like the other parts, before birth.

Should [the] routes for the passage of phlegm from the brain be blocked, the discharge enters the blood-vessels which I have described. This causes aphonia, choking, foaming at the mouth, clenching of the teeth and convulsive movements of the hands; the eyes are fixed, the patient becomes unconscious and, in some cases, passes a stool. . . . [T]he patient loses his voice and his wits. The hands become powerless and move convulsively for the blood can no longer maintain its customary flow. Divergence of the eyes takes place when the smaller blood-vessels supplying them are shut off and no longer provide an air supply; the vessels then pulsate. The froth which appears at the lips comes from the lungs for, when air no longer enters them, they produce froth which is expectorated as in the dying.

When the disease has been present from childhood, a habit develops of attacks occurring at any change of wind and specially when it is southerly. This is hard to cure because the brain has become more moist than normal and is flooded with phlegm. This renders discharges more frequent. The phlegm can no longer be completely separated out; neither can the brain, which remains wet and soaked, be dried up. This observation results specially from a study of animals, particularly of goats which are liable to this disease. Indeed, they are peculiarly susceptible to it. If you cut open the head you will find that the brain is wet, full of fluid and foul-smelling, convincing proof that disease and not the deity is harming the body. It is just the same with man, for when the malady becomes chronic, it becomes incurable.

Patients who suffer from this disease have a premonitory indication of an attack. In such circumstances they avoid company, going home if they are near enough, or to the loneliest spot they can find if they are not, so that as few people as possible will see them fall, and they at once wrap their heads up in their coats. This is the normal reaction to embarrassment and not, as most people suppose, from fear of the demon. Small children, from inexperience and being unaccustomed to the disease, at first fall down wherever they happen to be. Later, after a number of attacks, they run to their mothers or to someone whom they know well when they feel one coming on. This is through fear and fright at what they feel, for they have not yet learnt to feel ashamed.

The reasons for attacks occurring when there is a change of wind are, I believe, the following. Attacks are most likely to occur when the wind is southerly; less when it is northerly, less still when it is in any other quarter; for the South and North winds are the strongest of the winds and the most opposed in direction and in influence. The North wind precipitates the moisture in the air so that the cloudy and damp elements are separated out leaving the atmosphere clear and bright. It treats similarly all the other vapours which arise from the sea or from other stretches of water, distilling out from them the damp and dark elements. It does the same for human beings and it is therefore the healthiest wind. The South wind has just the opposite effect. . . . [S]outherly winds relax the brain and make it flabby, relaxing the blood-vessels at the same time. Northerly winds, on the other hand, solidify the healthy part of the brain while any morbid part is separated out and forms a fluid layer round the outside. Thus it is that discharges occur when the wind changes. It is seen, then, that this disease rises and flourishes according to changes we can see come and go. It is no more difficult to understand, nor is it any more divine than any other malady.

It ought to be generally known that the source of our pleasure, merriment, laughter and amusement, as of our grief, pain, anxiety and tears, is none other than the brain. It is specially the organ which enables us to think, see and hear, and to distinguish the ugly and the beautiful, the bad and the good, pleasant and unpleasant. Sometimes we judge according to convention; at other times according to the perceptions of expediency. It is the brain too which is the seat of madness and delirium, of the fears and frights which assail us, often by night, but sometimes even by day; it is there where lies the cause of insomnia and sleep-walking, of thoughts that will not come, forgotten duties and eccentricities. All such things result from an unhealthy condition of the brain; it may be warmer than it should be, or it may be colder, or moister or drier, or in any other abnormal state. Moistness is the cause of madness for when the brain is abnormally moist it is necessarily agitated and this agitation prevents sight or hearing being steady. Because of this, varying visual and acoustic sensations are produced, while the tongue can only describe things as they appear and sound. So long as the brain is still, a man is in his right mind.

The brain may be attacked both by phlegm and by bile and the two types of disorder which result may be distinguished thus: those whose madness results from phlegm are quiet and neither shout nor make a disturbance; those whose madness results from bile shout, play tricks and will not keep still but are always up to some mischief.

Warming of the brain also takes place when a plethora of blood finds its way to the brain and boils. It courses along the blood-vessels I have described in great quantity when a man is having a nightmare and is in a state of terror. He reacts in sleep in the same way that he would if he were awake; his face burns, his eyes are blood-shot as they are when scared or when the mind is intent upon the commission of a crime. All this ceases as soon as the man wakes and the blood is dispersed again into the blood vessels.

For these reasons I believe the brain to be the most potent organ in the body. So long as it is healthy, it is the interpreter which enables us to draw anything from the air. Consciousness is caused by air. The eyes, ears, tongue, hands and feet perform actions which are planned by the brain, for there is a measure of conscious thought throughout the body proportionate to the amount of air which it receives. The brain is also the organ of comprehension, for when a man draws in a breath it reaches the brain first, and thence is dispersed into the rest of the body having left behind in the brain its vigour and whatever pertains to consciousness and intelligence. If the air went first to the body and subsequently to the brain, the power of understanding would be left to the flesh and to the blood-vessels; it would only reach the brain hot and when it was no longer pure owing to admixture with fluid from the tissues and from the blood and this would blunt its keenness.

I therefore assert that the brain is the interpreter of comprehension. Accident and convention have falsely ascribed that function to the diaphragm which does not and could not possess it. I know of no way in which the diaphragm can think and be conscious, except that a sudden access of pleasure or of pain might make it jump and throb because it is so thin and is under greater tension than any other part of the body. Some say too that we think with our hearts and it is the heart which suffers pain and feels anxiety. There is no truth in this although it is convulsed as is the diaphragm and even more for the following reasons: blood-vessels from all parts of the body run to the heart and these connections ensure that it can feel if any pain or strain occurs in the body. Moreover, the body cannot help giving a shudder and a contraction when subjected to pain and the same effect is produced by an excess of joy, which heart and diaphragm feel most intensely. Neither of these organs takes any part in mental operations which are completely undertaken by the brain.

This so-called 'sacred disease' is due to the same causes as all other diseases, to the things we see come and go, the cold and the sun too, the changing and inconstant winds. These things are divine so that there is no need to regard this disease as more divine than any other; all are alike divine and all human. Each has its own nature and character and there is nothing in any disease which is unintelligible or which is insusceptible to treatment. The majority of maladies may be cured by the same things as caused them. One thing nourishes one thing, another another and sometimes destroys it too. The physician must know of these things in order to be able to recognize the opportune moment to nourish and increase one thing while robbing another of its sustenance and so destroy it.

A man with the knowledge of how to produce by means of a regimen dryness and moisture, cold and heat in the human body, could cure this disease too provided that he could distinguish the right moment for the application of the remedies. He would not need to resort to purifications and magic spells.

ST. AUGUSTINE (A.D. 354–430)

"The Creation of the Man's Soul"

Born in Tagaste, North Africa, Aurelius Augustinus was a philosopher, religious leader, and eventual saint who systematized the early teaching of
the Christian Church and assimilated classical traditions of thought to its
beliefs and doctrines. Augustine was converted to Christianity in 387, and
he was appointed Bishop of Hippo in 395 in an Empire coming apart at
the seams and a Church beset by heretics and schismatics. Principal among
these dangerous influences was the Manichean religion—a sect Augustine
had belonged to as a young man—whose adepts held that the power of evil
in the world was equal to that of good. *The Literal Meaning of Genesis* was,
in fact, first conceived by Augustine as a response to the Manichean claim
that Genesis misrepresented the nature of the created world. The problem
of explicating the creation narrative, however, would continue to haunt Augustine for the greater part of his adult life. Dissatisfied with his first two
works on the subject, he took it up yet a third time in 401, venturing on an
exhaustive twelve-book commentary on chapters 1 through 3 of Genesis—
little more than three hundred words—over the course of the next fourteen
years. Steeped in the intellectual traditions of classical learning, Augustine
brought to bear on the paradoxical nexus of body, mind, and soul the sum
of his knowledge of ancient philosophy, physics, natural history, medicine,
and psychology. Throughout his exegesis of Genesis, however, Augustine
made it eminently clear to his readers that the sacred text was to be taken
literally, not only as the epitome of the ultimate metaphysical questions of
human existence but as the report of historical fact, "a faithful record of
what happened" at the moment of Creation.

*The creation of the man's soul must now be considered
in the light of Gen. 2.7.*

*And God formed man of dust from the earth and breathed into his face the breath of
life; and man was made a living being.*

At the beginning of the preceding book I undertook to examine these words of Scripture; and I treated in a sufficiently thorough way, I believe, the creation of man, especially of his body, according to what seemed to me to be the meaning of Scripture.
But since it is no simple matter to understand the soul, I thought it wise to leave

From *St. Augustine: The Literal Meaning of Genesis,* Vol. 1, trans. and annot. John Hammond Tay-
lor, S.J. (New York and Ramsey, N.J.: Newman Press, 1982). Copyright 1982 by Rev. Johannes
Quasten and Rev. Walter J. Burghardt, S.J., and Thomas Comerford Lawler. Used by permission of
Paulist Press.

that question to this book, not knowing how much the Lord would help me in my desire to say the right thing. But I did know this much: that I was not going to say the right thing unless He helped me.

First, then, let us examine the statement in Scripture which says, *God breathed into his face the breath of life.*

We might say that the breath of God is not the soul of man but that God by breathing forth made the soul of man. But we must not think that the creatures He made by a word are better than what He made by a breath, in view of the fact that a word is better than a breath in us. Nevertheless, according to the account I have given above, there is no reason to hesitate to call the soul the breath of God, so long as we understand that it is not God's nature and substance, but simply that to breathe forth is to produce a breath, and that to produce a breath is to produce the soul.

Even one who holds that God is the world soul would not logically maintain that the breath of God is part of His substance.

If, then, we were to say that God is, so to speak, the soul of this corporeal world, and that the world itself is to Him a kind of body of one living being, we should not truly say that He made the soul of man by His breath, except in so far as we should speak of a material soul made from the surrounding air which, as part of His body, would be subject to Him. But what He would have given by breathing we should have to suppose He did not give from Himself but from the air subject to Him as part of His body, just as the soul produces breath not from itself but from something similarly subject to it, namely, its body.

When breathing the soul into Adam, did God create it out of nothing or form it from one previously created spiritual being?

What, then, are we to say about the creation of the soul?

We want to know whether God created from nothing the being which is called the soul and which before that moment was not existing, on the supposition that His breath would not come from some subordinate substance as is the case with the breath which the soul exhales from the body, as we have already pointed out. Was God's breath, then, quite simply made from nothing when it pleased Him to breathe forth and His breath became the soul of man? Or was there already existing some spiritual entity which, whatever its nature, was not yet soul, and from this entity was there made the breath of God, identified with the soul itself? There is a parallel with man's body, which was nonexistent before God formed it from the slime or dust of the earth. For dust or slime was not human flesh; nevertheless, it was something from which would be made a being which was not yet in existence.

Was there some previously created spiritual material for the soul as there was earth for the body?

Is it believable, then, that in the works of the first six days God created not only the causal reason of the future human body but also the material from which it would be made, namely, earth from whose slime or dust the body would be formed, whereas in the case of the soul He created only the causal reason according to which it would be made and not any kind of material *sui generis* from which it would be made?

For if the soul were something immutable, we should have no need to look for its own special kind of matter; however, its mutability shows it sometimes deformed by vice and deception and formed by virtue and true doctrine, its nature as soul meanwhile remaining, just as the flesh remains by nature flesh though it is glowing with health or disfigured by disease or wounds. But the flesh, before becoming flesh and having its natural beauty or deformity, also had the material, namely, earth, from which it was made into flesh. Perhaps, then, the soul, before it was made into the nature of soul, whose beauty is virtue and whose deformity is vice, could have had its own kind of spiritual material which was not yet soul, just as the earth from which the flesh was made was already something, although it was not flesh.

Difficulties connected with supposing that there was a spiritual material out of which the soul was made.

If there was any such thing as a spiritual material from which the soul was made, or if there is any such thing from which souls are now made, what precisely is it? What is its name, what is its form, what use does it have in the works of creation? Is it living or nonliving? If it lives, what does it do? What does it produce in the world? Does it live a happy life or a wretched life or neither? Does it give life to anything? Or is it without this function also, and does it rest quietly in some inmost recess of the universe without active perception and vital motion? For if there was no life whatsoever in it, how could it be some sort of incorporeal, nonliving material for life yet to come? The supposition, then, is false, or this is a mystery beyond our comprehension.

Difficulties in assuming an irrational soul as the material. Transmigration rejected.

But if an irrational soul is somehow the material from which the rational (namely, human) soul is made, again a question arises about the source from which this irrational soul comes. For it too can be made only by the Creator of all beings.

Was it made from corporeal matter? If so, why can we not say the same about the rational soul? Surely, if it is granted that a certain effect can be produced step by step, no one will deny that God can accomplish the same result even if He abridges the process. Consequently, whatever the intermediate steps, if a body is the material of an irrational soul, and the irrational soul is the material of the rational soul, there is no doubt that the body is the material of the rational soul. But I know of no one who has ever ventured such an opinion except a person who holds that the soul itself is nothing but a kind of body.

The human soul was not made of anything corporeal, not even of air or heavenly fire.

What, then, is the material out of which the soul was made by the breath of God? Was it a body of an earthly and humid nature? By no means! From these elements the flesh was made. For what else is slime than humid earth? And we must not suppose that the soul was made from moisture alone, as if the flesh was from earth and the soul from water. For it is utterly absurd to think that the soul of man was made of material from which the flesh of fish and birds was made.

Was the human soul, then, made out of air? For the breath belongs to this element— but our breath, not God's. Hence, I said above that this identification could be considered appropriate if we believed that God was the soul of the world (the world being considered as one large living being), so that He would have breathed the soul forth from the air of His body, just as our soul breathes its breath forth from the air of its body. But since it is clear that God is infinitely above every bodily creature in the world and above every spirit which He created, how can this explanation be seriously proposed?

Should we say that the more God is present to the whole of His creation by His unparalleled almighty power, the more He would have been able to make from air the breath which would be the soul of man? But the soul is not corporeal, and whatever comes from the corporeal elements of the world must necessarily be corporeal. Now, among the elements of the world we must include air; but even if the soul were said to have been made from the element of pure and heavenly fire, we ought not to believe it. There have been philosophers who maintained that all bodies are capable of being transformed into all other bodies. But that any body, earthly or heavenly, is changed into soul and becomes an incorporeal being is not to my knowledge held by anyone and is not part of our faith.

In the body the elements of fire and air, in addition to earth, are present according to the medical writers.

We should perhaps give some consideration to what the medical writers not only assert but also maintain that they can prove. They say that although all bodies obviously have the solidity proper to the element of earth, nevertheless they have in them also some air, which is in the lungs and is distributed from the heart through the veins, which they call arteries. Furthermore, as these writers have shown, bodies also have the warm quality of fire, which is situated in the liver, and its bright quality, which is made to flow and rise up to the highest place, namely, the brain, which is, as it were, the heaven of the body.

From this source come the rays which go forth out of the eyes, and from this center slender ducts go out not only to the eyes but also to the other senses, namely, to the ears, the nose, and the palate, making the sensations of hearing, smelling, and tasting possible. Moreover, they say that the sense of touch, which is all over the body, is directed from the brain also through the medulla of the neck and that of the bones to which the backbone is connected, and that from there tiny channels making sensation possible are spread throughout all parts of the body.

What the soul perceives by the intellect is far superior to what it perceives by the senses.

It is by these messengers, therefore, that the soul perceives whatever comes to its notice in the world of bodies. But the soul itself is of a quite different nature, so that when it wishes to understand the divine or God, or simply to understand itself and consider its own virtues, it turns away from this light of the eyes in order to have true and certain knowledge, and recognizing that this light is no help for its purpose, in fact is even something of an obstacle, it raises itself up to the vision of the mind. How could it belong to that lower order of being, since the summit of that order is merely the light that shines from the eyes, which is no help to the soul except for the perception of bodily forms and colors? The soul itself has innumerable objects utterly unlike every kind of body, and it sees these objects only with intellect and reason, a realm beyond the reach of the senses of the body.

The soul governs the body by means of light and air.

Hence, the human soul is not made of earth or of water or of air or of fire; but it is through the more subtle elements, namely, light and air, that it governs its material and grosser body, that is, moist earth which has been made into flesh. For without the two subtle elements there is no sensation in the body or any spontaneous bodily movement under the direction of the soul. And just as knowing must come before making, so sensing must come before moving. Since the soul, therefore, is incorporeal, it first acts upon a body which is akin to the incorporeal, that is, fire, or rather light and air; then through these it acts upon the grosser elements of the body, such as moisture and earth, which form the solid mass of the body and are more disposed to be acted upon than to act.

Bodily disorders which impair the activity of the soul in the body and eventually cause death.

In seeking for the source of the soul, that is, the quasi material out of which God made this breath which is called the soul, no corporeal material should be considered. As God by the excellence of His nature surpasses every creature, so does the soul surpass every corporeal creature. But light and air are bodies of a superior nature in this corporeal world, having a superiority in so far as they are more active than passive as contrasted with water and earth. The soul, therefore, governs the body by means of the two elements that have a kind of resemblance to the spirit.

Corporeal light, for example, announces something, and it announces it not to a being that is of the same nature as itself: it makes the announcement to the soul, but the light making the announcement is not soul. And when the soul is distressed because of a bodily affliction, it is discovered that its activity of ruling the body is impeded by reason of a rupture of the balance in the system, and this affliction is called pain. Moreover, the air which is diffused throughout the nerves obeys the will so as to move the members, but the air itself is not the will. Furthermore, the central part of the brain signals the motions in the body, which the memory is to retain, but it is not the memory. Finally, when these functions fail completely because of some affliction or disturbance, the messengers of sensation and the agents of motion cease to operate; and the soul, which seems to have no further reason for remaining, departs. But if they do not fail as completely as happens in death, the soul's attention is disturbed and it is like a man who tries unsuccessfully to put back things that keep falling. In this case, from the nature of the disturbance the physicians can know what part or the system is causing the dysfunction, so that, if possible, a remedy may be applied.

The soul is distinct from the organs of the body.

We must distinguish the soul itself from its corporeal agents, whether vessels or organs or whatever else they may be called. The difference is evident from the fact that the soul is frequently concentrated in thought and turns itself away from everything, so that it is ignorant of many things which are present before the eyes when they are wide open and able to see.

There are corporeal particles of the corporeal heaven, that is, particles of light and air, which are the first to receive the commands of the soul which vivifies the body because they are closer to an incorporeal substance than water and earth are. The soul, then, uses these finer elements in administering the mass of the body. Now, it is not clear whether God took the elements of light and air from the heavens which were round the earth and over it and mingled or joined them with the body of the living man, or whether He made them as He did flesh from the slime of the earth; but this question is not relevant to our enquiry. For it is believable that every bodily substance can be changed into every other bodily substance, but to believe that any bodily substance can be changed into soul is absurd.

The soul is incorporeal.

Therefore, no attention should be paid to the opinion of those who have said that the soul is from a fifth corporeal element, not earth or water or air or fire (whether earthly fire familiar to us, which is always in motion, or heavenly fire, which is pure and bright), but some other kind of being, without any established name, which is a body.

The soul does not think of itself in this manner, for it cannot be ignorant of itself even when it is seeking to know itself. For when it seeks itself, it knows that it seeks itself, a fact it would not know unless it knew itself. For the source in which it seeks itself is itself. When, therefore, it knows itself as seeking, it certainly knows itself. Now, in its entire being it knows all that it knows; and therefore, when it knows itself as seeking, in its entire being it knows itself; and therefore it knows itself entirely. For it is not something else but itself that it knows in its entire being.

My way of putting it is this: whatever the soul is, it is not one of the four familiar elements, which are obviously bodies; and on the other hand, it is not identified with God. The best words to designate it are "soul" or "life-spirit." I add the word "life" because the air is also usually called "spirit." However, men have called this same air "soul" (*anima*), so that it is impossible to find a word by which we can precisely distinguish this thing which is not a body, nor God, nor life without sensation (which apparently exists in trees), nor life without a rational mind (such as is found in beasts), but a life now inferior to that of the angels, but destined to be one with their life if in this world it lives according to the will of its Creator.

What, then, is the origin of the soul, that is, from what material was it made (if I may use the expression)? Or from what perfect and blessed substance did it emanate? Or was it simply made from nothing? Although we may have doubts about this problem and continue to search for a solution, there should be absolutely no doubt about the following: if it was something else before it became a soul, whatever it was, it was made by God; and in its present state it has been made by God to be a living soul. For either it was nothing or it was something other than what it now is.

MICHEL DE MONTAIGNE (1533–1592)

"On the Power of the Imagination"

Coming from a family of wine merchants in Bordeaux, Michel de Montaigne was sent to the prestigious Collège de Guienne at the age of six, having already mastered classical Latin. After graduating from Guienne, Montaigne took up the study of law, and in 1557 he became a member of the Bordeaux parliament, where he served for thirteen years in the midst of the great civil and religious strife stirred by Huguenot claims for freedom of conscience and worship. A supporter of the established order, Montaigne ardently sought the favor of the king, and when his efforts failed to secure him promotion, he resigned his office and retired to his "ancestral abode and sweet retreat," the Château at Montaigne. Here, between 1571 and 1580, he wrote a series of inquiries, or "essays"—a form he invented—expressing and exploring his attitudes and opinions on a vast range of social, political, and psychological topics. A year later, while traveling in Italy, Montaigne was elected mayor of Bordeaux at a time when plague and war were ravaging the area. By 1588, he had completed the third volume of his *Essais,* and to oversee its printing he returned to Paris, where he was welcomed at court by Henry of Navarre, now officially king of France in the wake of Henry III's assassination. A long-standing supporter of Navarre, Montaigne was asked to reside at court as his counselor, but this was not to be, for Montaigne died before the new king had moved his retinue to the capital. A selection from Montaigne's *Essais,* "On the Power of the Imagination" anticipates the intellectual agenda of the Enlightenment by naturalizing physical symptoms and responses commonly held to be of supernatural origin. In a series of vignettes or "case studies," Montaigne invokes the powerful influence of mind on body, rather than the sinister operations of witches and demons, to explain such phenomena as impotence, psychosomatic illness, and what today is called the "placebo effect."

"Fortis imaginatio generat casum," "a strong imagination begets the event," say the scholars. I am one of those who are very susceptible to the influence of imagination. Everyone feels its impact, but some are toppled over by it. Its impression on me is intense. My practice is to evade it rather than to resist it. I wish I could live in the company only of healthy and cheerful persons. The sight of another's anguish produces a real anguish in me, and my own sensations have often taken on the sensations of a third person. A perpetual cough in another irritates my lungs and throat. I more unwillingly visit the sick to whom I am bound by duty, than those who have less call upon me and about whom I am less concerned. I catch the disease I am

From *The Essays of Michel de Montaigne,* ed. and trans. Jacob Zeitlin (New York: Alfred A. Knopf, 1934).

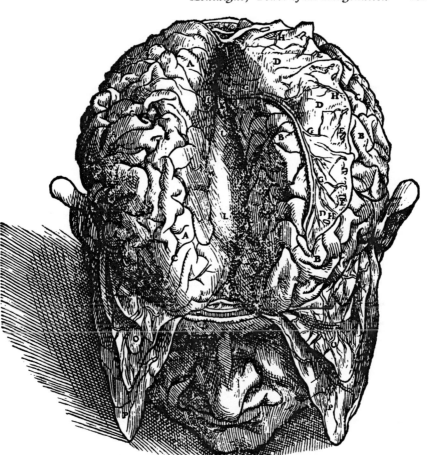

13. Woodcut of the brain from Andreas Vesalius, Suorum de Humani Corporis Fabrica Librorum Epitome *(Basle: Johannes Oporinus, 1543). Wellcome Institute Library, London. Vesalius starkly confronts us with the organ Hippocrates described as "the source of our pleasure, merriment, laughter, and amusement, as of our grief, pain, anxiety, and tears." In this dramatically foreshortened presentation of the brain, the viewer is compelled to gaze into its very core. Both the thin and dural membranes have been peeled off, revealing an intricate labyrinth of folds. The grave and bowed face of the figure, however, demands not only an act of physical inspection but also one of inner contemplation.*

contemplating and lodge it within myself. I am not surprised that the imagination should induce fevers and death in those who give it free rein and encourage it. Simon Thomas was a great physician of his time. I remember meeting him one day at the house of a rich old man who was troubled with weak lungs, and, discussing with the patient the means of curing him, he told him that one way would be to make me like his company, so that by fixing his eyes upon the freshness of my complexion, and his thoughts upon the sprightliness and vigour that exhaled from my youth, and by filling all his senses with the flourishing state I was in, his own condition might be amended. But he forgot to say that mine, at the same time, might be made worse.

Gallus Vibius strained his mind so much to grasp the nature and the motions of madness that he dragged his judgment from its seat and was never after able to put it back; he might boast of having become mad through wisdom. Some there are who through fear anticipate the hand of the hangman. And there was the man who, when his eyes were unbound to have his pardon read to him, was found stark dead upon the scaffold, killed only by the stroke of his imagination. We sweat copiously, we tremble, we turn pale and we blush under the thrusts of our imagination, and, plunged in our feather-beds, we feel our bodies agitated by its impulse, sometimes to the point of expiring. And boiling youth, when fast asleep, grows so warm with fancy as in a dream to satisfy its amorous desires:

> So that, as it were
> With all the matter acted duly out,
> They pour the billows of a potent stream
> And stain their garment.

Passing through Vitry le François, I might have seen a man to whom the Bishop of Soissons had given the name Germain at confirmation, and whom all the inhabits of the place had known and seen as a girl, called Marie till the age of twenty-two. He was now old, with a full beard, and not married. He says that straining himself while making a leap, his male member came forth; and there is still current among the girls of that place a song wherein they warn each other not to take too great strides for fear of turning into boys, like Marie Germain. It is no wonder if this sort of accident is frequently met with, for if the imagination has any power in such things, it is so continually and vigorously bent upon this subject that to keep it from so often relapsing into the same thought and sharpness of desire, it does better to incorporate this virile part in girls once for all.

It is probable that miracles, visions, enchantments, and the like extraordinary occurrences derive their credit principally from the power of imagination acting chiefly on the minds of the common people, which are more impressionable. Their belief has been so strongly seized that they think they see what they do not see. I am also of the opinion that those comic impediments, by which our society is so fettered that nothing else is talked about, are most likely the impressions of apprehension and fear. For I am personally acquainted with the case of a man for whom I can answer as for myself, on whom there could not fall the least suspicion of impotence, and as little of being under a spell, who, having heard a companion of his tell a story of an extraordinary loss of manhood that surprised him at a very inconvenient moment, and finding himself in a similar situation, his imagination all at once was struck so rudely by the horror of this story, that he suffered a similar fate; and from that time forward, the wretched remembrance of this misadventure so devoured and tyrannized over him that he was subject to relapse into it. He found some remedy for this fancy in another fancy: by himself confessing and declaring beforehand the weakness to which he was subject, the tension of his mind was relieved, in that, having raised an expectation of this mishap, his responsibility for it diminished and weighed less heavily upon him. When he had an opportunity of his own choosing (his thoughts being disengaged and free and his body in its normal state) to have it then first tried, seized, and taken by surprise, with the knowledge of the other party, he was completely cured of this infirmity. When a man has once been capable with a certain woman, he is with her never afterwards incapable, unless it be from real impotence.

This mischance is only to be feared in enterprises where our mind is immoderately tense with desire and respect, and especially where the opportunity is unforeseen and urgent; there is no way of recovering from this trouble. I know one who found it helpful to bring to it a body that had already begun to be sated elsewhere, in order to allay the ardour of this fury, and another who by reason of old age finds himself less impotent through being less potent. And I know a certain other who also found it helpful to be assured by a friend of his that he was supplied with a counter-battery of enchantments that was certain to save him. It is better for me to tell how this happened.

A count of very good family, with whom I was closely intimate, married a beautiful lady who had been courted by one who was present at the wedding feast. His friends were greatly distressed for him, and particularly an old lady, his kinswoman, who had the ordering of the nuptials and in whose house they were solemnized. She was very fearful of these sorceries and communicated her fears to me. I bade her rely upon me. I had by chance in my coffers a certain little flat piece of gold on which were engraved some celestial figures, good against sunstroke and for the relief of headache, if placed exactly upon the suture of the skull; and to hold it in its position it was sewed to a ribbon that could be tied under the chin. A fantastic notion, akin to the one of which we are speaking. Jacques Peletier had made me a present of this singular article. It occurred to me to make some use of it. So I said to the count that he might possibly suffer the same fate as others, there being men present who would be glad to play him a trick, but that he might go boldly to bed, for I would do him a friendly turn and would not, in his need, spare a miracle which it was in my power to perform, provided that he promised me, on his honour, to hold it a most faithful secret; he was only to give me a certain signal, when they came during the night to bring him his refreshment, if matters had not gone well with him. He had had his mind and his ears so battered, that he really found himself fettered with the trouble of his imagination, and at the time appointed gave me his signal. Thereupon I told him to rise under pretence of chasing us out of the room and to pull my night-robe from my shoulders as if in play (we were of much the same height) and wear it till he had carried out my instructions, which were, that when we were gone out of the chamber, he should withdraw to make water, should three times repeat certain prayers and go through certain motions, that each of the three times he should tie the ribbon I was putting into his hands about his middle, and place the medal that was fastened to it very carefully upon his kidneys with the figure in a particular position; this being done, and the ribbon so firmly tied that it could neither untie nor slip from its place, he might confidently return to his business, not forgetting to spread my robe over the bed so as to be sure to cover them both. These ape's tricks are the main part of the effect, our mind being unable to free itself from the thought that practices so strange must be based on some secret knowledge. Their inanity gives them weight and respect. In short, it is certain that my talisman proved itself more Venerian than Solar, more active than preventive. It was a sudden and curious whimsey that made me do a thing so alien to my nature. I am an enemy to all sudden and dissimulating actions and hate trickery, not only when it is in sport, but also when it is for some advantage. If the action is not wicked, the road to it is. Such as know their members to be naturally obedient, let them take care only to outwit their fancies.

Men have cause to remark the indocile liberty of this member, intruding so troublesomely when we have no need of it and failing us so troublesomely when we have most need of it, and so imperiously contesting in authority with our will and with so much haughtiness and obstinacy denying all solicitation both of mind and of hand. And yet if, on this accusation of rebelliousness and his condemnation on that account, this member had paid me to plead his cause, I should doubtless place our other members, his companions, under suspicion of having framed this fictitious charge against him out of pure envy at the importance and pleasure proper to his employment, and of having by a conspiracy armed the whole world against him by malevolently charging him alone with their common offence. For I ask you to consider if there is a single part of our bodies that does not often refuse its function in obedience to our will, and that does not often exercise it in opposition to our will. They have every one of them passions of their own that rouse them and put them to sleep without our leave. How often do the involuntary motions of the countenance discover the thoughts that we hold secret and betray us to the bystanders! The same cause that animates this member also animates, without our knowledge, the heart, the pulse, and the lungs, the sight of a pleasing object imperceptibly diffusing within us the flame of a feverish emotion.

Is there nothing but these veins and muscles that swell and subside without the consent, not only of our will, but even of our thoughts? We do not command our hairs to stand on end, nor our skin to quiver with desire or fear. The hand often moves where we do not send it. The tongue is paralyzed and the voice congealed in its own time. Even when, having nothing to put in the pot, we should like to restrain it, the appetite for food and drink does not cease to stir up the parts that are subject to it, neither more nor less than that other appetite, and in like manner it deserts us as unseasonably if it thinks fit. The vessels that serve to discharge the bowels have their own proper dilations and compressions, beyond and against our wishes, as well as those which are meant to purge the kidneys. And when, to vindicate the supremacy of the will, Saint Augustine alleges that he had known a man who could command his rear to break wind as often as he pleased, and when his commentator, Vives, improves upon it with another example of his own time, of a man that could break wind in harmony with the movement of any verses that were read, we are not to infer an absolute obedience in that organ; for is there any commonly more indiscreet or mutinous? To which let me add that I myself know one so turbulent and unruly that for forty years it has made its master vent with a continued and unintermitted compulsion, and so is bringing him to the grave.

But let us take our will, in whose behalf we prefer this accusation. With how much greater probability may we charge her with mutiny and sedition for her disorderliness and disobedience? Does she always will what we would have her to will? Does she not often will what we forbid her to will, and that to our manifest prejudice? Does she suffer herself more than the rest to be directed by the conclusions of our reason? In short, I should move, in behalf of Monsieur my client, that it please you to consider that in this matter, his cause being inseparably and indistinguishably conjoined with an accomplice, it is nevertheless he alone that is called in question, and that by arguments and accusations which, in view of the conditions of the parties, can in no wise pertain to or concern the said accomplice. Thus is the malice and injustice of his accusers manifestly apparent. But be it as it may, while protesting that advocates and judges wrangle and pass sentence to no purpose, Nature will in the meantime go her own way.

It is for this reason that in such cases one usually requires a mind that is prepared. Why do physicians work in advance upon the credulity of their patients with so many false promises of a cure, if not to enlist the imagination to mask the fraudulence of their potions? They know that one of the masters of their craft has handed down in writing that there are men on whom the mere sight of physic does the work.

And this whole whimsey has just come into my head through the remembrance of a story that was told me by an apothecary of my late father's, a simple man and a Swiss—a people not much addicted to vanity and lying—of a merchant he had long known at Toulouse, sickly and subject to the stone, who often made use of enemas; of these he had several sorts prescribed to him by the physicians according to the circumstances of his disease. When they were brought to him, none of the usual formalities were omitted; often he felt them to see if they were too hot. Behold him then lying upside down, with all the motions gone through, except that no injection was made! The apothecary having withdrawn after the ceremonial and the patient being accommodated as if he had really received an enema, he felt the same result as those do who have taken one. And if the physician did not find its effect sufficient, he would give him two or three more doses in the same manner. My informant swears that to save the expense (for he paid for them as if he had really taken them), the sick man's wife sometimes tried to make use of warm water only, but the result revealed the fraud, and this means having been found useless, it was necessary to return to the first method.

A woman, fancying she had swallowed a pin in a piece of bread, cried and suffered throes as though she had an intolerable pain in her throat, where she thought she felt it sticking; but an ingenious fellow, seeing there was no outward swelling or alteration and judging it to be only a notion or fancy caused by a crust of bread that had pricked her as it went down, made her vomit and by stealth threw a crooked pin into the basin. The women, believing she had thrown it up, immediately found herself eased of her pain. I know a gentleman who, having entertained a large company at his house, three or four days later bragged in jest (for there was nothing in it) that he had made them eat of a cat in a pastry, at which a gentlewoman of the party took such a horror, that she fell into a violent looseness of the bowels and fever, and it was impossible to save her. Even brute beasts are subject like ourselves to the force of imagination. Witness dogs, who die of grief for the loss of their masters. We also see them bark and tremble in their dreams, and horses whinny and kick.

But all this may be attributed to the close affinity between the soul and the body mingling their fortunes. It is another thing when the imagination works, as it sometimes does, not only upon one's own body, but upon that of another.

Magicians are no very good authority with me. Yet we see by experience that women impart the marks of their fancy to the bodies of children they carried in the womb; witness her that was brought to bed of a blackamoor. And there was presented to Charles, King of Bohemia and Emperor, a girl from near Pisa, all rough and hairy, whom her mother said to be so conceived by reason of a picture of Saint John the Baptist hanging in her bed. It is the same with animals, witness Jacob's sheep, and the hares and partridges that the snow turns white upon the mountains. There was seen recently at my house a cat watching a bird on the top of a tree, and the two for some time having fixed their eyes closely upon one another, the bird let herself drop as if dead into the cat's claws, being either dazed by its own imagination or drawn by some power of attraction in the cat. Those who like fowling have heard the story of the falconer who, having intently fixed his eyes upon a kite in the air, laid a wager that he would bring her down with the sole power of his sight, and did so, according to the story. The tales which I borrow I charge upon the consciences of those from whom I have them. The reflections are my own and depend upon the proofs of reason, not of experience; every one may adduce his own examples, and if he has none, let him not cease to believe that such exist, seeing the number and variety of occurrences is so great. If I do not apply my examples well, let another apply them for me.

ROBERT BURTON (1577–1640)

The Anatomy of Melancholy

Born on his father's estate in Leicestershire, England, Robert Burton entered Oxford at the age of sixteen, earning his Bachelor of Divinity in 1614. Two years later, he was appointed Vicar of St. Thomas, a parish in the suburbs of Oxford, where he undertook the writing of *The Anatomy of Melancholy, What it is. With all the Kindes, Causes, Symptoms, Prognostickes and severall Cures of it.* Published in 1621, *The Anatomy* went through seven editions in the next fifty years, becoming the most widely read work of its kind in England. Encyclopedic in its breadth of knowledge, *The Anatomy* surveys the views of both ancient and contemporary writers on a bewildering array of topics, ranging over sorcery, suicide, proper diet, demonic possession, the pleasures of hunting and traveling, lovesickness, jealousy, and the hard lot of scholars. In his preface to the book, Burton defends his right to take up the subject of melancholy, arguing that clergymen can speak of it with as much authority as can physicians, since it is an affliction of the soul as well as of the body. No one individual or group, Burton asserts, can claim to have divined its true causes or operations, for "the Tower of Babel never yielded such confusion of tongues as this Chaos of Melancholy doth of Symptoms." Whether the disorder could be brought on by demons was a matter of serious debate at the time, and in his efforts to elucidate such "mysteries," Burton compiled several reports that testified to the devil's power to induce fits of melancholy and to work extraordinary changes on the body and the mind.

[The Devil] can work both upon body and mind. Tertullian is of this opinion, that he can cause both sickness and health, and that secretly. Taurellus adds, by clancular poisons he can infect the bodies, & hinder the operations of the bowels, though we perceive it not, closely creeping into them, saith Lipsius, & so crucify our souls, and drive people mad by grievous melancholy. For being a spiritual body, he struggles with our spirits, saith Rogers, and suggests (according to Cardan), words without a voice, apparitions without sight, envy, lust, anger, &c., as he sees men inclined.

The manner how he performs it, Biarmannus, in his Oration against Bodine, sufficiently declares. *He begins first with the phantasy, & moves that so strongly, that no reason is able to resist.* Now he moves the *phantasy* by mediation of humours; although many Physicians are of the opinion, that the Devil can alter the mind, and produce this disease of himself. Of the same mind is Psellus, & Rhasis the Arab, *that this disease proceeds especially from the Devil, & from him alone.* Arculanus, Aelianus Montaltus, Daniel Sennertus, confirm as much, that the Devil can cause

From *The Anatomy of Melancholy,* ed. Floyd Dell and Paul Jordan-Smith (New York: Tudor Publishing Co., 1927).

this disease; by reason many times that the parties affected prophesy, speak strange language, but not without the humour, as he interprets himself; no more doth Avicenna, if contaminated by a daemon it is enough for us that it tends the whole system towards black bile; the immediate cause is choler adust, which Pomponatius likewise labours to make good: Galgerandus of Mantua, a famous Physician, so cured a daemoniacal woman in his time, that spake all languages, by purging black choler; and thereupon belike this humour of Melancholy is called the Devil's Bath; the Devil, spying his opportunity of such humours, drives them many times to despair, fury, rage, &c., mingling himself amongst these humours. This is that which Tertullian avers, they inflict shrewd and sudden turns on body and mind, and distort limbs, making their attack by stealth, &c., and which Lemnius goes about to prove, the bad Genii mix themselves with depraved humours and black bile, &c., and Jason Pratensis, *that the Devil, being a slender incomprehensible spirit, can easily insinuate and wind himself into human bodies, and cunningly couched in our bowels, vitiate our healths, terrify our souls with fearful dreams, and shake our mind with furies.* And in another place, *These unclean spirits settled in our bodies, and now mixed with our melancholy humours, do triumph as it were, and sport themselves as in another heaven.* Thus he argues, and that they go in and out of our bodies, as bees do in a hive, and so provoke and tempt us, as they perceive our temperature inclined of itself, and most apt to be deluded. Agrippa and Lavater are persuaded, that this humour invites the Devil to it, wheresoever it is in extremity, and, of all other, melancholy persons are most subject to diabolical temptations and illusions, and most apt to entertain them, and the Devil best able to work upon them; but whether by obsession, or possession, or otherwise, I will not determine; 'tis a difficult question. Delrio the Jesuit, Springer and his colleague, Thyreus the Jesuit, Hieronymus Mengus, and others of that rank of pontifical writers, it seems, by their exorcisms and conjurations approve of it, having forged many stories to that purpose. A nun did eat a lettuce *without grace, or without signing with the sign of the cross,* and was instantly possessed. Durand relates that he saw a wench possessed in Bononia with two devils, by eating an unhallowed pomegranate, as she did afterwards confess, when she was cured by exorcisms. And therefore our papists do sign themselves so often with the sign of the cross, that the daemon dare not enter, and exorcise all manner of meats, as being unclean or accursed otherwise, as Bellarmine defends. Many such stories I find amongst pontifical writers, to prove their assertions; let them free their own credits; some few I will recite in this kind out of most approved Physicians. Cornelius Gemma relates of a young maid, called Katherine Gualter, a cooper's daughter, in the year 1571, that had such strange passions and convulsions, three men could not sometimes hold her; she purged a live eel, which he saw, a foot and a half long, and touched himself, but the eel afterwards vanished; she vomited some 24 pounds of fulsome stuff of all colours twice a day for 14 days; and after that she voided great balls of hair, pieces of wood, pigeons' dung, parchment, goose dung, coals; and after them two pounds of pure blood, and then again coals and stones, of which some had inscriptions, bigger than a walnut, some of them pieces of glass, brass, &c. besides paroxysms of laughing, weeping and ecstasies, &c. And this (he says), I saw with horror. They could do no good on her by physick, but left her to the Clergy. Marcellus Donatus hath such another story of a country fellow, that had four knives in his belly, indented like a saw, every one a span long, with a wreath of hair like a globe, with much baggage of like sort, wonderful to behold. How it should come into his guts, he concludes, could only have been through the artifice and craft of a daemon. Langius hath many relations to this effect, and so hath Christopherus à Vega. Wierus, Sckenkius, Scribonius, all agree that they are done by the subtility and illusion of the Devil. If you shall ask a reason of this, 'tis to exercise our patience; for, as Tertullian holds, virtue is not virtue unless it has a foe by the conquering of which it shows its merit; 'tis to try us and our faith, 'tis for our offences, and for the punishment of our sins, by God's permission they do it, executioners of his will, as Tolosanus styles them; or rather as David, He cast upon them the fierceness of his anger, indignation, wrath, and vexation, by sending out of evil Angels. So did he afflict Job, Saul, the lunaticks and daemoniacal persons whom Christ cured. This, I say, happeneth for a punishment of sin, for their want of faith, incredulity, weakness, distrust, &c.

WILLIAM WORDSWORTH (1770–1850)

"Goody Blake and Harry Gill: A True Story"

An English Romantic poet raised in Cumberland and educated at Cambridge, William Wordsworth overturned the poetic conventions of the Augustan period by performing what he called "the experiment" of composing poetry based on the idioms of common speech. His extended autobiographical poem, *The Prelude,* traces his psychological, moral, and intellectual development as it was shaped by his childhood experiences of nature and by his entry into the social and political life of his day, primarily through the events and repercussions of the French Revolution. In 1798, Wordsworth published his first important collection of poems, *Lyrical Ballads,* which included several proto–case histories of men, women, and children from his native region. One of these ballads, "Goody Blake and Harry Gill," was based on a case of *mania mutabilis* in Erasmus Darwin's medical textbook, *Zoonomia.* As Wordsworth told his readers in a note to the poem, he recorded the incident in verse "to draw attention to the truth that the power of the human imagination is sufficient to produce changes even in our physical nature as might appear miraculous."

Oh ! what's the matter? what's the matter?
What is't that ails young Harry Gill?
That evermore his teeth they chatter,
Chatter, chatter, chatter still!
Of waistcoats Harry has no lack,
Good duffle grey, and flannel fine;
He has a blanket on his back,
And coats enough to smother nine.

In March, December, and in July,
'Tis all the same with Harry Gill;
The neighbours tell, and tell you truly,
His teeth they chatter, chatter still.
At night, at morning, and at noon,
'Tis all the same with Harry Gill;
Beneath the sun, beneath the moon,
His teeth they chatter, chatter still!

From *The Complete Poetical Works of Wordsworth* (Cambridge, Mass.: The Riverside Press, 1932).

Young Harry was a lusty drover,
And who so stout of limb as he?
His cheeks were red as ruddy clover;
His voice was like the voice of three.
Old Goody Blake was old and poor;
Ill fed she was, and thinly clad;
And any man who passed her door
Might see how poor a hut she had.

All day she spun in her poor dwelling:
And then her three hours' work at night,
Alas! 'twas hardly worth the telling,
It would not pay for candle-light.
Remote from sheltered village-green,
On a hill's northern side she dwelt,
Where from sea-blasts the hawthorns lean,
And hoary dews are slow to melt.

By the same fire to boil their pottage,
Two poor old Dames, as I have known,
Will often live in one small cottage;
But she, poor Woman! housed alone.
'Twas well enough, when summer came,
The long, warm, lightsome summer-day,
Then at her door the *canty* Dame
Would sit, as any linnet, gay.

But when the ice our streams did fetter,
Oh then how her old bones would shake!
You would have said, if you had met her,
'Twas a hard time for Goody Blake.
Her evenings then were dull and dead:
Sad case it was, as you may think,
For very cold to go to bed;
And then for cold not sleep a wink.

O joy for her! whene'er in winter
The winds at night had made a rout;
And scattered many a lusty splinter
And many a rotten bough about.
Yet never had she, well or sick,
As every man who knew her says,
A pile beforehand, turf or stick,
Enough to warm her for three days.

Now, when the frost was past enduring,
And made her poor old bones to ache,
Could any thing be more alluring
Than an old hedge to Goody Blake?
And, now and then, it must be said,
When her old bones were cold and chill,
She left her fire, or left her bed,
To seek the hedge of Harry Gill.

Now Harry he had long suspected
This trespass of old Goody Blake;
And vowed that she should be detected—
That he on her would vengeance take.
And oft from his warm fire he'd go,
And to the fields his road would take;
And there, at night, in frost and snow,
He watched to seize old Goody Blake.

And once, behind a rick of barley,
Thus looking out did Harry stand:
The moon was full and shining clearly,
And crisp with frost the stubble land.
—He hears a noise—he's all awake—
Again?—on tip-toe down the hill
He softly creeps—'tis Goody Blake;
She's at the hedge of Harry Gill!

Right glad was he when he beheld her:
Stick after stick did Goody pull:
He stood behind a bush of elder,
Till she had filled her apron full.
When with her load she turned about,
The by-way back again to take;
He started forward, with a shout,
And sprang upon poor Goody Blake.

And fiercely by the arm he took her,
And by the arm he held her fast,
And fiercely by the arm he shook her,
And cried, "I've caught you then at last!"
Then Goody, who had nothing said,
Her bundle from her lap let fall;
And, kneeling on the sticks, she prayed
To God that is the judge of all.

She prayed, her withered hand uprearing,
While Harry held her by the arm—
"God! who art never out of hearing,
O may he never more be warm!"
The cold, cold moon above her head,
Thus on her knees did Goody pray;
Young Harry heard what she had said:
And icy cold he turned away.

He went complaining all the morrow
That he was cold and very chill:
His face was gloom, his heart was sorrow,
Alas! that day for Harry Gill!
That day he wore a riding-coat,
But not a whit the warmer he:
Another was on Thursday brought,
And ere the Sabbath he had three.

'Twas all in vain, a useless matter,
And blankets were about him pinned;
Yet still his jaws and teeth they clatter,
Like a loose casement in the wind.
And Harry's flesh it fell away;
And all who see him say, 'tis plain,
That, live as long as live he may,
He never will be warm again.

No word to any man he utters,
A-bed or up, to young or old;
But ever to himself he mutters,
"Poor Harry Gill is very cold."
A-bed or up, by night or day;
His teeth they chatter, chatter still.
Now think, ye farmers all, I pray,
Of Goody Blake and Harry Gill!

PHILIPPE PINEL (1745–1826)

A Treatise on Insanity

The "father of modern psychiatry," Pinel is also one of the founders of moral treatment, which sought to cure insanity by engaging the patient's intellect and emotions rather than by purging and bleeding his body. Countering traditional views of madness as a disease caused by organic lesions in the brain, Pinel argued that it could also be brought on by "very vivid affections of the mind." Within five years of receiving his medical degree from the University of Toulouse in 1773, Pinel left for Paris, where he became editor of the *Gazette de Santé* and joined the intellectual life of the salons, which included such figures as Cabanis and Condorcet. Under the patronage of the leading medical revolutionaries of his day, Pinel assumed directorship of the Bicêtre in 1793. Convinced that the misfortunes suffered by patients played a role in imbalancing their minds, he endeavored to talk with them frequently and elicit their personal histories. In 1795, Pinel was transferred to the Salpêtrière—a medical warehouse for close to seven thousand destitute women—where he would practice and teach for the next thirty years. An advocate of the Enlightenment and its humanitarian reforms, Pinel brought a new order and sensibility to the treatment of the mad, freeing them from the brutal incursions of an ancient regimen and redefining them as individuals worthy of inclusion in the human fraternity.

Nothing has more contributed to the rapid improvement of modern natural history, than the spirit of minute and accurate observation which has distinguished its votaries. The habit of analytical investigation, thus adopted, has induced an accuracy of expression and a propriety of classification, which have themselves, in no small degree, contributed to the advancement of natural knowledge. Convinced of the essential importance of the same means in the illustration of a subject so new and so difficult as that of the present work, it will be seen that I have availed myself of their application, in all or most of the instances of this most calamitous disease, which occured in my practice at the Asylum de Bicêtre. On my entrance upon the duties of that hospital, every thing presented to me the appearance of chaos and confusion. Some of my unfortunate patients laboured under the horrors of a most gloomy and desponding melancholy. Others were furious, and subject to the influence of a perpetual delirium. Some appeared to possess a correct judgement upon most subjects, but were occasionally agitated by violent sallies of maniacal fury; while those of another class were sunk into a state of stupid ideotism and imbecility. Symptoms so different, and all comprehended under the general title of insanity, required, on my part, much study and discrimination; and to secure order in the establishment and

From *A Treatise on Insanity,* trans. D. D. Davis (Birmingham, Ala.: The Classics of Medicine Library, 1983).

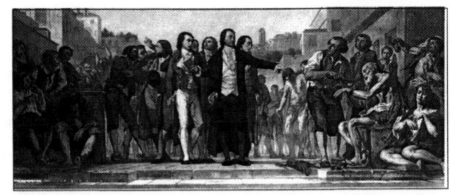

14. *"Pinel faisant ôter des chaînes aux aliénés de Bicêtre." by Charles Muller. Académie Nationale de Médecine, Paris. In authorizing that the inmates of Bicêtre be unshackled, Pinel extended to the insane the principles that guided the French Revolution. Pinel points in a gesture recalling Michelangelo's Creator awakening Adam, while the longtime manager of the asylum, Pussin, saws through the chains. The bringer of human reason and enlightenment to the brutal regime of madness, Pinel is represented as a figure of still repose, whose clean vertical and horizontal lines contrast eloquently with the contorted, almost writhing, bodies of the inmates. In the original color painting, Pinel is further set apart from the figures around him—all portrayed in red and sepia tones—by the dramatic black-and-white of his apparel.*

success to the practice, I determined upon adopting such a variety of measures, both as to discipline and treatment, as my patients required, and my limited opportunity permitted. From systems of nosology, I had little assistance to expect; since the arbitrary distributions of Sauvages and Cullen were better calculated to impress the conviction of their insufficiency than to simplify my labour. I, therefore, resolved to adopt that method of investigation which has invariably succeeded in all the departments of natural history, viz. to notice successively every fact, without any other object than that of collecting materials for future use; and to endeavour, as far as possible, to divest myself of the influence, both of my own prepossessions and the authority of others. With this view, I first of all took a general statement of the symptoms of my patients. To ascertain their characteristic peculiarities, the above survey was followed by cautious and repeated examinations into the condition of individuals. All our new cases were entered at great length upon the journals of the house. Due attention was paid to the changes of the seasons and the weather, and their respective influences upon the patients were minutely noticed. Having a peculiar attachment for the more general method of descriptive history, I did not confine myself to any exclusive mode of arranging my observations, nor to any one system of nosography. The facts which I have thus collected are now submitted to the consideration of the public, in the form of a regular treatise.

Few subjects in medicine are so intimately connected with the history and philosophy of the human mind as insanity. There are still fewer, where there are so many errors to rectify, and so many prejudices to remove. Derangement of the understanding is generally considered as an effect of an organic lesion of the brain, consequently as incurable; a supposition that is, in a great number of instances, contrary to anatomical fact. Public asylums for maniacs have been regarded as places of confinement for such of its members as are become dangerous to the peace of society. The managers of those institutions, who are frequently men of little knowledge and less humanity, have been permitted to exercise towards their innocent prisoners a most arbitrary system of cruelty and violence; while experience affords ample and daily proofs of the happier effects of a mild, conciliating treatment, rendered effective by steady and dispassionate firmness. Availing themselves of this consideration, many empirics have erected establishments for the reception of lunatics, and have practiced this very delicate branch of the healing heart with singular reputation. A great number of cures have undoubtedly been effected by those base born children of the profession; but, as might be expected, they have not in any degree contributed to the advancement of science by any valuable writings. It is on the other hand to be lamented, that regular physicians have indulged in a blind routine of inefficient treatment, and have allowed themselves to be confined within the fairy circle of antiphlogisticism, and by that means to be diverted from the more important management of the mind. Thus, too generally, has the philosophy of this disease, by which I mean the history of its symptoms, of its progress, of its varieties, and of its treatment in and out of hospitals, been most strangely neglected. The successful application of moral regimen exclusively, gives great weight to the supposition, that, in a majority of instances, there is no organic lesion of the brain nor of the cranium.

PERIODICAL INSANITY INDEPENDENT OF THE INFLUENCE OF THE SEASONS

From a general examination of the patients, at the Asylum de Bicêtre, in the second year of the republic, which was undertaken for the purpose of ascertaining the relative number of each variety of the disease; it appeared, that, out of two hundred maniacs, there were fifty-two of the class subject to paroxysms of insanity at irregular periods; and only six, whose periods of accession observed a regular intermission.

The peculiar character of those unfortunate cases consisted in a few but well marked circumstances. Their ideas were clear and connected;—they indulged in no extravagances of fancy;—they answered with great pertinence and precision to the questions that were proposed to them: but they were under the dominion of a most ungovernable fury, and of a thirst equally ungovernable for deeds of blood. In the mean time, they were fully aware of their horrid propensity, but absolutely incapable, without coercive assistance, of suppressing the atrocious impulse. How are we to reconcile these facts to the opinion which Locke and Condillac entertained with regard to the nature of insanity, which they made to consist exclusively in a disposition to associate ideas naturally incompatible, and to mistake ideas thus associated for real truths?

I cannot here avoid giving my most decided suffrage in favour of the moral qualities of maniacs. I have nowhere met, excepting in romances, with fonder husbands, more affectionate parents, more impassioned lovers, more pure and exalted patriots, than in the lunatic asylum, during their intervals of calmness and reason. A man of sensibility may go there every day of his life, and witness scenes of indescribable tenderness associated to a most estimable virtue.

DIFFERENT LESIONS OF THE FUNCTIONS OF THE UNDERSTANDING DURING PAROXYSMS OF INSANITY

The faculties of reflection and reasoning are visibly impaired or destroyed in the greatest number of cases. But I have seen some, where either or both of those faculties have retained all their energy, or have recovered themselves speedily upon an object presenting itself calculated to attract and to fix the attention. I engaged a person of this class, naturally of excellent parts, to write a letter for me at a time when he was maintaining very absurd and ridiculous positions. This letter, which I have still by me, is full of good reasoning and good sense. A silversmith, who had the extravagance to believe that he had exchanged his head, was at the same time infatuated with the chimera of perpetual motion. He got his tools and set to work with infinite resolution and obstinacy. It may be easily imagined that the discovery in question was not made. There resulted from it, however, several very ingenious pieces of machinery—such as must have been effects of the profoundest combinations. Do those facts consist with the doctrine of the unity and individuality of the seat and principle of the human mind? If not, what then must become of the thousands of volumes which have been written on metaphysics?

MANIACAL PAROXYSMS CHARACTERISED BY A HIGH DEGREE OF PHYSICAL AND MENTAL ENERGY

It is to be hoped, that the science of medicine will one day proscribe the very vague and inaccurate expressions of "images traced in the brain, the unequal determination of blood into different parts of this viscus, the irregular movements of the animal spirits," &c. expressions which are to be met with in the best writings that have appeared on the human understanding, but which do not accord with the origin, the causes, and the history of insanity. The nervous excitement, which characterises the greatest number of cases, affects not the system physically by increasing muscular power and action only, but likewise the mind, by exciting a consciousness of supreme importance and irresistible strength. Entertaining a high opinion of his capacity of resistance, a maniac often indulges in the most extravagant flights of fancy and caprice; and, upon attempts being made to repress or coerce him, aims furious blows at his keeper, and wages war against as many of the servants or attendants as he supposes he can well master. If met, however, by a force evidently and convincingly superior, he submits without opposition or violence. This is a great and invaluable secret in the management of well regulated hospitals. I have known it prevent many fatal accidents, and contribute greatly towards the cure of insanity. I have, however, seen the nervous excitement in question, in some few instances, become extremely obstinate and incoercible.

I have frequently stopt at the chamber door of a literary gentleman, who, during his paroxysms, appeared to soar above the mediocrity of intellect which was habitual to him, solely to admire his newly acquired powers of eloquence. He declaimed upon the events of the revolution with all the force, the dignity, and the purity of language that the very interesting subject could admit of. At other times, he was a man of very ordinary abilities. The elevation of mind, produced by the nervous excitement now under consideration, while it is associated with the chimerical consciousness of possessing supreme power or attributes of divinity, inspires the patient with the most extatic feelings, with a sort of inchantment or intoxication of happiness. A madman, who was confined at a pension-house in Paris, whenever his insane fits came on, believed himself to be the prophet Mahomet. He then assumed a commanding attitude and the tone of an embassador from the most high. His looks were penetrating and expressive, and his gait was that of majesty. One day, when there was a heavy cannonade at Paris, in celebration of some political event, he seemed firmly convinced that it was intended as a tribute of homage to himself. He enjoined silence around him, could not contain his joy, and he resembled the ancient prophets in their pretensions and manners.

ARE ALL LUNATICS EQUALLY CAPABLE OF SUPPORTING THE EXTREMES OF COLD AND HUNGER?

A great degree of muscular power, and a capacity of supporting with impunity the extremes of cold and hunger, are effects, or at least properties of the nervous excitement of maniacs, that are equally frequent and remarkable. This, however, like many other general truths, has been too frequently applied to all kinds and periods of insanity. I have seen some instances of muscular energy that impressed me with the idea of a strength almost supernatural. The strongest bands yielded to the efforts of the maniac, and the ease with which it was done, often surprised me more than the degree of resistance that was overcome. But this energy of muscular contraction is far from being common to all the species of insanity. In many instances, on the contrary, there is present a considerable degree of muscular debility. General propositions have, likewise, been too often advanced in regard to the capacity of maniacs to bear extreme hunger with impunity. I have known several, who were voracious to a great degree, and who languished even to fainting from want or deficiency of nourishment. It is said of an asylum at Naples, that a low spare diet is a fundamental principle of the institution. It would be difficult to trace the origin of so singular a prejudice. Unhappy experience, which I acquired during seasons of scarcity, has most thoroughly convinced me, that insufficiency of food, when it does not altogether extinguish the vital principle, is not a little calculated to exasperate and to prolong the disease.

THE VARIETY AND PROFUNDITY OF KNOWLEDGE REQUISITE ON THE PART OF THE PHYSICIAN, IN ORDER TO SECURE SUCCESS IN THE TREATMENT OF INSANITY

The time, perhaps, is at length arrived when medicine in France, now liberated from the fetters imposed upon it, by the prejudices of custom, by interested ambition, by its association with religious institutions, and by the discredit in which it has been held in the public estimation, will be able to assume its proper dignity, to establish its theories on facts alone, to generalise those facts, and to maintain its level with the other departments of natural history. The principles of free enquiry, which the revolution has incorporated with our national politics, have opened a wide field to the energies of medical philosophy. But, it is chiefly in great hospitals and asylums, that those advantages will be immediately felt, from the opportunities which are there afforded of making a great number of observations, experiments, and comparisons.

THE AUTHOR'S INDUCEMENTS TO STUDY THE PRINCIPLES OF MORAL TREATMENT

The administration of the civil hospitals, in Paris, opened to me in the second year of the republic a wide field of research, by my nomination to the office of chief physician to the national Asylum de Bicêtre, which I continued to fill for two years. In order, in some degree, to make up for the local disadvantages of the hospital, and the numerous inconveniences which arose from the instability and successive changes of the administration, I determined to turn my attention, almost exclusively, to the subject of moral treatment. The halls and the passages of the hospital were much confined, and so arranged as to render the cold of winter and the heat of summer equally intolerable and injurious. The chambers were exceedingly small and inconvenient. Baths we had none, though I made repeated applications for them; nor had we extensive liberties for walking, gardening or other exercises. So destitute of accommodations, we found it impossible to class our patients according to the varieties and degrees of their respective maladies. On the other hand, the gentleman, to whom was committed the chief management of the hospital, exercised towards all that were placed under his protection, the vigilance of a kind and affectionate parent. Accustomed to reflect, and possessed of great experience, he was not deficient either in the knowledge or execution of the duties of his office. He never lost sight of the principles of a most genuine philanthropy. He paid great attention to the diet of the house, and left no opportunity for murmur or discontent on the part of the most fastidious. He exercised a strict discipline over the conduct of the domestics, and punished, with severity, every instance of ill treatment, and every act of violence, of which they were guilty towards those whom it was merely their duty to serve. He was both esteemed and feared by every maniac; for he was mild, and at the same time inflexibly firm. In a word, he was master of every branch of his art, from its simplest to its most complicated principles. Thus was I introduced to a man, whose friendship was an invaluable acquisition to me. Our acquaintance matured into the closest intimacy. Our duties and inclinations concurred in the same object. Our conversation, which was almost exclusively professional, contributed to our mutual improvement. With those advantages, I devoted a great part of my time in examining for myself the various and numerous affections of the human mind in a state of disease. I regularly took notes of whatever appeared deserving of my attention; and compared what I thus collected, with facts analogous to them that I met with in books, or amongst my own memoranda of former dates. Such are the materials upon which my principles of moral treatment are founded.

A CASE OF INSANITY, IN WHICH IT IS PROBABLE, THAT MORAL TREATMENT WOULD HAVE BEEN ATTENDED WITH SUCCESS

A young gentleman, twenty-four years of age, endowed with a most vivid imagination, came to Paris to study the law, and flattered himself with the belief that nature had destined him for a brilliant station at the bar. An enthusiast for his own convictions, he was an inflexible disciple of Pythagoras in his system of diet: he secluded himself from society, and pursued, with the utmost ardour and obstinacy, his literary projects. Some months after his arrival, he was seized with great depression of spirits, frequent bleeding at the nose, spasmodic oppression of the chest, wandering pains of the bowels, troublesome flatulence and morbidly increased sensibility. Sometimes he came to me in a very cheerful state of mind, when he used to say, "How happy he was, and that he could scarcely express the supreme felicity which he experienced." At other times, I found him plunged in the horrors of consternation and despair. Thus, most acutely miserable, he frequently, and with great earnestness, intreated me to put an end to his sufferings. The characters of the profoundest hypochondriasis were now become recognisable in his feelings and conduct. I saw the approaching danger, and I conjured him to change his manner of life. My advice was unequivocally rejected. The nervous symptoms of the head, chest and bowels continued to be progressively exasperated. His intervals of complacency and cheerfulness were succeeded by extreme depression and pusillanimity and terror, and inexpressible anguish. Overpowered nearly by his apprehensions, he often and earnestly entreated me to rescue him from the arms of death. At those times I invited him to accompany me to the fields, and after walking for some time, and conversing together upon subjects likely to console or amuse him, he appeared to recover the enjoyment of his existence: but, upon returning to his chambers, his perplexities and terrors likewise returned. His despair was exasperated by the confusion of ideas to which he was constantly subject, and which interfered so much with his studies. But what appeared, altogether, to overwhelm him, was the distressing conviction that his pursuit of fame and professional distinction must be for ever abandoned. Complete lunacy, at length, established its melancholy empire. One night, he bethought himself that he would go to the play, to seek relief from his own too unhappy meditations. The piece which was presented, was the "Philosopher without knowing it." He was instantly seized with the most gloomy suspicions, and especially with a conviction, that the comedy was written on purpose and represented to ridicule himself. He accused me with having furnished materials for the writer of it, and the next morning he came to reproach me, which he did most angrily, for having betrayed the rights of friendship, and exposed him to public derision. His delirium observed no bounds. Every monk and priest he met with in the public walks, he took for comedians in disguise, dispatched there for the purpose of studying his gestures, and of discovering the secret operations of his mind. In the dead of night he gave way to the most terrific apprehensions,—believed himself to be attacked sometimes by spies, and at others, by robbers and assassins. He once opened his window with great violence and cried out murder and assistance with all his might. His relations, at length, determined tò have him put under a plan of treatment, similar to that which was adopted at the ci-de-vant Hôtel Dieu; and, with that view, sent him under the protection of a proper person, to a little village in the vicinity of the Pyrenees. Greatly debilitated both in mind and body, it was some time after agreed upon that he should return to his family residence, where, on account of his paroxysms of delirious extravagance, succeeded by fits of profound melancholy, he was insulated from society. Ennui and insurmountable disgust with life, absolute refusal of food, and dissatisfaction with every thing, and every body that came near him, were among the last ingredients of his bitter cup. To conclude our affecting history: he one day eluded the vigilance of his keeper; and, with no other garment on than his shirt, fled to a neighbouring wood, where he lost himself, and where, from weakness and inanition, he ended his miseries. Two days afterwards he was found a corpse. In his hand was found the celebrated work of Plato on the immortality of the soul.

THE ADVANTAGES OF RESTRAINT UPON THE IMAGINATION OF MANIACS ILLUSTRATED

A young religious enthusiast, who was exceedingly affected by the abolition of the catholic religion in France, became insane. After the usual treatment at the Hôtel Dieu, he was transferred to the Asylum de Bicêtre. His misanthropy was not to be equalled. His thoughts dwelled perpetually upon the torments of the other world; from which he founded his only chance of escaping, upon a conscientious adoption of the abstinences and mortifications of the ancient anchorites. At length, he refused nourishment altogether; and, on the fourth day after that unfortunate resolution was formed, a state of langour succeeded, which excited considerable apprehensions for his life. Kind remonstrances and pressing invitations proved equally ineffectual. He repelled, with rudeness, the services of the attendants, rejected, with the utmost pertinacity, some soup that was placed before him, and demolished his bed (which was of straw) in order that he might lie upon the boards. How was such a perverse train of ideas to be stemmed or counteracted? The excitement of terror presented itself as the only resource. For this purpose, Citizen Pussin appeared one night at the door of his chamber, and, with fire darting from his eyes, and thunder in his voice, commanded a group of domestics, who were armed with strong and loudly clanking chains, to do their duty. But the ceremony was artfully suspended;—the soup was placed before the maniac, and strict orders were left him to eat it in the course of the night, on pains of the severest punishment. He was left to his own reflections.

The night was spent (as he afterwards informed me) in a state of the most distressing hesitation, whether to incur the present punishment, or the distant but still more dreadful torments of the world to come. After an internal struggle of many hours, the idea of the present evil gained the ascendancy, and he determined to take the soup. From that time he submitted, without difficulty, to a restorative system of regimen. His sleep and strength gradually returned; his reason recovered its empire; and, after the manner above related, he escaped certain death. It was during his convalescence, that he mentioned to me the perplexities and agitations which he endured during the night of the experiment.

INTIMIDATION TOO OFTEN ASSOCIATED WITH VIOLENCE

In the preceding case of insanity, we trace the happy effects of intimidation, without severity; of oppression, without violence; and of triumph, without outrage. How different from the system of treatment, which is yet adopted in too many hospitals, where the domestics and keepers are permitted to use any violence that the most wanton caprice, or the most sanguinary cruelty may dictate. In the writings of the ancients, and especially of Celsus, a sort of intermediate and conditional mode of treatment is recommended, founded, in the first instance, upon a system of lenity and forbearance; and when that method failed, upon corporal and physical punishments, such as confinement, chains, flogging, spare diet, &c. Public and private madhouses, in more modern times, have been conducted on similar principles.

A HAPPY EXPEDIENT EMPLOYED IN THE CURE OF A MECHANICIAN

A celebrated watchmaker, at Paris, was infatuated with the chimera of perpetual motion, and to effect this discovery, he set to work with indefatigable ardour. From unremitting attention to the object of his enthusiasm coinciding with the influence of revolutionary disturbances, his imagination was greatly heated, his sleep was interrupted, and, at length, a complete derangement of the understanding took place. His case was marked by a most whimsical illusion of the imagination. He fancied that he had lost his head on the scaffold; that it had been thrown promiscuously among the heads of many other victims; that the judges, having repented of their cruel sentence, had ordered those heads to be restored to their respective owners, and placed upon their respective shoulders; but that, in consequence of an unfortunate mistake, the gentlemen, who had the management of that business, had placed upon his shoulders the head of one of his unhappy companions. The idea of this whimsical exchange of his head, occupied his thoughts night and day; which determined his relations to send him to the Hôtel Dieu. Thence he was transferred to the Asylum de Bicêtre. Nothing could equal the extravagant overflowings of his heated brain. He sung, cried, or danced incessantly; and, as there appeared no propensity in him to commit acts of violence or disturbance, he was allowed to go about the hospital without control, in order to expend, by evaporation, the effervescent excess of his spirits. "Look at these teeth," he constantly cried;—"Mine were exceedingly hand-some;—these are rotten and decayed. My mouth was sound and healthy: this is foul and diseased. What difference between this hair and that of my own head."

A keen and an unanswerable stroke of pleasantry seemed best adapted to correct this fantastic whim. Another convalescent of a gay and facetious humour, instructed in the part he should play in this comedy, adriotly turned the conversation to the subject of the famous miracle of Saint Denis. Our mechanician strongly maintained the possibility of the fact, and sought to confirm it by an application of it to his own case. The other set up a loud laugh, and replied with a tone of the keenest ridicule: "Madman as thou art, how could Saint Denis kiss his own head? Was it with his heels?" This equally unexpected and unanswerable retort, forcibly struck the maniac. He retired confused amidst the peals of laughter, which were provoked at his ex-pense, and never afterwards mentioned the exchange of his head. Close attention to his trade for some months, completed the restoration of his intellect. He was sent to his family in perfect health; and has, now for more than five years, pursued his busi-ness without a return of his complaint.

THE TREATMENT OF MANIACS TO BE VARIED ACCORDING TO THE SPECIFIC CHARACTERS OF THEIR HALLUCINATION

Of all the powers of the human mind, that of the imagination appears to be the most subject to injury. The fantastic illusions and ideal transformations, which are by far the most frequent forms of mental derangement, are solely ascribeable to le-sions of this faculty. Hence the expediency of a great variety of schemes and strata-gems for removing these prepossessions.

THE CONDUCT OF THE GOVERNOR OF BICÊTRE, UPON THE REVOLUTIONARY ORDERS HE RECEIVED TO DESTROY THE SYMBOLIC REPRESENTATIONS OF RELIGION

In the third year of the republic, the directors of the civil hospitals, in the excess of their revolutionary zeal, determined to remove from those places the external ob-jects of worship, the only remaining consolation of the indigent and the unhappy. A visit for this purpose was paid to the hospital de Bicêtre. The plunder, impious as it was and detestable, was begun in the dormitories of the old and the infirm, who were naturally struck at an instance of robbery so new and unexpected, some with astonishment, some with indignation, and others with terror. The first day of visita-tion being already far spent, it was determined to reserve the lunatic department of the establishment for another opportunity. I was present at the time, and seized the occasion to observe, that the unhappy residents of that part of the hospital required to be treated with peculiar management and address; and, that it would be much better to confide so delicate a business to the governor himself, whose character for pru-dence and firmness was well known. That gentleman, in order to prevent disturbance, and perhaps an insurrection in the asylum, wished to appear rather to submit to a measure so obnoxious than to direct it. Having purchased a great number of national cockades, he called a meeting of all the lunatics who could conveniently attend. When they were all arrived he took up the colours and said, "Let those who love liberty draw near and enrol themselves under the national colours." This invitation was accompanied by a most gracious smile. Some hesitated; but the greatest number complied. This moment of enthusiasm was not allowed to pass unimproved. The converts were instantly informed, that their new engagement required of them to remove from the chapel the image of the Virgin, with all the other appurtenances of the catholic worship. No sooner was this requisition announced than a great number of our new republicans set off for the chapel, and committed the desired depredation upon its sacred furniture. The images and paintings, which had been objects of reverence for so many years, were brought out to the court in a state of complete disorder and ruination. Consternation and terror seized the few devout but impotent witnesses of this scene of impiety. Murmurs, imprecations and threats expressed their honest feelings. The most exasperated amongst them prayed that fire from heaven might be poured upon the heads of the guilty, or believed that they saw the bottomless abyss opening to receive them. To convince them, however, that heaven was deaf equally to their imprecations and prayers, the governor ordered the holy things to be broken into a thousand pieces and to be taken away. The good-will and attachment, which he knew so well how to conciliate, ensured the execution of this revolutionary measure.

MANIACAL FURY TO BE REPRESSED; BUT NOT BY CRUEL TREATMENT

The lesions of the human intellect simply, embrace but a part of the object of the present treatise. The active faculties of the mind are not less subject to serious lesions and changes, nor less deserving of ample consideration. The diseased affections of the will—excessive or defective emotions, passions, &c. whether intermittent or continued, are sometimes associated with lesions of the intellect. At other times, however, the understanding is perfectly free in every department of its exercise. In all cases of excessive excitement of the passions, a method of treatment, simple enough in its application, but highly calculated to render the disease incurable, has been adopted from time immemorial:—that of abandoning the patient to his melancholy fate, as an untameable being, to be immured in solitary durance, loaded with chains, or otherwise treated with extreme severity, until the natural close of a life so wretched shall rescue him from his misery, and convey him from the cells of the mad-house to the chambers of the grave. But this treatment convenient indeed to a governor, more remarkable for his indolence and ignorance than for his prudence or humanity, deserves, at the present day, to be held up to public execration, and classed with the other prejudices which have degraded the character and pretensions of the human species. To allow every maniac all the latitude of personal liberty consistent with safety; to proportion the degree of coercion to the demands upon it from his extravagance of behaviour; to use mildness of manners or firmness as occasion may require,—the bland arts of conciliation, or the tone of irresistible authority pronouncing an irreversible mandate, and to proscribe, most absolutely, all violence and ill treatment on the part of the domestics, are laws of fundamental importance, and essential to the prudent and successful management of all lunatic institutions. But how many great qualities, both of mind and body, it is necessary that the governor should possess, in order to meet the endless difficulties and exigencies of so responsible a situation!

THE NECESSITY OF MAINTAINING CONSTANT ORDER IN LUNATIC ASYLUMS, AND OF STUDYING THE VARIETIES OF CHARACTER EXHIBITED BY THE PATIENTS

The extreme importance which I attach to the maintenance of order and moderation in lunatic institutions, and consequently to the physical and moral qualities requisite to be possessed by their governors, is by no means to be wondered at, since it is a fundamental principle in the treatment of mania to watch over the impetuosities of passion, and to order such arrangements of police and moral treatment as are favourable to that degree of excitement which experience approves as conducive to recovery. Unfortunate, indeed, is the fate of those maniacs who are placed in lunatic hospitals, where the basis of the practice is routine, and that perhaps under the direction of a governor devoid of the essential principles of morality; or where, which amounts to the same thing, they are abandoned to the savage and murderous cruelty of underlings. Great sagacity, ardent zeal, perpetual and indefatigable attention, are essential qualities of a governor who wishes to do his duty, in its various departments of watching the progress of every case, seizing the peculiar character of the hallucination, and meeting the numerous varieties of the disease depending upon temperament, constitution, ages and complications with other diseases. In some unusual or difficult cases, it requires great consideration to decide upon the treatment or experiment most eligible to be attempted. But in the greatest number of instances, especially of accidental mania originating in the depressing passions, the experience of every day attests the value of consolatory language, kind treatment, and the revival of extinguished hope. Severity in cases of this description can answer no other purpose than those of exasperating the disease, and of frequently rendering it incurable.

JOSEF BREUER (1842–1925)
AND SIGMUND FREUD (1856–1939)

Studies on Hysteria

A collaborative project by Josef Breuer and Sigmund Freud, *Studies on Hysteria* (1893–1895) is widely regarded as the founding document of psychoanalysis. Encompassing both technique and theory, the *Studies* contains "The Preliminary Communication," written jointly by Breuer and Freud, the case of "Anna O." by Breuer, four case histories by Freud, a section on theory by Breuer, and another on psychotherapy by Freud. Breuer and Freud's longstanding friendship began in the late 1870s, when they met at Ernst Brücke's Institute for Physiology in Vienna, where Freud was working as a medical student. Sharing common interests and viewpoints, the two men soon became intimate friends, and when Freud undertook private practice in 1886, it was the older Breuer who sent him patients of considerable social prominence and great wealth, two of whom appear as cases in the *Studies*. "The Preliminary Communication," originally published as a separate paper in 1893, introduced Breuer's cathartic therapy—a treatment that required the patient to be placed under hypnosis, during which she was asked to remember the traumatic event that had precipitated her hysterical symptoms and to "abreact," to discharge the affect associated with them by putting it into words. Conscious verbal expression of the affect was, therefore, substituted for its unconscious semiological enactment through bodily symptoms. By 1895, Freud's views on hysteria had diverged significantly from Breuer's. Whereas Breuer continued to believe that it was caused by the chance entry of a traumatic idea into the patient's unconscious during a "hypnoid," or dissociated, state of mind, Freud became convinced that hysteria resulted from the patient's active, although unconscious, repression of the traumatic idea for reasons that remained beyond her conscious awareness. The therapist's job was to bring these reasons to light and to interpret the unconscious resistance that kept them in the dark. Such work, however, could be carried out only if the patient were in a conscious state, for hypnosis obliterated resistance, the very phenomenon that needed to be analyzed. By the time Freud had completed the final section of the *Studies,* he had sketched out the mechanisms of repression, defense, and transference, and had moved away from hypnosis and Breuer's cathartic treatment toward "free association" and a method he had newly named "psychical analysis."

From *The Standard Edition of the Complete Psychological Works of Sigmund Freud,* ed. and trans. James Strachey, Vol. 2: *Studies on Hysteria* (London: The Hogarth Press, 1955).

PRELIMINARY COMMUNICATION (1893)
I

A chance observation has led us, over a number of years, to investigate a great variety of different forms and symptoms of hysteria, with a view to discovering their precipitating cause—the event which provoked the first occurrence, often many years earlier, of the phenomenon in question. In the great majority of cases it is not possible to establish the point of origin by a simple interrogation of the patient, however thoroughly it may be carried out. This is in part because what is in question is often some experience which the patient dislikes discussing; but principally because he is genuinely unable to recollect it and often has no suspicion of the causal connection between the precipitating event and the pathological phenomenon. As a rule it is necessary to hypnotize the patient and to arouse his memories under hypnosis of the time at which the symptom made its first appearance; when this has been done, it becomes possible to demonstrate the connection in the clearest and most convincing fashion.

This method of examination has in a large number of cases produced results which seem to be of value alike from a theoretical and a practical point of view.

They are valuable theoretically because they have taught us that external events determine the pathology of hysteria to an extent far greater than is known and recognized. It is of course obvious that in cases of 'traumatic' hysteria what provokes the symptoms is the accident. The causal connection is equally evident in hysterical attacks when it is possible to gather from the patient's utterances that in each attack he is hallucinating the same event which provoked the first one. The situation is more obscure in the case of other phenomena.

Our experiences have shown us, however, that the most various symptoms, which are ostensibly spontaneous and, as one might say, idiopathic products of hysteria, are just as strictly related to the precipitating trauma as the phenomena to which we have just alluded and which exhibit the connection quite clearly. The symptoms which we have been able to trace back to precipitating factors of this sort include neuralgias and anaesthesias of very various kinds, many of which had persisted for years, contractures and paralyses, hysterical attacks and epileptoid convulsions, which every observer regarded as true epilepsy, *petit mal* and disorders in the nature of *tic*, chronic vomiting and anorexia, carried to the pitch of rejection of all nourishment, various forms of disturbance of vision, constantly recurrent visual hallucinations, etc. The disproportion between the many years' duration of the hysterical symptom and the single occurrence which provoked it is what we are accustomed invariably to find in traumatic neuroses. Quite frequently it is some event in childhood that sets up a more or less severe symptom which persists during the years that follow.

The connection is often so clear that it is quite evident how it was that the precipitating event produced this particular phenomenon rather than any other. In that case the symptom has quite obviously been determined by the precipitating cause. We may take as a very commonplace instance a painful emotion arising during a meal but suppressed at the time, and then producing nausea and vomiting which persists for months in the form of hysterical vomiting. A girl, watching beside a sickbed in a torment of anxiety, fell into a twilight state and had a terrifying hallucination, while her right arm, which was hanging over the back of her chair, went to sleep; from this there developed a paresis of the same arm accompanied by contracture and anaesthesia. She tried to pray but could find no words; at length she succeeded in repeating a children's prayer in English. When subsequently a severe and highly complicated hysteria developed, she could only speak, write and understand English, while her native language remained unintelligible to her for eighteen months.

In other cases the connection is not so simple. It consists only in what might be called a 'symbolic' relation between the precipitating cause and the pathological phenomenon—a relation such as healthy people form in dreams. For instance, a neuralgia may follow upon mental pain or vomiting upon a feeling of moral disgust. We have studied patients who used to make the most copious use of this sort of symbolization.

Observations such as these seem to us to establish an analogy between the pathogenesis of common hysteria and that of traumatic neuroses, and to justify an extension of the concept of traumatic hysteria. In traumatic neuroses the operative cause of the illness is not the trifling physical injury but the affect of fright—the psychical trauma. In an analogous manner, our investigations reveal, for many, if not for most, hysterical symptoms, precipitating causes which can only be described as psychical traumas. Any experience which calls up distressing affects—such as those of fright, anxiety, shame or physical pain—may operate as a trauma of this kind; and whether it in fact does so depends naturally enough on the susceptibility of the person affected (as well as on another condition which will be mentioned later). In the case of common hysteria it not infrequently happens that, instead of a single, major trauma, we find a number of partial traumas forming a *group* of provoking causes. These have only been able to exercise a traumatic effect by summation and they belong together in so far as they are in part components of a single story of suffering.

But the causal relation between the determining psychical trauma and the hysterical phenomenon is not of a kind implying that the trauma merely acts like an *agent provocateur* in releasing the symptom, which thereafter leads an independent existence. We must presume rather that the psychical trauma—or more precisely the memory of the trauma—acts like a foreign body which long after its entry must continue to be regarded as an agent that is still at work; and we find the evidence for this in a highly remarkable phenomenon which at the same time lends an important *practical* interest to our findings.

For we found, to our great surprise at first, that *each individual hysterical symptom immediately and permanently disappeared when we had succeeded in bringing clearly to light the memory of the event by which it was provoked and in arousing its accompanying affect, and when the patient had described that event in the greatest possible detail and had put the affect into words.* Recollection without affect almost invariably produces no result. The psychical process which originally took place must be repeated as vividly as possible; it must be brought back to its *status nascendi* and then given verbal utterance. Where what we are dealing with are phenomena involving stimuli (spasms, neuralgias and hallucinations) these re-appear once again with the fullest intensity and then vanish for ever. Failures of function, such as paralyses and anaesthesias, vanish in the same way, though, of course, without the temporary intensification being discernible.

We may reverse the dictum *'cessante causa cessat effectus'* ['when the cause ceases the effect ceases'] and conclude from these observations that the determining process continues to operate in some way or other for years—not indirectly, through a chain of intermediate causal links, but as a *directly* releasing cause—just as a psychical pain that is remembered in waking consciousness still provokes a lachrymal secretion long after the event. *Hysterics suffer mainly from reminiscences.*

II

At first sight it seems extraordinary that events experienced so long ago should continue to operate so intensely—that their recollection should not be liable to the wearing away process to which, after all, we see all our memories succumb. The following considerations may perhaps make this a little more intelligible.

The fading of a memory or the losing of its affect depends on various factors. The most important of these is *whether there has been an energetic reaction to the event that provokes an affect.* By 'reaction' we here understand the whole class of voluntary and involuntary reflexes—from tears to acts of revenge—in which, as experience shows us, the affects are discharged. If this reaction takes place to a sufficient amount a large part of the affect disappears as a result. Linguistic usage bears witness to this fact of daily observation by such phrases as 'to cry oneself out' [*'sich ausweinen'*], and to 'blow off steam' [*'sich austoben'*, literally 'to rage oneself out']. If the reaction is suppressed, the affect remains attached to the memory. An injury that has been repaid, even if only in words, is recollected quite differently from one that has had to be accepted. Language recognizes this distinction, too, in its mental and physical consequences; it very characteristically describes an injury that has been suffered in silence as 'a mortification' [*'Kränkung'*, lit. 'making ill'].—The injured person's reaction to the trauma only exercises a completely 'cathartic' effect if it is an *adequate* reaction—as, for instance, revenge. But language serves as a substitute for action; by its help, an affect can be 'abreacted' almost as effectively. In other cases speaking is itself the adequate reflex, when, for instance, it is a lamentation or giving utterance to a tormenting secret, e.g. a confession. If there is no such reaction, whether in deeds or words, or in the mildest cases in tears, any recollection of the event retains its affective tone to begin with.

'Abreaction,' however, is not the only method of dealing with the situation that is open to a normal person who has experienced a psychical trauma. A memory of such a trauma, even if it has not been abreacted, enters the great complex of associations, it comes alongside other experiences, which may contradict it, and is subjected to rectification by other ideas. In this way a normal person is able to bring about the disappearance of the accompanying affect through the process of association.

Our observations have shown . . . that the memories which have become the determinants of hysterical phenomena persist for a long time with astonishing freshness and with the whole of their affective colouring. We must, however, mention another remarkable fact, which we shall later be able to turn to account, namely, that these memories, unlike other memories of their past lives, are not at the patients' disposal. On the contrary, *these experiences are completely absent from the patients' memory when they are in a normal psychical state, or are only present in a highly summary form.* Not until they have been questioned under hypnosis do these memories emerge with the undiminished vividness of a recent event.

It appears, that is to say, that these memories correspond to traumas that have not been sufficiently abreacted; and if we enter more closely into the reasons which have prevented this, we find at least two sets of conditions under which the reaction to the trauma fails to occur.

In the first group are those cases in which the patients have not reacted to a psychical trauma because the nature of the trauma excluded a reaction, as in the case of the apparently irreparable loss of a loved person or because social circumstances made a reaction impossible or because it was a question of things which the patient wished to forget, and therefore intentionally repressed from his conscious thought and inhibited and suppressed. It is precisely distressing things of this kind that, under hypnosis, we find are the basis of hysterical phenomena (e.g. hysterical deliria in saints and nuns, continent women and well-brought-up children).

The second group of conditions are determined, not by the content of the memories but by the psychical states in which the patient received the experiences in question. For we find, under hypnosis, among the causes of hysterical symptoms ideas which are not in themselves significant, but whose persistence is due to the fact that they originated during the prevalence of severely paralysing affects, such as fright, or during positively abnormal psychical states, such as the semi-hypnotic twilight state of day-dreaming, auto-hypnoses, and so on. In such cases it is the nature of the states which makes a reaction to the event impossible.

Both kinds of conditions may, of course, be simultaneously present, and this, in fact, often occurs.

It may therefore be said that the ideas which have become pathological have persisted with such freshness and affective strength because they have been denied the normal wearing-away processes by means of abreaction and reproduction in states of uninhibited association.

III

We have stated the conditions which, as our experience shows, are responsible for the development of hysterical phenomena from psychical traumas. In so doing, we have already been obliged to speak of abnormal states of consciousness in which these pathogenic ideas arise, and to emphasize the fact that the recollection of the operative psychical trauma is not to be found in the patient's normal memory but in his memory when he is hypnotized.

We should like to balance the familiar thesis that hypnosis is an artificial hysteria by another—the basis and *sine qua non* of hysteria is the existence of hypnoid states. These hypnoid states share with one another and with hypnosis, however much they may differ in other respects, one common feature: the ideas which emerge in them are very intense but are cut off from associative communication with the rest of the content of consciousness. Associations may take place between these hypnoid states, and their ideational content can in this way reach a more or less high degree of psychical organization.

If hypnoid states of this kind are already present before the onset of the manifest illness, they provide the soil in which the affect plants the pathogenic memory with its consequent somatic phenomena.

We have nothing new to say on the question of the origin of these . . . hypnoid states. They often, it would seem, grow out of the day-dreams which are so common even in healthy people and to which needlework and similar occupations render women especially prone.

Our observations contribute nothing fresh on this subject. But they throw a light on the contradiction between the dictum 'hysteria is a psychosis' and the fact that among hysterics may be found people of the clearest intellect, strongest will, greatest character and highest critical power. This characterization holds good of their waking thoughts; but in their hypnoid states they are insane, as we all are in dreams. Whereas, however, our dream-psychoses have no effect upon our waking state, the products of hypnoid states intrude into waking life in the form of hysterical symptoms.

IV

What we have asserted of chronic hysterical symptoms can be applied almost completely to hysterical *attacks.* Charcot, as is well known, has given us a schematic description of the 'major' hysterical attack, according to which four phases can be distinguished in a complete attack: (1) the epileptoid phase, (2) the phase of large movements, (3) the phase of *'attitudes passionnelles'* (the hallucinatory phase), and (4) the phase of terminal delirium. Charcot derives all those forms of hysterical attack which are in practice met with more often than the complete *'grande attaque,'* from the abbreviation, absence or isolation of these four distinct phases.

Thus, a little girl suffered for years from attacks of general convulsions which could well be, and indeed were, regarded as epileptic. She was hypnotized with a view to a differential diagnosis, and promptly had one of her attacks. She was asked what she was seeing and replied 'The dog! the dog's coming!'; and in fact it turned out that she had had the first of her attacks after being chased by a savage dog. The success of the treatment confirmed the choice of diagnosis.

Again, an employee who had become a hysteric as a result of being ill-treated by his superior, suffered from attacks in which he collapsed and fell into a frenzy of rage, but without uttering a word or giving any sign of a hallucination. It was possible to provoke an attack under hypnosis, and the patient then revealed that he was living through the scene in which his employer had abused him in the street and hit him with a stick. A few days later the patient came back and complained of having had another attack of the same kind. On this occasion it turned out under hypnosis that he had been re-living the scene to which the actual onset of the illness was related: the scene in the law-court when he failed to obtain satisfaction for his maltreatment.

In all other respects, too, the memories which emerge, or can be aroused, in hysterical attacks correspond to the precipitating causes which we have found at the root of *chronic* hysterical symptoms. Like these latter causes, the memories under-lying hysterical attacks relate to psychical traumas which have not been disposed of by abreaction or by associative thought-activity. Like them, they are, whether com-pletely or in essential elements, out of reach of the memory of normal conscious-ness and are found to belong to the ideational content of hypnoid states of consciousness with restricted association. Finally, too, the therapeutic test can be applied to them. Our observations have often taught us that a memory of this kind which had hitherto provoked attacks, ceases to be able to do so after the process of reaction and associative correction have been applied to it under hypnosis.

Hysterical attacks, furthermore, appear in a specially interesting light if we bear in mind a theory that we have mentioned above, namely, that in hysteria groups of ideas originating in hypnoid states are present and that these are cut off from asso-ciative connection with the other ideas, but can be associated among themselves, and thus form the more or less highly organized rudiment of a second conscious-ness, a *condition seconde.*

V

It will now be understood how it is that the psychotherapeutic procedure which we have described in these pages has a curative effect. *It brings to an end the op-erative force of the idea which was not abreacted in the first instance, by allowing its strangulated affect to find a way out through speech; and it subjects it to asso-ciative correction by introducing it into normal consciousness (under light hypno-sis) or by removing it through the physician's suggestion, as is done in somnambulism accompanied by amnesia.*

In our opinion the therapeutic advantages of this procedure are considerable. . . . [I]t seems to us far superior in its efficacy to removal through direct suggestion, as it is practised to-day by psychotherapists.

In 1895, when *Studies on Hysteria* appeared, Breuer was one of the most esteemed internists in all of Vienna. It was said that he needed only to set foot in a patient's home for her hysterical symptoms to improve. From De-cember of 1880 to June of 1882, Breuer treated Bertha Pappenheim (1859–1936), the patient who was to become known as "Anna O." When Breuer first saw her, she had been through a grueling period of nursing her dying father. Completely bedridden, she was suffering from disturbances in her vision and speech, bizarre states of consciousness, and varying degrees of pain, paralysis, contracture, and numbness in different parts of her body. As treatment proceeded, Bertha Pappenheim manifested severe "absences," periods of dissociation in which she seemed to become a different person—her "bad self," as she called it. Although she was not able to recall in her normal state what she had experienced during these absences, Pappenheim began to speak of them during the periods of autohypnosis into which she would lapse every evening. In his determination to uncover the precipitat-ing causes of her scores of symptoms, Breuer spent hours with Pappenheim day and night, encouraging her to recollect the terrifying details of her afternoon deliriums during her hypnoid states in the evening. Astonishingly, this procedure, which Breuer named "catharsis" and Pappenheim called "chimney sweeping" or "the talking cure," worked time and again to dispel her symptoms and to relieve her emotional distress. Although Bertha Pappenheim suffered several setbacks in the years following her treatment, she eventually recovered full health and went on to become one of Vienna's most prominent figures. Author, social worker, reformer, and a leader of the women's movement in Germany, Pappenheim directed a Frankfurt orphanage from 1895 to 1907, founded a home for unwed mothers, started the League of Jewish Women, and traveled widely to investigate the problems of homelessness, prostitution, and the white slavery trade.

FRÄULEIN ANNA O.

At the time of her falling ill (in 1880) Fräulein Anna O. was twenty-one years old. She may be regarded as having had a moderately severe neuropathic heredity, since some psychoses had occurred among her more distant relatives. Her parents were normal in this respect. She herself had hitherto been consistently healthy and had shown no signs of neurosis during her period of growth. She was markedly intelligent, with an astonishingly quick grasp of things and penetrating intuition. She possessed a powerful intellect which would have been capable of digesting solid mental pabulum and which stood in need of it—though without receiving it after she had left school. She had great poetic and imaginative gifts, which were under the control of a sharp and critical common sense. Owing to this latter quality she was *completely unsuggestible;* she was only influenced by arguments, never by mere assertions. Her willpower was energetic, tenacious and persistent; sometimes it reached the pitch of an obstinacy which only gave way out of kindness and regard for other people.

One of her essential character traits was sympathetic kindness. Even during her illness she herself was greatly assisted by being able to look after a number of poor, sick people, for she was thus able to satisfy a powerful instinct. Her states of feeling always tended to a slight exaggeration, alike of cheerfulness and gloom; hence she was sometimes subject to moods. The element of sexuality was astonishingly undeveloped in her. The patient, whose life became known to me to an extent to which one person's life is seldom known to another, had never been in love; and in all the enormous number of hallucinations which occurred during her illness that element of mental life never emerged.

This girl, who was bubbling over with intellectual vitality, led an extremely monotonous existence in her puritanically-minded family. She embellished her life in a manner which probably influenced her decisively in the direction of her illness, by indulging in systematic day-dreaming, which she described as her 'private theatre'. While everyone thought she was attending, she was living through fairy tales in her imagination; but she was always on the spot when she was spoken to, so that no one was aware of it. She pursued this activity almost continuously while she was engaged on her household duties, which she discharged unexceptionably. I shall presently have to describe the way in which this habitual day-dreaming while she was well passed over into illness without a break.

The course of the illness fell into several clearly separable phases:

(*A*) Latent incubation. From the middle of July, 1880, till about December 10. This phase of an illness is usually hidden from us; but in this case, owing to its peculiar character, it was completely accessible; and this in itself lends no small pathological interest to the history. I shall describe this phase presently.

(*B*) The manifest illness. A psychosis of a peculiar kind, paraphasia, a convergent squint, severe disturbances of vision, paralyses (in the form of contractures), complete in the right upper and both lower extremities, partial in the left upper extremity, paresis of the neck muscles. A gradual reduction of the contracture to the right-hand extremities. Some improvement, interrupted by a severe psychical trauma (the death of the patient's father) in April, after which there followed

(*C*) A period of persisting somnambulism, subsequently alternating with more normal states. A number of chronic symptoms persisted till December, 1881.

(*D*) Gradual cessation of the pathological states and symptoms up to June, 1882.

In July, 1880, the patient's father, of whom she was passionately fond, fell ill of a peripleuritic abscess which failed to clear up and to which he succumbed in April, 1881. During the first months of the illness Anna devoted her whole energy to nursing her father, and no one was much surprised when by degrees her own health greatly deteriorated. No one, perhaps not even the patient herself, knew what was happening to her; but eventually the state of weakness, anaemia and distaste for food became so bad that to her great sorrow she was no longer allowed to continue nursing the patient. The immediate cause of this was a very severe cough, on account of which I examined her for the first time. It was a typical *tussis nervosa*. She soon began to display a marked craving for rest during the afternoon, followed in the evening by a sleep-like state and afterwards a highly excited condition.

At the beginning of December a convergent squint appeared. An ophthalmic surgeon explained this (mistakenly) as being due to paresis of one abducens. On December 11 the patient took to her bed and remained there until April 1.

There developed in rapid succession a series of severe disturbances which were *apparently* quite new: left-sided occipital headache; convergent squint (diplopia), markedly increased by excitement; complaints that the walls of the room seemed to be falling over (affection of the obliquus); disturbances of vision which it was hard to analyse; paresis of the muscles of the front of the neck, so that finally the patient could only move her head by pressing it backwards between her raised shoulders and moving her whole back; contracture and anaesthesia of the right upper, and, after a time, of the right lower extremity. The latter was fully extended, adducted and rotated inwards. Later the same symptom appeared in the left lower extremity and finally in the left arm, of which, however, the fingers to some extent retained the power of movement. So, too, there was no complete rigidity in the shoulder-joints. The contracture reached its maximum in the muscles of the upper arms. In the same way, the region of the elbows turned out to be the most affected by anaesthesia when, at a later stage, it became possible to make a more careful test of this. At the beginning of the illness the anaesthesia could not be efficiently tested, owing to the patient's resistance arising from feelings of anxiety.

It was while the patient was in this condition that I undertook her treatment, and I at once recognized the seriousness of the psychical disturbance with which I had to deal. Two entirely distinct states of consciousness were present which alternated very frequently and without warning and which became more and more differentiated in the course of the illness. In one of these states she recognized her surroundings; she was melancholy and anxious, but relatively normal. In the other state she hallucinated and was 'naughty'—that is to say, she was abusive, used to throw the cushions at people, so far as the contractures at various times allowed, tore buttons off her bed-clothes and linen with those of her fingers which she could move, and so on. At this stage of her illness if something had been moved in the room or someone had entered or left it [during her other state of consciousness] she would complain of having 'lost' some time and would remark upon the gap in her train of conscious thoughts. Since those about her tried to deny this and to soothe her when she complained that she was going mad, she would, after throwing the pillows about, accuse people of doing things to her and leaving her in a muddle, etc.

These *'absences'* had already been observed before she took to her bed; she used then to stop in the middle of a sentence, repeat her last words and after a short pause go on talking. These interruptions gradually increased till they reached the dimensions that have just been described; and during the climax of the illness, when the contractures had extended to the left side of her body, it was only for a short time during the day that she was to any degree normal. But the disturbances invaded even her moments of relatively clear consciousness. There were extremely rapid changes of mood leading to excessive but quite temporary high spirits, and at other times severe anxiety, stubborn opposition to every therapeutic effort and frightening hallucinations of black snakes, which was how she saw her hair, ribbons and similar things. At the same time she kept on telling herself not to be so silly: what she was seeing was really only her hair, etc. At moments when her mind was quite clear she would complain of the profound darkness in her head, of not being able to think, of becoming blind and deaf, of having two selves, a real one and an evil one which forced her to behave badly, and so on.

In the afternoons she would fall into a somnolent state which lasted till about an hour after sunset. She would then wake up and complain that something was tormenting her—or rather, she would keep repeating in the impersonal form 'tormenting, tormenting.' For alongside of the development of the contractures there appeared a deep-going functional disorganization of her speech. It first became noticeable that she was at a loss to find words, and this difficulty gradually increased. Later she lost her command of grammar and syntax; she no longer conjugated verbs, and eventually she used only infinitives, for the most part incorrectly formed from weak past participles; and she omitted both the definite and indefinite article. In the process of time she became almost completely deprived of words. She put them together laboriously out of four or five languages and became almost unintelligible. When she tried to write (until her contractures entirely prevented her doing so) she employed the same jargon. For two weeks she became completely dumb and in spite of making great and continuous efforts to speak she was unable to say a syllable. And now for the first time the psychical mechanism of the disorder became clear. As I knew, she had felt very much offended over something and had determined not to speak about it. When I guessed this and obliged her to talk about it, the inhibition, which had made any other kind of utterance impossible as well, disappeared.

This change coincided with a return of the power of movement to the extremities of the left side of her body, in March, 1881. Her paraphasia receded; but thenceforward she spoke only in English—apparently, however, without knowing that she was doing so. She had disputes with her nurse who was, of course, unable to understand her. It was only some months later that I was able to convince her that she was talking English. Nevertheless, she herself could still understand the people about her who talked German. Only in moments of extreme anxiety did her power of speech desert her entirely, or else she would use a mixture of all sorts of languages. At times when she was at her very best and most free, she talked French and Italian. There was complete amnesia between these times and those at which she talked English. At this point, too, her squint began to diminish and made its appearance only at moments of great excitement. She was once again able to support her head. On the first of April she got up for the first time.

On the fifth of April her adored father died. During her illness she had seen him very rarely and for short periods. This was the most severe psychical trauma that she could possibly have experienced. A violent outburst of excitement was succeeded by profound stupor which lasted about two days and from which she emerged in a greatly changed state. At first she was far quieter and her feelings of anxiety were much diminished. The contracture of her right arm and leg persisted as well as their anaesthesia, though this was not deep. There was a high degree of restriction of the field of vision: in a bunch of flowers which gave her much pleasure she could only see one flower at a time. She complained of not being able to recognize people. Normally, she said, she had been able to recognize faces without having to make any deliberate effort; now she was obliged to do laborious 'recognizing work' and had to say to herself 'this person's nose is such-and-such, his hair is such-and-such, so he must be so-and-so.' All the people she saw seemed like wax figures without any connection with her. She found the presence of some of her close relatives very distressing and this negative attitude grew continually stronger. If someone whom she was ordinarily pleased to see came into the room, she would recognize him and would be aware of things for a short time, but would soon sink back into her own broodings and her visitor was blotted out. I was the only person whom she always recognized when I came in; so long as I was talking to her she was always in contact with things and lively, except for the sudden interruptions caused by one of her hallucinatory 'absences.'

She now spoke only English and could not understand what was said to her in German. Those about her were obliged to talk to her in English; even the nurse learned to make herself to some extent understood in this way. She was, however, able to read French and Italian. If she had to read one of these aloud, what she produced, with extraordinary fluency, was an admirable extempore English translation.

She began writing again, but in a peculiar fashion. She wrote with her left hand, the less stiff one, and she used Roman printed letters, copying the alphabet from her edition of Shakespeare.

She had eaten extremely little previously, but now she refused nourishment altogether. However, she allowed me to feed her, so that she very soon began to take more food. But she never consented to eat bread. After her meal she invariably rinsed out her mouth and even did so if, for any reason, she had not eaten anything—which shows how absent-minded she was about such things.

Her somnolent states in the afternoon and her deep sleep after sunset persisted. If, after this, she had talked herself out (I shall have to explain what is meant by this later) she was clear in mind, calm and cheerful.

This comparatively tolerable state did not last long. Some ten days after her father's death a consultant was brought in, whom, like all strangers, she completely ignored while I demonstrated all her peculiarities to him. 'That's like an examination,' she said, laughing, when I got her to read a French text aloud in English. The other physician intervened in the conversation and tried to attract her attention, but in vain. It was a genuine 'negative hallucination' of the kind which has since so often been produced experimentally. In the end he succeeded in breaking through it by blowing smoke in her face. She suddenly saw a stranger before her, rushed to the door to take away the key and fell unconscious to the ground. There followed a short fit of anger and then a severe attack of anxiety which I had great difficulty in calming down. Unluckily I had to leave Vienna that evening, and when I came back several days later I found the patient much worse. She had gone entirely without food the whole time, was full of anxiety and her hallucinatory *absences* were filled with terrifying figures, death's heads and skeletons. Since she acted these things through as though she was experiencing them and in part put them into words, the people around her became aware to a great extent of the content of these hallucinations.

The regular order of things was: the somnolent state in the afternoon, followed after sunset by the deep hypnosis for which she invented the technical name of 'clouds.' If during this she was able to narrate the hallucinations she had had in the course of the day, she would wake up clear in mind, calm and cheerful. She would sit down to work and write or draw far into the night quite rationally. At about four she would go to bed. Next day the whole series of events would be repeated. It was a truly remarkable contrast: in the day-time the irresponsible patient pursued by hallucinations, and at night the girl with her mind completely clear.

In spite of her euphoria at night, her psychical condition deteriorated steadily. Strong suicidal impulses appeared which made it seem inadvisable for her to continue living on the third floor. Against her will, therefore, she was transferred to a country house in the neighbourhood of Vienna (on June 7, 1881). I had never threatened her with this removal from her home, which she regarded with horror, but she herself had, without saying so, expected and dreaded it. This event made it clear once more how much the affect of anxiety dominated her psychical disorder. Just as after her father's death a calmer condition had set in, so now, when what she feared had actually taken place, she once more became calmer. Nevertheless, the move was immediately followed by three days and nights completely without sleep or nourishment, by numerous attempts at suicide (though, so long as she was in a garden, these were not dangerous), by smashing windows and so on, and by hallucinations unaccompanied by *absences*—which she was able to distinguish easily from her other hallucinations. After this she grew quieter, let the nurse feed her and even took chloral at night.

Before continuing my account of the case, I must go back once more and describe one of its peculiarities which I have hitherto mentioned only in passing. I have already said that throughout the illness up to this point the patient fell into a somnolent state every afternoon and that after sunset this period passed into a deeper sleep—'clouds.' (It seems plausible to attribute this regular sequence of events merely to her experience while she was nursing her father, which she had had to do for several months. During the nights she had watched by the patient's bedside or had been awake anxiously listening till the morning; in the afternoons she had lain down for a short rest, as is the usual habit of nurses. This pattern of waking at night and sleeping in the afternoons seems to have been carried over into her own illness and to have persisted long after the sleep had been replaced by a hypnotic state.) After the deep sleep had lasted about an hour she grew restless, tossed to and fro and kept repeating 'tormenting, tormenting,' with her eyes shut all the time. It was also noticed how, during her *absences* in day-time she was obviously creating some situation or episode to which she gave a clue with a few muttered words. It happened then—to begin with accidentally but later intentionally—that someone near her repeated one of these phrases of hers while she was complaining about the 'tormenting.' She at once joined in and began to paint some situation or tell some story, hesitatingly at first and in her paraphasic jargon; but the longer she went on the more fluent she became, till at last she was speaking quite correct German. (This applies to the early period before she began talking English only.) The stories were always sad and some of them very charming, in the style of Hans Andersen's *Picture-book without Pictures,* and, indeed, they were probably constructed on that model. As a rule their starting-point or central situation was of a girl anxiously sitting by a sickbed. But she also built up her stories on quite other topics.—A few moments after she had finished her narrative she would wake up, obviously calmed down, or, as she called it, *'gehäglich.'* During the night she would again become restless, and in the morning, after a couple of hours' sleep, she was visibly involved in some other set of ideas.—If for any reason she was unable to tell me the story during her evening hypnosis she failed to calm down afterwards, and on the following day she had to tell me *two* stories in order for this to happen.

The essential features of this phenomenon—the mounting up and intensification of her *absences* into her auto-hypnosis in the evening, the effect of the products of her imagination as psychical stimuli and the easing and removal of her state of stimulation when she gave utterance to them in her hypnosis—remained constant throughout the whole eighteen months during which she was under observation.

The stories naturally became still more tragic after her father's death. It was not, however, until the deterioration of her mental condition, which followed when her state of somnambulism was forcibly broken into in the way already described, that her evening narratives ceased to have the character of more or less freely-created poetical compositions and changed into a string of frightful and terrifying hallucinations. (It was already possible to arrive at these from the patient's behaviour during the day.) I have already described how completely her mind was relieved when, shaking with fear and horror, she had reproduced these frightful images and given verbal utterance to them.

While she was in the country, when I was unable to pay her daily visits, the situation developed as follows. I used to visit her in the evening, when I knew I should find her in her hypnosis, and I then relieved her of the whole stock of imaginative products which she had accumulated since my last visit. It was essential that this should be effected completely if good results were to follow. When this was done she became perfectly calm, and next day she would be agreeable, easy to manage, industrious and even cheerful; but on the second day she would be increasingly moody, contrary and unpleasant, and this would become still more marked on the third day. When she was like this it was not always easy to get her to talk, even in her hypnosis. She aptly described this procedure, speaking seriously, as a 'talking cure,' while she referred to it jokingly as 'chimney-sweeping.' She knew that after she had given utterance to her hallucinations she would lose all her obstinacy and what she described as her 'energy'; and when, after some comparatively long interval, she was in a bad temper, she would refuse to talk, and I was obliged to overcome her unwillingness by urging and pleading and using devices such as repeating a formula with which she was in the habit of introducing her stories. But she would never begin to talk until she had satisfied herself of my identity by carefully feeling my hands. On those nights on which she had not been calmed by verbal utterance it was necessary to fall back upon chloral. I had tried it on a few earlier occasions, but I was obliged to give her 5 grammes, and sleep was preceded by a state of intoxication which lasted for some hours. When I was present this state was euphoric, but in my absence it was highly disagreeable and characterized by anxiety as well as excitement. (It may be remarked incidentally that this severe state of intoxication made no difference to her contractures.) I had been able to avoid the use of narcotics, since the verbal utterance of her hallucinations calmed her even though it might not induce sleep; but when she was in the country the nights on which she had not obtained hypnotic relief were so unbearable that in spite of everything it was necessary to have recourse to chloral. But it became possible gradually to reduce the dose.

The persisting somnambulism did not return. But on the other hand the alternation between two states of consciousness persisted. She used to hallucinate in the middle of a conversation, run off, start climbing up a tree, etc. If one caught hold of her, she would very quickly take up her interrupted sentence without knowing anything about what had happened in the interval. All these hallucinations, however, came up and were reported on in her hypnosis.

A year had now passed since she had been separated from her father and had taken to her bed, and from this time on her condition became clearer and was systematized in a very peculiar manner. Her alternating states of consciousness, which were characterized by the fact that, from morning onwards, her *absences* (that is to say, the emergence of her *condition seconde*) always became more frequent as the day advanced and took entire possession by the evening—these alternating states had differed from each other previously in that one (the first) was normal and the second alienated; now, however, they differed further in that in the first she lived, like the rest of us, in the winter of 1881–2, whereas in the second she lived in the winter of 1880–1, and had completely forgotten all the subsequent events. The one thing that nevertheless seemed to remain conscious most of the time was the fact that her father had died. She was carried back to the previous year with such intensity that in the new house she hallucinated her old room, so that when she wanted to go to the door she knocked up against the stove which stood in the same relation to the window as the door did in the old room. . . . [S]he lived through the previous winter day by day. I should only have been able to *suspect* that this was happening, had it not been that every evening during the hypnosis she talked through whatever it was that had excited her on the same day in 1881, and had it not been that a private diary kept by her mother in 1881 confirmed beyond a doubt the occurrence of the underlying events. This re-living of the previous year continued till the illness came to its final close in June, 1882.

Her evening hypnosis was thus heavily burdened, for we had to talk off not only her contemporary imaginative products but also the events and 'vexations' of 1881.

But in addition to all this the work that had to be done by the patient and her physician was immensely increased by a third group of separate disturbances which had to be disposed of in the same manner. These were the psychical events involved in the period of incubation of the illness between July and December, 1880; it was they that had produced the whole of the hysterical phenomena, and when they were brought to verbal utterance the symptoms disappeared.

When this happened for the first time—when, as a result of an accidental and spontaneous utterance of this kind, during the evening hypnosis, a disturbance which had persisted for a considerable time vanished—I was greatly surprised. It was in the summer during a period of extreme heat, and the patient was suffering very badly from thirst; for, without being able to account for it in any way, she suddenly found it impossible to drink. She would take up the glass of water she longed for, but as soon as it touched her lips she would push it away like someone suffering from hydrophobia. As she did this, she was obviously in an *absence* for a couple of seconds. She lived only on fruit, such as melons, etc., so as to lessen her tormenting thirst. This had lasted for some six weeks, when one day during hypnosis she grumbled about her English lady-companion whom she did not care for, and went on to describe, with every sign of disgust, how she had once gone into that lady's room and how her little dog—horrid creature!—had drunk out of a glass there. The patient had said nothing, as she had wanted to be polite. After giving further energetic expression to the anger she had held back, she asked for something to drink, drank a large quantity of water without any difficulty and woke from her hypnosis with the glass at her lips; and thereupon the disturbance vanished, never to return. A number of extremely obstinate whims were similarly removed after she had described the experiences which had given rise to them. She took a great step forward when the first of her chronic symptoms disappeared in the same way—the contracture of her right leg, which, it is true, had already diminished a great deal. These findings—that in the case of this patient the hysterical phenomena disappeared as soon as the event which had given rise to them was reproduced in her hypnosis—made it possible to arrive at a therapeutic technical procedure which left nothing to be desired in its logical consistency and systematic application. Each individual symptom in this complicated case was taken separately in hand; all the occasions on which it had appeared were described in reverse order, starting before the time when the patient became bed-ridden and going back to the event which had led to its first appearance. When this had been described the symptom was permanently removed.

In this way her paralytic contractures and anaesthesias, disorders of vision and hearing of every sort, neuralgias, coughing, tremors, etc., and finally her disturbances of speech were 'talked away.' Amongst the disorders of vision, the following, for instance, were disposed of separately: the convergent squint with diplopia; deviation of both eyes to the right, so that when her hand reached out for something it always went to the left of the object; restriction of the visual field; central amblyopia; macropsia; seeing a death's head instead of her father; inability to read. Only a few scattered phenomena (such, for instance, as the extension of the paralytic contractures to the left side of her body) which had developed while she was confined to bed, were untouched by this process of analysis, and it is probable, indeed, that they had in fact no immediate psychical cause.

It turned out to be quite impracticable to shorten the work by trying to elicit in her memory straight away the first provoking cause of her symptoms. She was unable to find it, grew confused, and things proceeded even more slowly than if she was allowed quietly and steadily to follow back the thread of memories on which she had embarked. Since the latter method, however, took too long in the evening hypnosis, owing to her being over-strained and distraught by 'talking out' the two other sets of experiences—and owing, too, to the reminiscences needing time before they could attain sufficient vividness—we evolved the following procedure. I used to visit her in the morning and hypnotize her. (Very simple methods of doing this were arrived at empirically.) I would next ask her to concentrate her thoughts on the symptom we were treating at the moment and to tell me the occasions on which it had appeared. The patient would proceed to describe in rapid succession and under brief headings the external events concerned and these I would jot down. During her subsequent evening hypnosis she would then, with the help of my notes, give me a fairly detailed account of these circumstances.

The work of remembering was not always an easy matter and sometimes the patient had to make great efforts. On one occasion our whole progress was obstructed for some time because a recollection refused to emerge. It was a question of a particularly terrifying hallucination. While she was nursing her father she had seen him with a death's head. She and the people with her remembered that once, while she still appeared to be in good health, she had paid a visit to one of her relatives. She had opened the door and all at once fallen down unconscious. In order to get over the obstruction to our progress she visited the same place again and, on entering the room, again fell to the ground unconscious. During her subsequent evening hypnosis the obstacle was surmounted. As she came into the room, she had seen her pale face reflected in a mirror hanging opposite the door; but it was not herself that she saw but her father with a death's head.—We often noticed that her dread of a memory, as in the present instance, inhibited its emergence, and this had to be brought about forcibly by the patient or physician.

Since this laborious analysis for her symptoms dealt with the summer months of 1880, which was the preparatory period of her illness, I obtained complete insight into the incubation and pathogenesis of this case of hysteria, and I will now describe them briefly.

In July, 1880, while he was in the country, her father fell seriously ill of a sub-pleural abscess. Anna shared the duties of nursing him with her mother. She once woke up during the night in great anxiety about the patient, who was in a high fever; and she was under the strain of expecting the arrival of a surgeon from Vienna who was to operate. Her mother had gone away for a short time and Anna was sitting at the bedside with her right arm over the back of her chair. She fell into a waking dream and saw a black snake coming towards the sick man from the wall to bite him. (It is most likely that there were in fact snakes in the field behind the house and that these had previously given the girl a fright; they would thus have provided the material for her hallucination.) She tried to keep the snake off, but it was as though she was paralysed. Her right arm, over the back of the chair, had gone to sleep and had become anaesthetic and paretic; and when she looked at it the fingers turned into little snakes with death's heads (the nails). (It seems probable that she had tried to use her paralysed right arm to drive off the snake and that its anaesthesia and paralysis had consequently become associated with the hallucination of the snake.) When the snake vanished, in her terror she tried to pray. But language failed her: she could find no tongue in which to speak, till at last she thought of some children's verses in English and then found herself able to think and pray in that language. The whistle of the train that was bringing the doctor whom she expected broke the spell.

Next day, in the course of a game, she threw a quoit into some bushes; and when she went to pick it out, a bent branch revived her hallucination of the snake, and simultaneously her right arm became rigidly extended. Thenceforward the same thing invariably occurred whenever the hallucination was recalled by some object with a more or less snake-like appearance. This hallucination, however, as well as the contracture only appeared during the short *absences* which became more and more frequent from that night onwards.

Some of her symptoms, however, seem not to have emerged in her *absences* but merely in an affect during her waking life; but if so, they recurred in just the same way. Thus we were able to trace back all of her different disturbances of vision to different, more or less clearly determining causes. For instance, on one occasion, when she was sitting by her father's bedside with tears in her eyes, he suddenly asked her what time it was. She could not see clearly; she made a great effort, and brought her watch near to her eyes. The face of the watch now seemed very big—thus accounting for her macropsia and convergent squint. Or again, she tried hard to suppress her tears so that the sick man should not see them.

A dispute, in the course of which she suppressed a rejoinder, caused a spasm of the glottis, and this was repeated on every similar occasion.

I cannot feel much regret that the incompleteness of my notes makes it impossible for me to enumerate all the occasions on which her various hysterical symptoms appeared. She herself told me them in every single case, with the one exception I have mentioned; and, as I have already said, each symptom disappeared after she had described its first occurrence.

In this way, too, the whole illness was brought to a close. The patient herself had formed a strong determination that the whole treatment should be finished by the anniversary of the day on which she was moved into the country. At the beginning of June, accordingly, she entered into the 'talking cure' with the greatest energy. On the last day—by the help of re-arranging the room so as to resemble her father's sickroom—she reproduced the terrifying hallucination which I have described above and which constituted the root of her whole illness. During the original scene she had only been able to think and pray in English; but immediately after its reproduction she was able to speak German. She was moreover free from the innumerable disturbances which she had previously exhibited. After this she left Vienna and travelled for a while; but it was a considerable time before she regained her mental balance entirely. Since then she has enjoyed complete health.

Although I have suppressed a large number of quite interesting details, this case history of Anna O. has grown bulkier than would seem to be required for a hysterical illness that was not in itself of an unusual character. It was, however, impossible to describe the case without entering into details, and its features seem to me of sufficient importance to excuse this extensive report. The interest of the present case seems to me above all to reside in the extreme clarity and intelligibility of its pathogenesis.

There were two psychical characteristics present in the girl while she was still completely healthy which acted as predisposing causes for her subsequent hysterical illness:

(1) Her monotonous family life and the absence of adequate intellectual occupation left her with an unemployed surplus of mental liveliness and energy, and this found an outlet in the constant activity of her imagination.

(2) This led to a habit of day-dreaming (her 'private theatre'), which laid the foundations for a dissociation of her mental personality. Nevertheless a dissociation of this degree is still within the bounds of normality. Reveries and reflections during a more or less mechanical occupation do not in themselves imply a pathological splitting of consciousness, since if they are interrupted—if, for instance, the subject is spoken to—the normal unity of consciousness is restored; nor, presumably, is any amnesia present. In the case of Anna O., however, this habit prepared the ground upon which the affect of anxiety and dread was able to establish itself in the way I have described, when once that affect had transformed the patient's habitual day-dreaming into a hallucinatory *absence*. But hitherto this only occurred for fleeting moments. Before the patient took permanently to her bed she had already developed

the whole assemblage of hysterical phenomena, without anyone knowing it. It was only after the patient had broken down completely owing to exhaustion brought about by lack of nourishment, insomnia and constant anxiety, and only after she had begun to pass more time in her *condition seconde* than in her normal state, that the hysterical phenomena extended to the latter as well and changed from intermittent acute symptoms into chronic ones.

The question now arises how far the patient's statements are to be trusted and whether the occasions and mode of origin of the phenomena were really as she represented them. So far as the more important and fundamental events are concerned, the trustworthiness of her account seems to me to be beyond question. As regards the symptoms disappearing after being 'talked away,' I cannot use this as evidence; it may very well be explained by suggestion. But I always found the patient entirely truthful and trustworthy. The things she told me were intimately bound up with what was most sacred to her. Whatever could be checked by other people was fully confirmed.

. . . [I]n the present case, too, the story of the development of the illness would have remained completely unknown alike to the patient and the physician if it had not been for her peculiarity of remembering things in hypnosis, as I have described, and of relating what she remembered. While she was in her waking state she knew nothing of all this. Thus it is impossible to arrive at what is happening in other cases from an examination of the patients while in a waking state, for with the best will in the world they can give one no information. And I have already pointed out how little those surrounding the present patient were able to observe of what was going on. Accordingly, it would only be possible to discover the state of affairs in other patients by means of some such procedure as was provided in the case of Anna O. by her auto-hypnoses.

Throughout the entire illness her two states of consciousness persisted side by side: the primary one in which she was quite normal psychically, and the secondary one which may well be likened to a dream in view of its wealth of imaginative products and hallucinations, its large gaps of memory and the lack of inhibition and control in its associations. In this secondary state the patient was in a condition of alienation. The fact that the patient's mental condition was entirely dependent on the intrusion of this secondary state into the normal one seems to throw considerable light on at least one class of hysterical psychosis. Every one of her hypnoses in the evening afforded evidence that the patient was entirely clear and well-ordered in her mind and normal as regards her feeling and volition so long as none of the products of her secondary state was acting as a stimulus 'in the unconscious.'

It is hard to avoid expressing the situation by saying that the patient was split into two personalities of which one was mentally normal and the other insane. The sharp division between the two states in the present patient only exhibits more clearly, in my opinion, what has given rise to a number of unexplained problems in many other hysterical patients. It was especially noticeable in Anna O. how much the products of her 'bad self,' as she herself called it, affected her moral habit of mind. If these products had not been continually disposed of, we should have been faced by a hysteric of the malicious type—refractory, lazy, disagreeable and ill-natured; but, as it was, after the removal of those stimuli her true character, which was the opposite of all these, always reappeared at once.

Nevertheless, though her two states were thus sharply separated, not only did the secondary state intrude into the first one, but—and this was at all events frequently true, and even when she was in a very bad condition—a clear-sighted and calm observer sat, as she put it, in a corner of her brain and looked on at all the mad business. This persistence of clear thinking while the psychosis was actually going on found expression in a very curious way. At a time when, after the hysterical phenomena had ceased, the patient was passing through a temporary depression, she brought up a number of childish fears and self-reproaches, and among them the idea that she had not been ill at all and that the whole business had been simulated. Similar observations, as we know, have frequently been made. When a disorder of this kind has cleared up and the two states of consciousness have once more become merged into one, the patients, looking back to the past, see themselves as the single undivided personality which was aware of all the nonsense; they think they could have prevented it if they had wanted to, and thus they feel as though they had done all the mischief deliberately.

I have already described the astonishing fact that from beginning to end of the illness all the stimuli arising from the secondary state, together with their consequences, were permanently removed by being given verbal utterance in hypnosis, and I have only to add an assurance that this was not an invention of mine which I imposed on the patient by suggestion. It took me completely by surprise, and not until symptoms had been got rid of in this way in a whole series of instances did I develop a therapeutic technique out of it.

Darkness Visible: A Memoir of Madness

Born in Newport News, Virginia, William Styron served as first lieutenant in the United States Marine Corps during World War II and received his B.A. from Duke University in 1947. Shortly after this, he moved to New York City to take the post of associate editor at McGraw-Hill and to study writing at the New School for Social Research, publishing his first novel, *Lie Down in Darkness,* in 1951. Two years later, he married Rose Burgunder, starting a family that would grow to include four children. In 1967, he published his Pulitzer Prize–winning novel, *The Confessions of Nat Turner,* a "meditation on history" based on the transcript of a slave's testimony that recounted the short-lived revolt he had led against his Virginia owners. Styron's next success came with *Sophie's Choice,* a novel set in post–World War II Brooklyn that examined the insidious reverberations set off by the Holocaust in the emotional lives and relationships of several characters. These two novels exemplify Styron's focus on the psychodynamics of suffering, a subject he explores with devastating force and clarity in *Darkness Visible: A Memoir of Madness* (1990). An account of a serious depressive illness that overtook him in October of 1985, the memoir describes what Styron calls his psychic "meltdown," from its early signs in June of that year to his hospitalization in December and his recovery in February of 1986. Beginning as a lecture Styron gave at a symposium on affective disorders organized by the Department of Psychiatry at the Johns Hopkins University School of Medicine, *Darkness Visible* evolved into the retelling of an ageless story: the hero's descent into the infernal regions of the underworld. Continuing this tradition, Styron's memoir takes its place in a narrative continuum that has shaped the individual's quest for self-understanding since the beginnings of Western civilization.

The storm which swept me into a hospital in December began as a cloud no bigger than a wine goblet the previous June. And the cloud—the manifest crisis—involved alcohol, a substance I had been abusing for forty years. Like a great many American writers, whose sometimes lethal addiction to alcohol has become so legendary as to provide in itself a stream of studies and books, I used alcohol as the magical conduit to fantasy and euphoria, and to the enhancement of the imagination. There is no need to either rue or apologize for my use of this soothing, often sublime agent, which had contributed greatly to my writing; although I never set down a line while under its influence, I did use it—often in conjunction with music—as a means to let my mind conceive visions that the unaltered, sober brain has no access to. Alcohol

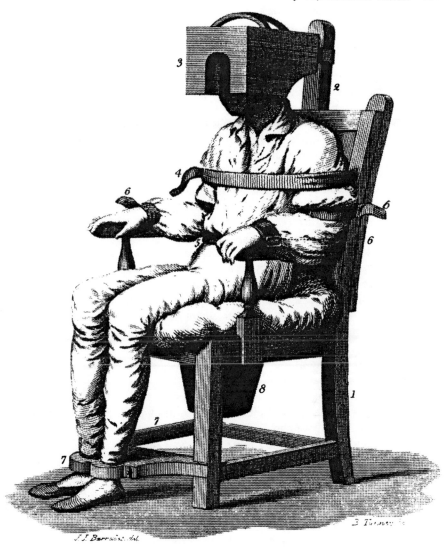

Rush's "Tranquillizer"

15. Engraving of Benjamin Rush's restraint chair from J. J. Barralet and Del. B. Tanner, Observations on the Tranquillizer *(Philadelphia, 1811). Designed to calm the madman, the "tranquillizer" virtually immobilized and literally effaced the patient. Among the most famous icons of restraint in the nineteenth-century treatment of the insane, Rush's chair was one of many devices, including the "maniac's bed" and the "English camisole" or straitjacket, that replaced the use of chains.*

was an invaluable senior partner of my intellect, besides being a friend whose ministrations I sought daily—sought also, I now see, as a means to calm the anxiety and incipient dread that I had hidden away for so long somewhere in the dungeons of my spirit.

The trouble was, at the beginning of this particular summer, that I was betrayed. It struck me quite suddenly, almost overnight: I could no longer drink. It was as if my body had risen up in protest, along with my mind, and had conspired to reject this daily mood bath which it had so long welcomed and, who knows? perhaps even come to need. Many drinkers have experienced this intolerance as they have grown older. I suspect that the crisis was at least partly metabolic—the liver rebelling, as if to say, "No more, no more"—but at any rate I discovered that alcohol in minuscule amounts, even a mouthful of wine, caused me nausea, a desperate and unpleasant wooziness, a sinking sensation and ultimately a distinct revulsion. The comforting friend had abandoned me not gradually and reluctantly, as a true friend might do, but like a shot—and I was left high and certainly dry, and unhelmed.

It was not really alarming at first, since the change was subtle, but I did notice that my surroundings took on a different tone at certain times: the shadows of nightfall seemed more somber, my mornings were less buoyant, walks in the woods became less zestful, and there was a moment during my working hours in the late afternoon when a kind of panic and anxiety overtook me, just for a few minutes, accompanied by a visceral queasiness—such a seizure was at least slightly alarming, after all. As I set down these recollections, I realize that it should have been plain to me that I was already in the grip of the beginning of a mood disorder, but I was ignorant of such a condition at that time.

By now I had moved back to my house in Connecticut. It was October, and one of the unforgettable features of this stage of my disorder was the way in which my old farmhouse, my beloved home for thirty years, took on for me at that point when my spirits regularly sank to their nadir an almost palpable quality of ominousness. The fading evening light—akin to that famous "slant of light" of Emily Dickinson's, which spoke to her of death, of chill extinction—had none of its familiar autumnal loveliness, but ensnared me in a suffocating gloom. I wondered how this friendly place, teeming with such memories of (again in her words) "Lads and Girls," of "laughter and ability and Sighing, / And Frocks and Curls," could almost perceptibly seem so hostile and forbidding. Physically, I was not alone. As always Rose was present and listened with unflagging patience to my complaints. But I felt an immense and aching solitude. I could no longer concentrate during those afternoon hours, which for years had been my working time, and the act of writing itself, becoming more and more difficult and exhausting, stalled, then finally ceased.

There were also dreadful, pouncing seizures of anxiety. One bright day on a walk through the woods with my dog I heard a flock of Canada geese honking high above trees ablaze with foliage; ordinarily a sight and sound that would have exhilarated me, the flight of birds caused me to stop, riveted with fear, and I stood stranded there, helpless, shivering, aware for the first time that I had been stricken by no mere pangs of withdrawal but by a serious illness whose name and actuality I was able finally to acknowledge. Going home, I couldn't rid my mind of the line of

Baudelaire's, dredged up from the distant past, that for several days had been skittering around at the edge of my consciousness: "I have felt the wind of the wing of madness."

Our perhaps understandable modern need to dull the sawtooth edges of so many of the afflictions we are heir to has led us to banish the harsh old-fashioned words: madhouse, asylum, insanity, melancholia, lunatic, madness. But never let it be doubted that depression, in its extreme form, is madness. The madness results from an aberrant biochemical process. It has been established with reasonable certainty (after strong resistance from many psychiatrists, and not all that long ago) that such madness is chemically induced amid the neurotransmitters of the brain, probably as the result of systemic stress, which for unknown reasons causes a depletion of the chemicals norepinephrine and serotonin, and the increase of a hormone, cortisol. With all of this upheaval in the brain tissues, the alternate drenching and deprivation, it is no wonder that the mind begins to feel aggrieved, stricken, and the muddied thought processes register the distress of an organ in convulsion. Sometimes, though not very often, such a disturbed mind will turn to violent thoughts regarding others. But with their minds turned agonizingly inward, people with depression are usually dangerous only to themselves. The madness of depression is, generally speaking, the antithesis of violence. It is a storm indeed, but a storm of murk. Soon evident are the slowed-down responses, near paralysis, psychic energy throttled back close to zero. Ultimately, the body is affected and feels sapped, drained.

That fall, as the disorder gradually took full possession of my system, I began to conceive that my mind itself was like one of those outmoded small-town telephone exchanges, being gradually inundated by floodwaters: one by one, the normal circuits began to drown, causing some of the functions of the body and nearly all of those of instinct and intellect to slowly disconnect. My few hours of sleep were usually terminated at three or four in the morning, when I stared up into yawning darkness, wondering and writhing at the devastation taking place in my mind, and awaiting the dawn, which usually permitted me a feverish, dreamless nap. I'm fairly certain that it was during one of these insomniac trances that there came over me the knowledge—a weird and shocking revelation, like that of some long-beshrouded metaphysical truth—that this condition would cost me my life if it continued on such a course.

I had now reached that phase of the disorder where all sense of hope had vanished, along with the idea of a futurity; my brain, in thrall to its outlaw hormones, had become less an organ of thought than an instrument registering, minute by minute, varying degrees of its own suffering. The mornings themselves were becoming bad now as I wandered about lethargic, following my synthetic sleep, but afternoons were still the worst, beginning at about three o'clock, when I'd feel the horror, like some poisonous fogbank, roll in upon my mind, forcing me into bed. There I would lie for as long as six hours, stuporous and virtually paralyzed, gazing at the ceiling and waiting for that moment of evening when, mysteriously, the crucifixion would ease up just enough to allow me to force down some food and then, like an automaton, seek an hour or two of sleep again. Why wasn't I in a hospital?

When we endure severe discomfort of a physical nature our conditioning has taught us since childhood to make accommodations to the pain's demands—to accept it, whether pluckily or whimpering and complaining, according to our personal degree of stoicism, but in any case to accept it. Except in intractable terminal pain, there is almost always some form of relief; we look forward to that alleviation, whether it be through sleep or Tylenol or self-hypnosis or a change of posture or, most often, through the body's capacity for healing itself, and we embrace this eventual respite as the natural reward we receive for having been, temporarily, such good sports and doughty sufferers, such optimistic cheerleaders for life at heart.

In depression this faith in deliverance, in ultimate restoration, is absent. The pain is unrelenting, and what makes the condition intolerable is the foreknowledge that no remedy will come—not in a day, an hour, a month, or a minute. If there is mild relief, one knows that it is only temporary; more pain will follow. It is hopelessness even more than pain that crushes the soul. So the decision-making of daily life involves not, as in normal affairs, shifting from one annoying situation to another less annoying—or from discomfort to relative comfort, or from boredom to activity—but moving from pain to pain. One does not abandon, even briefly, one's bed of nails, but is attached to it wherever one goes. And this results in a striking experience—one which I have called, borrowing military terminology, the situation of the walking wounded. For in virtually any other serious sickness, a patient who felt similar devastation would be lying flat in bed, possibly sedated and hooked up to the tubes and wires of life-support systems, but at the very least in a posture of repose and in an isolated setting. His invalidism would be necessary, unquestioned and honorably attained. However, the sufferer from depression has no such option and therefore finds himself, like a walking casualty of war, thrust into the most intolerable social and family situations. There he must, despite the anguish devouring his brain, present a face approximating the one that is associated with ordinary events and companionship. He must try to utter small talk, and be responsive to questions, and knowingly nod and frown and, God help him, even smile. But it is a fierce trial attempting to speak a few simple words.

That December evening, for example, I could have remained in bed as usual during those worst hours, or agreed to the dinner party my wife had arranged downstairs. But the very idea of a decision was academic. Either course was torture, and I chose the dinner not out of any particular merit but through indifference to what I knew would be indistinguishable ordeals of fogbound horror. At dinner I was barely able to speak, but the quartet of guests, who were all good friends, were aware of my condition and politely ignored my catatonic muteness. Then, after dinner, sitting in the living room, I experienced a curious inner convulsion that I can describe only as despair beyond despair. It came out of the cold night; I did not think such anguish possible.

A phenomenon that a number of people have noted while in deep depression is the sense of being accompanied by a second self—a wraithlike observer who, not sharing the dementia of his double, is able to watch with dispassionate curiosity as his companion struggles against the oncoming disaster, or decides to embrace it. There is a theatrical quality about all this, and during the next several days, as I went about stolidly preparing for extinction, I couldn't shake off a sense of melodrama— a melodrama in which I, the victim-to-be of self-murder, was both the solitary actor and lone member of the audience. I had not as yet chosen the mode of my departure, but I knew that that step would come next, and soon, as inescapable as nightfall.

Late one bitterly cold night, when I knew that I could not possibly get myself through the following day, I sat in the living room of the house bundled up against the chill; something had happened to the furnace. My wife had gone to bed, and I had forced myself to watch the tape of a movie in which a young actress, who had been in a play of mine, was cast in a small part. At one point in the film, which was set in late-nineteenth-century Boston, the characters moved down the hallway of a music conservatory, beyond the walls of which, from unseen musicians, came a contralto voice, a sudden soaring passage from the Brahms *Alto Rhapsody.*

This sound, which like all music—indeed, like all pleasure—I had been numbly unresponsive to for months, pierced my heart like a dagger, and in a flood of swift recollection I thought of all the joys the house had known: the children who had rushed through its rooms, the festivals, the love and work, the honestly earned slumber, the voices and the nimble commotion, the perennial tribe of cats and dogs and birds, "laughter and ability and Sighing, / And Frocks and Curls." All this I realized was more than I could ever abandon, even as what I had set out so deliberately to do was more than I could inflict on those memories, and upon those, so close to me, with whom the memories were bound. And just as powerfully I realized I could not commit this desecration on myself. I drew upon some last gleam of sanity to perceive the terrifying dimensions of the mortal predicament I had fallen into. I woke up my wife and soon telephone calls were made. The next day I was admitted to the hospital.

I'm convinced I should have been in the hospital weeks before. For, in fact, the hospital was my salvation, and it is something of a paradox that in this austere place with its locked and wired doors and desolate green hallways—ambulances screeching night and day ten floors below—I found the repose, the assuagement of the tempest in my brain, that I was unable to find in my quiet farmhouse.

This is partly the result of sequestration, of safety, of being removed to a world in which the urge to pick up a knife and plunge it into one's own breast disappears in the newfound knowledge, quickly apparent even to the depressive's fuzzy brain, that the knife with which he is attempting to cut his dreadful Swiss steak is bendable plastic. But the hospital also offers the mild, oddly gratifying trauma of sudden stabilization—a transfer out of the too familiar surroundings of home, where all is anxiety and discord, into an orderly and benign detention where one's only duty is to try to get well. For me the real healers were seclusion and time.

Until the onslaught of my own illness and its denouement, I never gave much thought to my work in terms of its connection with the subconscious—an area of investigation belonging to literary detectives. But after I had returned to health and was able to reflect on the past in the light of my ordeal, I began to see clearly how depression had clung close to the outer edges of my life for many years. Suicide has been a persistent theme in my books—three of my major characters killed themselves. In rereading, for the first time in years, sequences from my novels—passages where my heroines have lurched down pathways toward doom—I was stunned to perceive how accurately I had created the landscape of depression in the minds of these young women, describing with what could only be instinct, out of a subconscious already roiled by disturbances of mood, the psychic imbalance that led them to destruction. Thus depression, when it finally came to me, was in fact no stranger, not even a visitor totally unannounced; it had been tapping at my door for decades.

The morbid condition proceeded, I have come to believe, from my beginning years—from my father, who battled the gorgon for much of his lifetime, and had been hospitalized in my boyhood after a despondent spiraling downward that in retrospect I saw greatly resembled mine. The genetic roots of depression seem now to be beyond controversy. But I'm persuaded that an even more significant factor was the death of my mother when I was thirteen; this disorder and early sorrow—the death or disappearance of a parent, especially a mother, before or during puberty—appears repeatedly in the literature on depression as a trauma sometimes likely to create nearly irreparable emotional havoc. The danger is especially apparent if the young person is affected by what has been termed "incomplete mourning"—has, in effect, been unable to achieve the catharsis of grief, and so carries within himself through later years an insufferable burden of which rage and guilt, and not only dammed-up sorrow, are a part, and become the potential seeds of self-destruction.

So if this theory of incomplete mourning has validity, and I think it does, and if it is also true that in the nethermost depths of one's suicidal behavior one is still subconsciously dealing with immense loss while trying to surmount all the effects of its devastation, then my own avoidance of death may have been belated homage to my mother. I do know that in those last hours before I rescued myself, when I listened to the passage from the *Alto Rhapsody*—which I'd heard her sing—she had been very much on my mind.

Since antiquity—in the tortured lament of Job, in the choruses of Sophocles and Aeschylus—chroniclers of the human spirit have been wrestling with a vocabulary that might give proper expression to the desolation of melancholia. Through the course of literature and art the theme of depression has run like a durable thread of woe.... The vast metaphor which most faithfully represents this fathomless ordeal, however, is that of Dante, and his all-too-familiar lines still arrest the imagination with their augury of the unknowable, the black struggle to come:

> In the middle of the journey of our life
> I found myself in a dark wood,
> For I had lost the right path.

One can be sure that these words have been more than once employed to conjure the ravages of melancholia, but their somber foreboding has often overshadowed the last lines of the best-known part of that poem, with their evocation of hope. To most of those who have experienced it, the horror of depression is so overwhelming as to be quite beyond expression, hence the frustrated sense of inadequacy found in the work of even the greatest artists.

But one need not sound the false or inspirational note to stress the truth that depression is not the soul's annihilation; men and women who have recovered from the disease—and they are countless—bear witness to what is probably its only saving grace: it is conquerable.

For those who have dwelt in depression's dark wood, and known its inexplicable agony, their return from the abyss is not unlike the ascent of the poet, trudging upward and upward out of hell's black depths and at last emerging into what he saw as "the shining world." There, whoever has been restored to health has almost always been restored to the capacity for serenity and joy, and this may be indemnity enough for having endured the despair beyond despair.

And so we came forth, and once again beheld the stars.

PART 5

The Contaminated and the Pure

"The Symptoms of Lepers"

The scant information we have about Jordan of Turre indicates that he was master of medicine at the University of Montpellier during the 1320s and that, as consulting physician there, he helped to draw up a regimen for a bishop in failing health. Jordan's treatise on leprosy borrows from past knowledge but also adds new information to the clinical "picture" of the disease. Although various aspects of leprosy were mentioned in early Latin commentaries, the first complete description of it in the West was given by Gilbert the Englishman in the mid–thirteenth century. Jordan's discussion of the condition also cites Arabic authorities but, unlike Gilbert's, focuses on identifying "universal signs" and diagnostic procedures rather than on cataloguing the various forms the disease was believed to take. Jordan's account of leprosy bears little resemblance to that of the condition depicted in the Bible, where "leprosy" is regarded as the bodily manifestation of sin, the visitation of God's punishment on the morally unclean. The model for many medical treatises on the subject, Leviticus, chapters 13 and 14, gives an exhaustive set of instructions for the proper detection and management of the affliction, but with one crucial difference: In ancient Jewish culture it was the priest, not the physician, who made the diagnosis and dictated the course of treatment.

Lepers can be recognized by five signs: by the urine, by the pulse, by the blood, by the voice, and by the different members. Whoever wants to determine whether someone has leprosy should first make him sing: If his voice is harsh, it may be a sign of leprosy, but if it is clear, it is a good sign. (Proceed as follows: take a tablet and write the good signs on one side and the bad signs on the other, and you will not become confused.)

It is also possible to judge by the urine, and this in four ways. First, the urine of lepers must be white with a certain transparency. Moreover, it must be clear and thin. As for the contents, they will be clotted and should look like flour or ground bran. Finally, if the urinal is shaken, it should make a sound; the reason is that while with fevered patients there would be no noise, because of the oiliness removed from the body, with lepers there will be, thanks to the earthiness and dryness of the matters contained in it.

It is also possible to recognize lepers by the pulse, which should be weak. Avicenna gives the reason for this, that it has little force because of the resistance of the artery, which is almost entirely dried up.

Similarly, they can be recognized by the blood. You should bleed the patient from

---

From *A Source Book in Medieval Science,* ed. Edward Grant (Cambridge, Mass.: Harvard University Press, 1974). Reprinted by permission.

a vein in any part of the body so that the blood is collected in a clean vessel; leave it until a residue is formed, which should be put into a linen cloth and shaken in fresh water; squeeze it gently until the water is no longer appreciably tinted. Then take what is left in the cloth after the squeezing, and if you see brilliant white corpuscles there, looking like millet or panicum, it is a sign of leprosy. Or put a large lump of salt in the liquid extracted from the blood; if it melts or dissolves, this is a good sign, but if not, if it remains whole, it is a sign of leprosy. The reason for this is that in leprous blood there is no good warm moistness able to dissolve it, only a thick earthiness by which it cannot be dissolved. Or pour strong vinegar onto the blood; if the vinegar foams, it is a sign of leprosy, just as when you pour it on the ground it foams, because of its dryness. Finally, you can pour urine onto the blood; if it sinks and mixes, it is a sign of leprosy, and if not, not. The reason for using urine and not some other liquid is that urine is a very subtle, penetrating substance and also has a greater suitability for use with blood, being its filtrate.

It is also possible to recognize lepers by examining the different members. First, because lepers have thin, fine hairs, so that they thicken at the roots; moreover, their hairs are pale and grey. This is due to the fact that the material from which the hairs are formed is lacking and cannot be exhaled through the pores, and because the pores are [almost] closed. It is advisable to examine the hairs in sunlight, to see if they are thin and straight, like pigs' bristles.

They are also recognized by the skin of the head, which is lumpy, so that one area is higher than the next; and by the lack of hair on the eyebrows, since lepers have no hair there, particularly at the corners; their brows have a curvature, seeming almost round and spherical. They are recognized, too, by the roundness of the eyeballs, which seem to be starting from their sockets, so that a leper's face is horrible to see; its natural expression being distorted, it is a terrible sight. These are the most obvious signs.

But it can also be recognized by a wound in the nostrils, which can be examined in the following manner. Cut a small wooden wand and fork it like tongs and introduce it into the nose, expanding it; then examine the interior with a lighted candle. If you see within an ulceration or excoriation in the deepest part of the nose, it is a sign of leprosy itself; this is a sign which is known not to all but to the wise only. Or it can be recognized by the bridge of the nose, where there should be a depression like a thread stretched lengthwise along it; for the cartilage which joins the two parts is eaten away, leaving a furrow.

They can also be recognized by the veins around the eyes and by the veins of the chest, which are very red, since the veins and arteries are bleached out by desiccation, while the blood is red, so that their red color is seen; for contraries stand out when juxtaposed. Or they can be recognized by the tongue. Draw out the tongue, using a cloth, and if you see white corpuscles at its root, like grains of millet, it is a sure sign of leprosy.

Having done all these things, you must examine the patient completely naked, to see whether his skin is darkened, and to see if its surface feels rough with a certain smoothness at the same time; if so, it is a sign of leprosy. Then sprinkle cold water on the shoulders; if it is not retained, it is a sign of leprosy. The reason is that the oiliness of the skin is weakened by the excess heat beneath the skin [in healthy people?], and the water will not stay on this oiliness; and so it is a sign.

Or make the patient cover his eyes so that he cannot see, and say, "Look out, I'm going to prick you!" and do not prick him. Then say, "I pricked you on the foot"; and if he agrees, it is a sign of leprosy. Likewise, prick him with a needle, from the little finger and the flesh next to it up to the arm. The reason for doing it in these fingers rather than others is that they are the weakest and therefore the ones which are first lost to the natural state.

These are the universal signs of leprosy, which are not dependent on any of its forms. But any of the latter can be known, [for example,] whether it is leonine, by using the signs listed above with those given by Avicenna in Book I, Fen 2, of the *Canon*: "Cuiuslibet humor, scil. sanguinis, flegmatis, etc." If you find signs of blood, you are dealing with the variety called "alopecia," for there their hair falls and they seem flayed like a fox, whence the name. If you find signs of phlegm, it is the variety called "tyria," whose name comes from the serpent "tyro." If you find signs of choler, it is the leonine variety, which gets its name because the face [of the patient] looks like that of a lion. But if symptoms of melancholy are found, it is the variety called "elephantia," in which the skin seems flayed away.

ULRICH VON HUTTEN (1488–1523)

"Of the Beginning of the French Pox, and the Several Names by Which It Has Been Called"

A poet and reformer, Ulrich von Hutten came from a family of German knights but was compelled to enter the Benedictine Monastery near Fulda because of poor health. Although he developed his great love of learning there, von Hutten found cloistered life intolerably dull and fled, ending any chance of his preferment within the Church. After nine years of roaming through Germany and Italy, von Hutten found a patron in Albert, Archbishop of Brandenburg, who admired his poetic gifts and to whom he dedicated *De morbo Gallico* in 1519. When von Hutten began to dispute the papacy's claims in Germany and to champion Luther's cause, Pope Leo X issued orders for his arrest and sent assassins to dispatch him. Pursued on all sides, von Hutten finally found refuge with the reformer Zwingli on the island of Ufnau, where he died at the age of thirty-five. Having endured nine years of various "cures" for syphilis, von Hutten wrote his treatise to foster understanding of the disease, but also to protest—in an age of protestors, or "protestants"—a regimen of treatment that sometimes seemed more like torture than therapy.

It hath pleased God, that in our time, Sicknesses should arise, unknown to our Forefathers, as we have Cause to surmise.

In the Year of Christ 1493, or thereabouts, this Evil began amongst the People, not only of *France,* but originally at *Naples* in the *French* Camp, who under King *Charles* were set down before that Place, and where it was taken notice of, before it came elsewhere; upon which account the French, disdaining that it should be called of their Country, gave it the Name of *Neopolitane,* or the Evil of *Naples*; reckoning, it is before observed, a Scandal to them to have it called by that of the *French* Pox. However the Consent of all Nations hath obtained, and we also in this Book, shall so call it, not out of Envy to that noble and courteous People, but to prevent a Misunderstanding among some, should we give it any other Appellation.

At the time of its first Appearance, some Men superstitiously named it the Sickness of *Mevin,* from I know not what holy Man of that Name. Some again accounted it of kin to *Job's* Scab, whom this Likeness I think also hath brought into the Number of *Saints*.

From *Classic Descriptions of Disease: With Biographical Sketches of Authors,* by Ralph H. Major (Springfield, Ill.: Charles C. Thomas, 1932). Used by permission of Blackwell Scientific Publications Ltd.

The *Divines* imputed this Disease to the Wrath of God, sent from Heaven as a Scourge for our Wickedness, and took upon them thus to preach openly, as if they had been admitted to Council with God, and came to understand thereby, that Men never lived worse, or so bad as we; or as if in the Golden Age of *Augustus* and *Tiberius,* when Christ was here on Earth, no such Evil could have happened; as if Nature had no Power to usher in any new Diseases, which in all other things bringeth forth great Changes and Alterations. As well may they prattle that of late in our times, because Men are grown better in their Lives, therefore is the Remedy of *Guajacum* found out as a Cure for this Sickness: So well do these things accord, which these Pretenders to the Oracles of God do thus deliver to us.

Now also began the Enquiry of the Physicians, who searched not so much for proper Remedy, as for the Cause; for they cared not even to behold it, much less at the first to touch the infected; for truly when it first began, it was so horrible to behold, that one would scarce think the Disease that now reigneth to be of the same kind. They had *Boils* that stood out like Acorns, from whence issued such filthy stinking Matter, that whosoever came within the Scent, believed himself infected. The Colour of these was of a dark Green and the very Aspect as shocking as the Pain itself, which yet was as if the Sick had lain upon a Fire.

Not long after its beginning, it made a Progress into *Germany,* where it hath wander'd more largely than in any other Place; which I ascribe to our greater intemperance than that of other Nations.

There were some who having taken Counsel of the Stars, prophesy'd that this Sickness should not endure more than Seven Years, in which they were out, if they meant the same of the Evil in general, and all the subsequent Symptoms; but if they interpreted concerning the foresaid most outrageous kind thereof, which cometh of itself, and not barely by Infection, Corruption of the Atmosphere, or of divine Appointment, they were then, I say, not deceived; for it tarried not long above the Seventh Year before the Disease abated of its Fierceness, and that the succeeding one, which yet remaineth, became not so filthy. The Sores being now less, neither so high, nor yet so hard, though there is often a broad creeping Scab, under which the Poison lurketh, and bringeth forth farther Mischiefs; and it is thought this Disease in our Days ariseth not, unless by infection from carnal Contact, as in copulating with a diseased Person, since it appears now that young Children, old Men and others, not given to Fornication or bodily lust, are very rarely diseased: Also the more a Man is addicted to these Pleasures, the sooner he catcheth it, and as they manage themselves after, either temperately or otherwise, so it the sooner leaves them, holds them a long time, or utterly consumes them. Thus is it more easy to the *Italians* and *Spaniards* as well as others, living soberly, but through our surfeiting and Intemperance it doth longer hold, and more grievously vex us.

OF THE CAUSES OF THIS DISEASE

The Physicians have not yet certainly discovered the secret Cause of this Disease, although they have long and diligently enquired after the same. In this all agree, which is very evident, that through some unwholesome Blasts of the Air, which happen[ed] about that time, the Lakes, Fountains, and even the Waters of the Sea were corrupted, and the Earth for a large Tract, as it were poisoned thereby: The Pastures were infected, and venomous, Streams filled the whole Air, which living Creatures took in with their Breath; for this Distemper at first was found among the Cattle as well as among Men.

The *Astrologers* deriving the Cause from the Stars, said, That it proceeded from the Conjunction of *Saturn* and *Mars,* which happened not long before, and of two Eclipses of the Sun; affirming, that hence they perceived were like to ensue many *cholerick* as well as *phlegmatick* Distempers, which would long continue, and slowly depart; such as *Elephantiasis, Lepra, Impetigo,* and all kinds of Scabs and Boils, with whatever could afflict Man's Body, as the *Gout, Palsy, Sciatic* or *Joynt-Ach,* and the like Infirmities; and that these should chance rather in the North, by reason of the Sign *Aquarius,* wherein fell the first Eclipse, and in the West from *Piscis,* in which happened the last.

But the Physicians concluded this to arise from ill Humours abounding in Men's Bodies, as black, adust or yellow Choler; salt Phlegm; of one of these alone, or mix'd together with the rest, and thrown out to the Skin, which is covered over with Scabs; whilst that which proceedeth of raw, heavy and gross Humour, is cast upon the Joints, causing great Pain therein, raising also Swellings with hard Knobs, or Knots, and shriveling of the Skin, with stubborn Headaches also, strangely altering the Complection of the Sick. Some briefly concluding say, it arose from a corrupt, burnt or adust, and infected Blood, and these Disputes held doubtful for a long time, the Nature of the Disease not rightly known; but now it is generally believed, and my self do verily think it to be no other, than the Effect of an aprostemated, rotten or corrupted Blood, which beginning to dry, turneth into these hard Swellings or Knobs, the Spring or Source of which is in the Liver corrupted.

To enquire farther after the Nature and Quality of this sickness would be tiresome and uncertain; for we see in our times diverse Opinions very confidently held forth, and much Pains in the Physicians have taken therein, since it came among us. Those of *Germany,* for the Space of two Years, were employed in such like disputations; and when I was yet a Child, they undertook to heal me: . . . I remember among others, they forbid me to eat Peas, for in some Places, there were found certain Worms therein, which had Wings; of the which Hogs Flesh also was thought to be infected, because that Creature especially was found diseased, either with this, or some other like it.

OF THE SYMPTOMS ATTENDING THIS DISEASE

Though this Distemper singly may be lightly accounted, yet doth it soon convert itself into many others; and indeed whatever Pains affect a Man's Joints, may seem to arise hence; for first there is a sharp Ache in these Parts, and yet nothing to be seen; but afterwards a Flux of Humours falls down, occasioning a Swelling, which beginning to harden about the Part, a most vehement Pain ariseth: which is the first Appearance of the Distemper when it begins to fortify itself as in a Castle, there resting for a long time, and thence to disperse its Emissaries into every part of the

Body, kindling therein all sorts of Aches and Dolors; when the longer the Swellings are before they ripen, the more Pain is the Patient to suffer, and truly of all others, this is the most intolerable. I myself had such a Knob or hard Swelling above my left heel on the inside, the which after it was indurated for the Space of seven Years, could by no Application be softened or brought to Matter, but still continued like a Bone, till by the help of *Guajacum* it gradually vanished.

In Women the Disease resteth in their secret Places, wherein are little pretty Sores, full of venomous Poison, being very dangerous for such as unknowingly meddle with them; the which Sickness, when contracted from these infected Women, is so much the more grievous, by how much they are more inwardly corrupted and polluted therewith. By this a Man's Sinews are sometimes relaxed, and again grow hard, and contract themselves. Sometimes the Disease transforms itself into the Gout; at others, into a *Palsy* and *Apoplexy,* and infecteth many also with a *Leprosy*; for it is thought these Diseases are Neighbours each to the other by reason of some Affinity there appears between them; those which are seized with the *Pox,* frequently becoming *Lepers,* and through the acuteness of the Pain, Men will shake and quiver as in a Fever.

After this there will appear small Holes and Sores, turning *cankerous* and *fistulous,* which the more putrid they grow, the more they will eat into the Bones, and when they have been long corrupted the Sick grows lean, his Flesh wasting away, so that there remaineth only the Skin as a Cover for them: And by this many fall into Consumptions, having their inward Parts corrupted.

HOW MEN AT FIRST ATTEMPTED THE CURE OF THIS DISEASE

Whilst the Physicians were thus confounded like Men amazed, the Surgeons as wretchedly lent a helping Hand to the same Error, and first began to burn the Sores with hot Irons. But for as much, as there seemed no end of this Cruelty, they endeavoured now to avoid the same with their *Ointments,* but all in vain, unless they added *Quick-Silver* thereunto. To this purpose they used the Powders of *Myrrh, Mastich, Ceruse, Bayberries, Allum, Bole Armoniac, Cinnabar, Vermillion, Coral, burnt salt, rust of Brass, Litharge, Rust of Iron, Refine of Turpentine,* and all manner of the best Oils, as of *Bay, Roses, Turpentine, Juniper,* (and of yet greater Power) the Oil of *Spike;* also *Hogs-Lard, Neats-Foot Oil, May Butter, Goats* and *Deers Suet, Virgin Honey,* red *Worms* dried to Powder or boiled up with Oil, *Camphire, Euphorbium, Castor.*

With these, fewer or more, they anointed the sick Man's Joints, his Arms, Thighs, his Neck and Back, with other parts of his Body. Some using these Anointings once a Day, some twice, others three times, and four times, others; the Patient being shut up in a Stove, with continual and fervent Heat, some twenty, some thirty, whole days. Some lying in Bed within the Stove were thus anointed, and covered with many Clothes, being compelled to Sweat; Part at the second anointing began to faint; yet was the Ointment of such Strength, that whatsoever Distemper was in the upper Parts it drew it into the Stomach, and thence to the Brain; and so the Disease was voided both by the Nose and Mouth, and put the Patient to so great Pain, that except they took good heed, their Teeth fell out, and their Throats, their Lungs, with the Roofs of their Mouths, were full of Sores; their Jaws did swell, their Teeth loosen'd, and a stinking Matter continually was voided from these places. What Part soever it touched, the same was strait corrupted thereby, so that not only their Lips, but the inside of their Cheeks, were grievously pained, and made the place where they were, stink most abominably; which sort of Cure was indeed so terrible, that many chose rather to die than to be eased thus of their Sickness. However, scarce one Sick Person in a hundred could be cured in this Way, but quickly after relapsed, so that the Cure held but for a few Days. Whereby may be infer'd what I suffered in the same Disease, who underwent the same in this Fashion for eleven times, with great Peril and Jeopardy of Life, struggling with the Disease nine Years together, taking all the time whatever was thought proper to withstand the Disease; such as *Baths with Herbs, Drinks* and *Corrosives,* of which kind we had *Arnick, Ink, Calcantum, Verdegraese* and *Aquasortis,* which occasioned such bitter Pains, that those might be thought very desirous of Life, who had not rather die than thus to prolong it. . . . [N]ot only the Surgeons, but every bold Fellow played the Physician in this Business, and these *Men Tormentors* were suffered thus to practice on all Persons as they were minded, whilst the Physicians were as Men struck dumb, not knowing what Course to take; and thus without Rule or Order, with torment of Heat, and plenty of Sweat, all were set upon after one Fashion, without regard of Time, Habit or Complection.

EDWIN CHADWICK (1800–1890)

Report on the Sanitary Condition of the Labouring Population of Great Britain

Educated as a lawyer, Edwin Chadwick early on served as assistant to Jeremy Bentham and remained a Benthamite all his life, profoundly committed to the idea that society should be rationally organized and administered. England's first full-time civil servant, Chadwick was the chief architect of the 1834 Poor Law, which attempted to replace an indiscriminate system of local parish relief with a centralized government bureaucracy. More importantly, the law redefined the poor, placing them for the first time into two distinct categories: the "deserving" and the "undeserving." In undertaking a report on the sanitary conditions of Britain's working classes, Chadwick invented a new method of public inquiry and investigation, gathering the immense amount of national data that would lay the groundwork for the Sanitary Reform Act of 1848. Along with his cadre of young lawyers and physicians, Chadwick gathered information from more than two thousand individuals, distributing questionnaires to commissioners, physicians, clerks, and inspectors, who were asked to assess the living conditions of local laborers and their families. Upon the project's completion, Chadwick issued his *Report* in "blue books" that were widely available to the general public. Among the estimated 100,000 copies that were sold or distributed, several were destined to fall into key hands, including those of John Stuart Mill, Thomas Carlyle, Charles Dickens, and Friedrich Engels, who would use Chadwick's data in his revolutionary book, *The Condition of the Working Class in England in 1844.*

London, May 1842.

GENTLEMEN,—Since my special attention was directed to the inquiry as to the chief removable circumstances affecting the health of the poorer classes of the population, I have availed myself of every opportunity to collect information respecting them. In company with Dr. Arnott I visited Edinburgh and Glasgow, and inspected those residences that were pointed out by the local authorities as the chief seats of disease. I also visited Dumfries. An inspection of similar districts in Spitalfields, Manchester, Leeds, and Macclesfield, and inquiries formerly made under the Commission of Poor Law Inquiry, and inspections of the condition of the residences of the poorer classes in parts of Berkshire, Sussex, and Hertfordshire, had supplied me with means of comparison. Abandoning any inquiries as to remedies, strictly so called,

From *Report on the Sanitary Condition of the Labouring Population of Great Britain,* ed. M. W. Flinn (1842; reprint, Edinburgh: Edinburgh University Press, 1965).

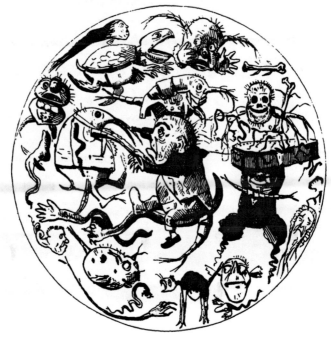

A DROP OF LONDON WATER.

16. A newspaper illustration of "A Drop of London Water" from Punch *18 (1850). Wellcome Institute Library, London. By 1850, images of contaminated water began to appear in the press, helping to spearhead the first public health movement. The caption accompanying this "molecular magnification" of a drop of water claims that it is representative of the water found in the Thames and in the wells of London "when the former has received the contents of the sewers, and the latter the oozings of intramural graveyards." There was a political message in the imagery as well. Among the curious creatures swimming in the drop can be found "aldermen, deputies, common councilmen," and even undertakers—all "disporting in the liquid dirt as in their native element."*

or the treatment of diseases after their appearance, I have directed the examinations of witnesses and the reports of medical officers chiefly to collect information of the best means available as preventives of the evils in question. On the documentary evidence of the medical officers, and on the examinations of witnesses, aided by personal inspections, I have the honour to report as follows:—

Partial descriptions of the condition of the labouring classes, in respect to their residences and the habits which influence their health, afford but a faint conception of the evils which are the subject of inquiry. If only particular instances, or some groups of individual cases be adduced, the erroneous impression might be created that they were cases of comparatively infrequent occurrence.

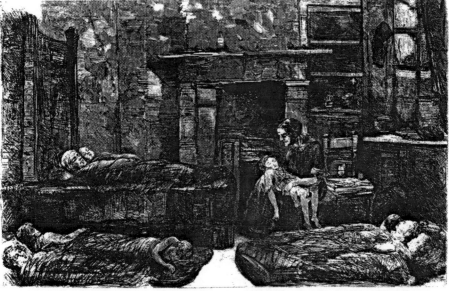

ATTIC OCCUPIED BY A FAMILY OF TEN PERSONS.

17. A newspaper illustration of an attic occupied by a family of ten persons from Illustrated Times *(1863). Wellcome Institute Library, London. The execrable housing conditions of the London poor finally became visible and gained public attention by the second half of the nineteenth century. In this newspaper illustration, the family's plight is presented simply and sympathetically. The room is clean and tidy and the mother weary but loving, suggesting that the misery of the poor is not to be blamed on their lax moral habits but on inadequate social and legislative policies. Not all such representations, however, were as sensitive to the sufferings of the poor.*

GENERAL CONDITION OF THE RESIDENCES OF THE LABOURING CLASSES WHERE DISEASE IS FOUND TO BE THE MOST PREVALENT

The following extracts will serve to show, in the language chiefly of eye-witnesses, the varied forms in which disease attendant on removable circumstances appears from one end of the island to the other amidst the population of rural villages, and of the smaller towns, as well as amidst the population of the commercial cities and the most thronged of the manufacturing districts—in which last pestilence is frequently supposed to have its chief and almost exclusive residence.

The state of the dwellings of many of the agricultural labourers in Dorset, where the deaths from the four classes of disease bear a similar proportion to those in Devon, is described in the return of *Mr. John Fox*, the medical officer of the Cerne union, who, remarking upon some cases of disease among the poor whom he had attended, says:

'In my district I do not think there is *one* cottage to be found consisting of a day-room, three bed-rooms, scullery, pantry, and convenient receptacles for refuse and for fuel in the occupation of a labourer, but there are many consisting of a day-room and two bed-rooms, constructed with a due regard to ventilation and warmth, pantry, and fuel house, with a small garden and pig-sty adjoining, and the labourers occupying such cottages, generally speaking, are far superior to others less advantageously situated. Their persons and cottages are always neater and cleaner, they are less disposed to frequent the beer-houses or to engage in poaching, whilst their children are generally sent daily to some school, in many instances chiefly supported by the clergyman of the parish. As a corroboration of my opinion, I need only state that I am frequently employed by the labourers in the good cottages to attend their wives during their confinement, and generally receive my guinea before I leave the house, whilst the labourer less favourably situated invariably applies to his parish for medical relief under such circumstances. I think there cannot be a doubt if the whole of the wretched hovels were converted into good cottages, with a strict attention to warmth, ventilation, and drainage, and a receptacle for filth of every kind placed at a proper distance, it would not only improve the health of the poor by removing a most prolific source of disease, and thereby most sensibly diminish the rates, but I am convinced it would also tend most materially to raise the moral character of the poor man, and render him less susceptible to the allurements of the idle and wicked.'

The following extract from the report of *Mr. Aaron Little,* the medical officer of the Chippenham union, affords a specimen of the frequent condition of rural villages which have apparently the most advantageous sites:

'The parish of Colerne, which, upon a cursory view, any person (unacquainted with its peculiarities) would pronounce to be the most healthy village in England, is in fact the most unhealthy. From its commanding position (being situated upon a high hill) it has an appearance of health and cheerfulness which delight the eye of the traveller, who commands a view of it from the Great Western road, but this impression is immediately removed on entering at any point of the town. The filth, the dilapidated buildings, the squalid appearance of the majority of the lower orders, have a sickening effect upon the stranger who first visits this place. During three years' attendance on the poor of this district, I have never known the small-pox, scarlatina, or the typhus fever to be absent. The situation is damp, and the buildings unhealthy, and the inhabitants themselves inclined to be of dirty habits. There is also a great want of drainage.'

Mr. Weale reports instances of the condition of large proportions of the agricultural population in the counties of Bedford, Northampton, and Warwick. The medical officer of the Woburn union states, in respect to Toddington, that:

'In this town fever prevailed during the last year, and, from the state of the dwellings of the persons I called on, this could not be wondered at. Very few of the cottages were furnished with privies that could be used, and contiguous to almost every door a dung heap was raised on which every species of filth was accumulated, either for the purpose of being used in the garden allotments of the cottagers, or to be disposed of for manure. Scarcely any cottage was provided with a pantry, and I found the provisions generally kept in the bed-rooms. In several instances I found whole families, comprising adult and infant children with their parents, sleeping in one room.'

Mr. J. S. Nott, the medical officer of the Witham union, states:

'As medical officer of my district, I am glad to have an opportunity of recording my opinion of many of the causes of fever that uniformly prevails in the autumn and spring in this neighbourhood. I must first state that the situation of the town is exceedingly low, with two small rivers passing through it, and numerous open sewers intersecting the town and its environs, the effluvia of which is frequently exceedingly offensive, and at all times prejudicial to the general health, and calculated to create, by its malaria, the various kinds of fevers, (typhus and remittent). Part of the town is subject to floods; added to which, the cottages are small and crowded together. A great number of the inhabitants accumulate filth and manure for the purpose of sale. There are also many open slaughter-houses, where the refuse and filth is allowed to accumulate for weeks together without removal; and innumerable pigs are kept and fattened on the back of the premises of a great number of the inhabitants; and altogether it would be difficult to find any town of its size where so little regard is paid to cleanliness and ventilation; but where we do find the exception, roomy and well-ventilated cottages, (and they are but few,) the cases of fever are more manageable, and recover sooner.'

Mr. Harding, medical officer of the Epping union, states:

'The state of some of the dwellings of the poor is most deplorable as it regards their health, and also in a moral point of view. As it relates to the former, many of their cottages are neither wind nor water tight. It has often fallen to my lot to be called on to attend a labour where the wet has been running down the walls, and light to be distinguished through the roof, and this in the winter season, with no fire-place in the room. As it relates to the latter, in my opinion a great want of accommodation for bed-rooms often occurs, so that you may frequently find the father, mother, and children all sleeping in the same apartment, and in some instances the children having attained the age of 16 or 17 years, and of both sexes; and if a death occurs in the house, let the person die of the most contagious disease, they must either sleep in the same room, or take their repose in the room they live in, which most frequently is a stone or brick floor, which must be detrimental to health.'

In the month of December, 1839, an application was made to the Board for advice and aid to meet the emergencies created by an epidemic which had broken out in the parish of Breadsall in the Shardlow union (Derbyshire). Mr. Senior, the Assistant Commissioner for the district, accompanied Dr. Kennedy to the spot where the fever was prevalent, and that report may be submitted to attention, as containing a picture of the habits of a large proportion of the population of that part of the country, and an exemplification in a group of individual cases of the common causes and effects of such calamities on the labouring population.

The report from Dr. Baker, of Derby, and Mr. Senior's report, comprising the returns from the medical officers of Nottingham, Lincoln, and other rural and town unions within his district, portray the sanitary condition of a large proportion of the population included in them.

Proceeding northward, a report from *Mr. Bland,* the medical officer of the Macclesfield union, gives the following description of the state of the residences occupied by many of the labourers of that town:

> 'In a part of the town called the Orchard, Watercoates, there are 34 houses without back doors, or other complete means of ventilation; the houses are chiefly small, damp, and dark; they are rendered worse with respect to dampness perhaps than they would be from the habit of the people closing their windows to keep them warm. To these houses are three privies uncovered; here little pools of water, with all kinds of offal, dead animal and vegetable matter are heaped together, a most foul and putrid mass, disgusting to the sight, and offensive to the smell; the fumes of contagion spreads periodically itself in the neighbourhood, and produces different types of fever and disorder of the stomach and bowels. The people inhabiting these abodes are pale and unhealthy, and in one house in particular are pale, bloated, and rickety.'

Mr. William Rayner, the medical officer of the Heaton Norris district of the Stockport union describes the condition of a part of the population of that place:

> 'The localities in which fever mostly prevails in my district, are Shepherd's Buildings and Back Water Street, both in the township of Heaton Norris. Shepherd's Buildings consist of two rows of houses with a street seven yards wide between them; each row consists of what are styled back and front houses—that is two houses placed back to back. There are no yards or out-conveniences; the privies are in the centre of each row, about a yard wide; over them there is part of a sleeping-room; there is no ventilation in the bedrooms; each house contains two rooms, viz., a house place and sleeping room above; each room is about three yards wide and four long. In one of these houses there are nine persons belonging to one family, and the mother on the eve of her confinement. There are 44 houses in the two rows, and 22 cellars, all of the same size. The cellars are let off as separate dwellings; these are dark, damp, and very low, not more than six feet between the ceiling and floor. The street between the two rows is seven yards wide, in the centre of which is the common gutter, or more properly sink, into which all sorts of refuse is thrown; it is a foot in depth. Thus there is always a quantity of putrefying matter contaminating the air. At the end of the rows is a pool of water very shallow and stagnant, and a few yards further, a part of the town's gas works. In many of these dwellings there are four persons in one bed.
>
> 'Backwater-street, the other locality of fever, is proverbially the most filthy street in the town, contains a number of lodging-houses and Irish, who mostly live in dark damp cellars, in which the light can scarcely penetrate.'

The report of Dr. Baron Howard, on the condition of the population of Manchester, and that of Dr. Duncan, on the condition of the population of Liverpool, will make up a progressive view of the condition of the labouring population in those parts of the country. The Report of one of the medical officers of the West Derby union, with relation to the condition of the labouring population connected with Liverpool, will serve to show that the evils in question are not confined to the labouring population of the town properly so called.

'The locality of the residences of the labouring classes are in respect to the surrounding atmosphere favourably situated, but their internal structure and economy the very reverse of favourable. The cottages are in general built more with a view to the per centage of the landlord than to the accommodation of the poor. The joiner's work is ill performed; admitting by the doors, windows, and even floors, air in abundance, which, however, in many cases, is not disadvantageous to the inmates. The houses generally consist of three apartments, viz., the day-room, into which the street-door opens, and two bedrooms, one above the other. There is likewise beneath the day-room a cellar, let off either by the landlord or tenant of the house, to a more improvident class of labourers; which cellar, in almost all cases, is small and damp, and often crowded with inhabitants to excess. These cellars are, in my opinion, the source of many diseases, particularly catarrh, rheumatic affections, and tedious cases of typhus mitior, which, owing to the over-crowded state of the apartment, occasionally pass into typhus gravior. I need scarcely add that the furniture and bedding are in keeping with the miserable inmates. The rooms above the day-room are often let separately by the tenant to lodgers, varying in number from one or two, to six to eight individuals in each, their slovenly habits, indolence, and consequent accumulation of filth go far to promote the prevalence of contagious and infectious diseases.

'The houses already alluded to front the street, but there are houses in back courts still more unfavourably placed, which also have their cellars, and their tenants of a description worse, if possible. There is commonly only one receptacle for refuse in a court of eight, ten, or twelve densely crowded houses. In the year 1836–7, I attended a family of 13, twelve of whom had typhus fever, without a bed in the *cellar*, without straw or timber shavings—frequent substitutes. They lay on the floor, and so crowded, that I could scarcely pass between them. In another house I attended 14 patients; there were only two beds in the house. All the patients, as lodgers, lay on the boards, and during their illness, never had their clothes off. I met with many cases in similar conditions, yet amidst the great destitution and want of domestic comfort, I have never heard during the course of twelve years' practice, a complaint of inconvenient accommodation.'

The following is a brief notice of the condition of the residences of the population amidst which the cholera first made its appearance in this country.

Mr. Robert Atkinson, Gateshead, states, that:

'It is impossible to give a proper representation of the wretched state of many of the inhabitants of the indigent class, situated in the confined streets called Pipewellgate and Killgate, which are kept in a most filthy state, and to a stranger would appear inimical to the existence of human beings, where each small, ill ventilated apartment of the house contained a family with lodgers in number from seven to nine, and seldom more than two beds for the whole. The want of convenient offices in the neighbourhood is attended with many very unpleasant circumstances, as it induces the lazy inmates to make use of chamber utensils, which are suffered to remain in the most offensive state for several days, and are then emptied out of the windows. The writer had occasion a short time ago to visit a person ill of the cholera; his lodgings were in a room of a miserable house situated in the very filthiest part of Pipewellgate, divided into six apartments, and occupied by different families to the number of 26 persons in all. The room contained three wretched beds with two persons sleeping in each; it measured about 12 feet in length and 7 in breadth, and its greatest height would not admit of a person's standing erect; it received light from a small window, the sash of which was fixed. Two of the number lay ill of the cholera, and the rest appeared afraid of the admission of pure air, having carefully closed up the broken panes with plugs of old linen.'

The most wretched of the stationary population of which I have been able to obtain any account, or that I have ever seen, was that which I saw in company with *Dr. Arnott,* and others, in the wynds of Edinburgh and Glasgow.

I prefer citing his description of the residences we visited:

'We entered a dirty low passage like a house door, which led from the street through the first house to a square court immediately behind, which court, with the exception of a narrow path around it leading to another long passage through a second house, was occupied entirely as a dung receptable of the most disgusting kind. Beyond this court the second passage led to a second square court, occupied in the same way by its dunghill; and from this court there was yet a third passage leading to a third court, and third dungheap. There were no privies or drains there, and the dungheaps received all filth which the swarm of wretched inhabitants could give; and we learned that a considerable part of the rent of the houses was paid by the produce of the dungheaps. Thus, worse off than wild animals, many of which withdraw to a distance and conceal their ordure, the dwellers in these courts had converted their shame into a kind of money by which their lodging was to be paid. The interiors of these houses and their inmates corresponded with the exteriors. We saw half-dressed wretches crowding together to be warm; and in one bed, although in the middle of the day, several women were imprisoned under a blanket, because as many others who had on their backs all the articles of dress that belonged to the party were then out of doors in the streets. This picture is so shocking that, without ocular proof, one would be disposed to doubt the possibility of the facts; and yet there is perhaps no old town in Europe that does not furnish parallel examples. London, before the great fire of 1666, had few drains and had many such scenes, and the consequence was, a pestilence occurring at intervals of about 12 years, each destroying at an average about a fourth of the inhabitants.

'Edinburgh stands on a site beautifully varied by hill and hollow, and owing to this, unusual facilities are afforded for perfect drainage; but the old part of the town was built long before the importance of drainage was understood in Britain, and in the unchanged parts there is none but by the open channels in the streets, wynds, and closes or courts. To remedy the want of covered drains, there is in many neighborhoods a very active service of scavengers to remove everything which open drains cannot be allowed to carry; but this does not prevent the air from being much more contaminated by the frequent stirring and sweeping of impurities than if the transport were effected under ground; and there are here and there enclosed spaces between houses too small to be used for any good purpose but not neglected for bad, and to which the scavengers have not access.'

It might admit of dispute, but, on the whole, it appeared to us that both the structural arrangements and the condition of the population in Glasgow was the worst of any we had seen in any part of Great Britain.

PUBLIC ARRANGEMENTS EXTERNAL TO THE RESIDENCES BY WHICH THE SANITARY CONDITION OF THE LABOURING POPULATION IS AFFECTED

I now propose to bring under consideration those parts of the various local reports and communications which most prominently set forth special defects that apparently admit of specific remedies.

The defects which are the most important, and which come most immediately within practical legislative and administrative control, are those chiefly *external* to the dwellings of the population, and principally arise from the neglect of drainage. The remedies include the means for drainage simply, *i.e.,* the means for the removal of an excess of moisture; and

The means for the removal of the noxious refuse of houses, streets, and roads, by sewerage, by supplies of water, and by the service of scavengers and sweepers.

The following is the comparison of the different mortality in a drained and an undrained district, made by *Mr. Crowfoot,* surgeon, of Beccles, one of the most eminent of the medical practitioners in Suffolk. In a letter to Mr. Twisleton, the Assistant Commissioner, he states:

'You are aware that these two towns of nearly equal population are nearly alike as to natural advantages of situation, &c., except that Bungay, having a larger proportion of rural population inhabiting the district called Bungay Uplands, ought to be more healthy than Beccles, which has nearly its whole population confined to the town. About 30 years since, Beccles began a system of drainage, which it has continued to improve, till at the present time every part of the town is well drained, and I am not aware of a single open drain in the place. Bungay, on the contrary, with equally convenient opportunities for drainage, has neglected its advantages in that respect, has one or two large reservoirs for filth in the town itself, and some of its principal drains are open ones. The result you will see is, that Bungay, with a smaller proportion of town inhabitants, has become of late years less healthy than Beccles. I have carefully taken the number of burials from the parish registers of each town for the last 30 years, and dividing them into decennial periods, I have calculated the proportion which the deaths bore to the mean population, between one census and the other, during each 10 years; the only possible source of fallacy is the want of the census for 1841; but in its absence I have supposed the same rate of increase as took place between that of 1821 and that of 1831 for each place. Sinking fractions, the following has been the proportion of deaths to the population in the two towns:—

		Beccles	Bungay
Between the years	1811 and 1821	1 in 67	1 in 69
"	1821 and 1831	1 in 72	1 in 67
"	1831 and 1841	1 in 71	1 in 59

You will therefore see that the rate of mortality has gradually diminished in Beccles since it has been drained, whilst in Bungay, notwithstanding its larger proportion of rural population, it has considerably increased.'

The condition of the labouring population of Liverpool, in respect to drainage, is thus described in the report of *Dr. Duncan*:

'The sewerage of Liverpool was so very imperfect, that about 10 years ago a local Act was procured, appointing commissioners with power to levy a rate on the parish for the construction of sewers. Under this Act, which expires next year, about 100,000*l.* have been expended in the formation of sewers along the main streets, but many of these are still unsewered; and with regard to the streets inhabited by the working classes, I believe that the great majority are without sewers, and that where they do exist they are of a very imperfect kind unless where the ground has a natural inclination, therefore the surface water and fluid refuse of every kind stagnate in the street, and add, especially in hot weather, their pestilential influence to that of the more solid filth already mentioned. With regard to the courts, I doubt whether there is a single court in Liverpool which communicates with the street by an underground drain, the only means afforded for carrying off the fluid dirt being a narrow, open, shallow gutter, which sometimes exists, but even this is very generally choked up with stagnant filth.

'There can be no doubt that the emanations from this pestilential surface, in connexion with other causes, are a frequent source of fever among the inhabitants of these undrained localities. I may mention two instances in corroboration of this assertion:—In consequence of finding that not less than 63 cases of fever had occurred in one year in Union-court Banastre-street, (containing 12 houses,) I visited the court in order to ascertain, if possible, their origin, and I found the whole court inundated with fluid filth which had oozed through the walls from two adjoining ash-pits or cess-pools, and which had no means of escape in consequence of the court being below the level of the street, and having no drain. The court was owned by two different landlords, one of whom had offered to construct a drain provided the other would join him in the expense; but this offer having been refused, the court had remained for two or three years in the state in which I saw it; and I was informed by one of the inhabitants that the fever was constantly occurring there. The house nearest the ash-pit had been untenanted for nearly three years in consequence of the filthy matter oozing up through the floor, and the occupiers of the adjoining houses were unable to take their meals without previously closing the doors and windows. Another court in North-street, consisting of only four small houses I found in a somewhat similar condition, the air being contaminated by the emanations from two filthy ruinous privies, a large open ash-pit and a stratum of semi-fluid abomination covering the whole surface of the court.

'From the absence of drains and sewers, there are of course few cellars entirely free from damp; many of those in low situations are literally inundated after a fall of rain. To remedy the evil, the inhabitants frequently make little holes or wells at the foot of the cellar steps on in the floor itself; and notwithstanding these contrivances, it has been necessary in some cases to take the door off its hinges and lay it on the floor supported by bricks, in order to protect the inhabitants from the wet. Nor is this the full extent of the evil; the fluid matter of the court privies sometimes oozes through into the adjoining cellars, rendering them uninhabitable by any one whose olfactories retain the slightest sensibility. In one cellar in Lace-street I was told that the filthy water thus collected measured not less than two feet in depth; and in another cellar, a well, four feet deep, into which this stinking fluid was allowed to drain, was discovered below the bed where the family slept!'

Internal Economy and Domestic Habits
Domestic mismanagement, a predisposing cause of disease

The subsequent examples relate chiefly to the effects of general domestic mismanagement as a concurrent cause of disease.

Dr. Baker, in his report on the sanitary condition of the population of Derby, states that:

'There is also another cause of sickness to be found in their houses, and which, like the former, *i.e.,* the external circumstances, is in constant operation: I mean the want of domestic comforts, a want which the wages they earn would, in many instances, enable them to remove if their means were not, as too often happens, expended viciously or improvidently. It is with regret that I speak unfavourably of the poor, whilst my whole aim, in this communication, has been to awaken a sympathy towards those sufferings of which I have been so often a witness. But several years' experience of the habits of the poor, derived from my situation as an hospital physician, and backed by the additional evidence I have obtained by acting for three years as a guardian of the poor in this large town, has, I am sorry to say, served but to confirm me in the opinion I have just now expressed; and in support of which I shall instance the family of the Slaters mentioned at No. 12, in Short-street.

'The earnings of four members of this family were as follows:—

	s.	*d.*		
The father	.14	0	per week	at gardening, &c.
The eldest son, aged 20	.12	0	"	at a brewery.
Daughter, ... { Twins }	.6	0	"	at a factory
Son, ... { aged 18 }	.9	0	"	at the same factory.
	£2 1	0	per week.	

'The mother of this family, it appears, is left disengaged from all but her household duties and the care of the younger children; the house, nevertheless, is nearly destitute of furniture, and presents a picture of disorder and want. On the other hand, at No. 15, (Briggs) although the husband has for some years past been a weak and ailing man, the family is well ordered and cleanly; and to this fact I mainly attribute the milder and modified form of fever which affected the children.'

The Committee of Physicians and Surgeons at Birmingham, in their report, indicate the powerful operation of depraved domestic habits as a predisposing cause to disease:

'It cannot,' they say, 'be doubted that whilst the arts and manufactures of the place prove in some instances injurious to health, and in a few possibly destructive to life, these evil consequences, as well as hereditary predisposition to disease, are promoted by intemperance, not that intemperance is an infinitely more frequent cause of disease and death amongst the artisans than all the various employments of all the manufactories combined.

'In the expenditure of their weekly earnings, improvidence and thoughtless extravagance prevail to a lamentable degree. The observations upon which this opinion is formed are made upon the habits of the people themselves, confirmed by extensive and recent inquiries among the shopkeepers with whom they deal. Tea, coffee, sugar, butter, cheese, bacon, (of which a great deal is consumed in this town,) and other articles, the working people purchase in small quantities from the hucksters, who charge an enormous profit upon them, being, as they state, compelled to do so to cover the losses which they frequently sustain by bad debts. Huckster dealing is a most extravagant mode of dealing; there were in this town, in 1834, 717 of these shops, and the number has greatly increased since that time. Meat is purchased in the same improvident manner; the working men generally contrive to have a good joint of meat upon the Sunday; the dinner on the other days of the week is made from steaks or chops, which is the most extravagant mode either of purchasing or cooking meat.

'The improvidence of this class of persons arises in many instances from the indulgence of vicious propensities. Drunkenness, with all its attendant miseries, prevails to a great extent, though it is by no means to be regarded as a characteristic feature of the mechanic of this town in particular. It most generally prevails among that class of workmen who obtain the highest wages, but who are often found in the most deplorable and abject condition. The improvidence of which we are speaking is to be traced in very many instances to extreme ignorance on the part of the wives of these people. The females are from necessity bred up from their youth in the workshops, as the earnings of the younger members contribute to the support of the family. The minds and morals of the girls become debased, and they marry totally ignorant of all those habits of domestic economy which tend to render a husband's home comfortable and happy; and this is very often the cause of the man being driven to the alehouse to seek that comfort after his day of toil which he looks for in vain by his own fireside. The habit of a manufacturing life being once established in a woman, she continues it, and leaves her home and children to the care of a neighbour or of a hired child, sometimes only a few years older than her own children, whose services cost her probably as much as she obtains for her labour. To this neglect on the part of their parents is to be traced the death of many children; they are left in the house with a fire before they are old enough to know the danger to which they are exposed, and are often dreadfully burnt.'

Mr. Mott's report on the sanitary condition of the population of his district presents parallel instances of the different economy prevalent amongst these classes:

Contrast in the Economy of Families

1

Cellar in Wellington-court, Chorlton-upon-Medlock; a man, his wife and seven children; income per week, 1*l.* 11*s.*; rent 1*s.* 6*d.* per week; three beds for seven, in a dark, unventilated back room, bed-covering of the meanest and scantiest kind—the man and wife occupying the front room as a sleeping-room for themselves, in which the whole family take their food and spend their leisure time; here the family, in a filthy destitute state, with an income averaging 3*s.* 5$^1/_4$*d.* each per week, four being children under 11 years of age.

1

In a dwelling-house in Chorlton Union, containing one sitting-room and two bedrooms; a man, his wife and three children; rent 2*s.* 6*d.* per week; income per week 12*s.* 6*d.,* being an average of 2*s.* 6*d.* per week for each person. Here, with a sickly man, the house presented an appearance of comfort in every part, as also the bedding was in good order.

2

Cellar in York-street, Chorlton-upon-Medlock; a man—a hand-loom weaver—his wife and family (one daughter married, with her husband forms part of the family), comprising altogether seven persons; income 2*l.* 7*s.,* or 6*s.* 8$^1/_2$*d.* per head; rent 2*s.* Here, with the largest amount of income, the family occupy two filthy, damp, unwholesome cellars, one of which is a back place without pavement or flooring of any kind, occupied by the loom of the family, and used as a sleeping-room for the married couple and single daughter.

2

In a dwelling-house, Stove-street, one sitting-room, one kitchen and two bedrooms, rent 4*s.* per week. A poor widow, with a daughter also a widow, with ten children, making together 13 in family; income 1*l.* 6*s.* per week, averaging 2*s.* per head per week. Here there is every appearance of cleanliness and comfort.

3

John Salt, of Carr Bank (labourer), wages 12*s.* per week; a wife, and one child aged 15: he is a drunken, disorderly fellow, and very much in debt.

3

George Hall, of Carr Bank (labourer), wages 10*s.* per week; has reared ten children; he is in comfortable circumstances.

4

William Haynes, of Oakamoore (wire-drawer), wages 1*l.* per week; he has a wife and five children; he is in debt, and his family is shamefully neglected.

4

John Hammonds, of Woodhead (collier), wages 18*s.* per week; has six children to support; he is a steady man and saving money.

5

George Locket, of Kingsley (boatman), wages 18*s.* per week, with a wife and seven children; his family are in a miserable condition.

5

George Mosley, of Kingsley (collier), wages 18*s.* per week; he has a wife and seven children; he is saving money.

6

John Banks, of Cheadle (collier), wages 18*s.* per week; wife and three children; his house is in a filthy state, and the furniture not worth 10*s.*

6

William Faulkner, of Tean (tape-weaver), wages 18*s.* per week; supports his wife and seven children without assistance.

7

William Weaver, of Kingsley (boatman), wages 18*s.* per week; wife and three children; he is a drunken, disorderly fellow, and his family entirely destitute.

7

Charles Rushton, of Lightwoodfields, wages 14*s.* per week; he supports his wife and five children in credit.

8

Richard Barlow, of Cheadle (labourer), wages 12*s.* per week; wife and five children, in miserable circumstance, not a bed to lie on.

8

William Sargeant, of Lightwoodfields (labourer), wages 13*s.* a-week; he has a wife and six children, whom he supports comfortably.

9

Thomas Bartlem, of Tean (labourer), wages 14*s.* per week; his wife earns 7*s.* per week; five children; he is very much in debt; home neglected.

9

William Box, of Tean (tape-weaver), wages 18*s.* or 20*s.* per week; supports his wife in bad health, and five children.

10

Thomas Johnson, of Tean (blacksmith), wages 18*s.* per week; his wife earns 7*s.* per week; three children; he is very much in debt, and his family grossly neglected.

10

Ralph Faulkner, of Tean (tape-weaver), wages 18*s.* or 20*s.* per week; supports a wife and five children, three of them are deaf and dumb.

These descriptions are not confined to the English towns. Mr. Jupp and others cite instances from the rural districts. They are similarly prevalent in Scotland. As an example I would refer to the description given by Dr. Scott Alison, of the condition of the highly-paid collier population of Tranent. Take another instance of the condition of the same class, the colliers at Ayr, given by *Dr. Sym,* in his report on the sanitary condition of the population of that town:

> 'Although the colliers have large wages, they are, from their want of economy and their dissolute habits, uniformly in poverty; and their families, though well fed, are miserably clothed, ill lodged, uneducated, and less industrious than the families of the weavers; the females of which work with great constancy at hand-sewing. The modes of living of these two classes are very different. The weaver is not intemperate, because he cannot afford to purchase ardent spirits, and the nature of his employment prevents him from having those hours of idleness during the day which the collier is so apt to consume in dissipation. He lives on very innutritious food, seldom eats butchers' meat, and the most indigent, who are generally Irishmen, subsist chiefly on potatoes. The collier, on the other hand, indulges to excess in ardent spirits, and both he and his family partake of animal food every day. In short, the colliers live better than any of the other labouring classes in Ayr.'

The domestic condition of this population admits of a contrast with the condition of individuals of their own description of employment, or with the condition of other classes of miners who receive no higher wages, but whose condition is highly superior, to show that the depraved habits and condition are not the necessary result of the employment. He contrasts the condition of the colliery population of Tranent with the condition of the agriculture labourers in the immediate vicinity of the town:

> 'With very few exceptions, the condition of the interior of the houses of the hind population is excellent, most pleasing to the eye, and comfortable. These respectable people, in spite of the defective construction of their cottages, manage to throw an air of comfort, plenty, neatness, and order around their homes. I have often been delighted to observe these characteristics, and not less so to mark the co-existence of pure, moral, and religious principles in the inmates, the presence of practical religion and practical morals.'

The like contrast, derived from an intimate knowledge of the population of another class, in presented in the following portions of a report from *Mr. Wood,* of Dundee:

> 'There are many families among the working class who are in the receipt of from 15*s.* to 22*s.* per week, who are insufficiently clothed, and irregularly and poorly fed, and whose houses as well as their persons appear filthy, disorderly, and uncomfortable. There are other families among them, containing the same number of persons, whose incomes average from 10*s.* to 14*s.* a-week, who are neatly, cleanly, and sufficiently clothed, regularly and suitably fed, and whose houses appear orderly and comfortable. The former class care little for the physical comfort, and far less for the intellectual, moral, and religious education of their children; in many cases, indeed, they neglect the education of their offspring

when it is offered to them gratuitously, and in place of sending them to school, where they might be fitted for the duties and disappointments of life, they send them at a very early age to some employment, where they will earn the poor pittance of 1s. 6d. to 3s. a-week. The latter class, on the contrary, are most anxious to give their children a good education: they study to obtain it for them by every means in their power, and they pay for it most cheerfully. The former class again grasp at every benefit which the charitable institutions of the place have provided for the poor. When, for example, medical attendance is given them gratuitously, they not unfrequently despise and refuse it, unless medicines are given them gratuitously also. Whereas the latter description of families are not only ready and willing to pay for medicines when prescribed to them, but they generally manifest much gratitude, and very often present their medical attendant with a small fee.

'Now it is among the former class of families where generally there appears to me to be a deficiency of wholesome food and of warm clothing; where contagious, febrile diseases are most commonly found; and from whence they are most extensively propagated. Fever is no doubt found among the latter, more frugal, and therefore better conditioned families, but seldom of that malignant, contagious character which it invariably assumes among the other class of families. Here, then, we have on the one hand, filth, destitution, and disease, associated with good wages; and on the other, cleanliness, comfort, and comparative good health, in connexion with wages which are much lower. The difference in the amount of their incomes does not account for the difference in the amount of comfort which is found existing among the working classes. The statements just made make known the fact, that above a certain amount, say 12s. or 14s. of weekly income, wages *alone,* without intelligence and good habits, contribute nothing towards the comfort, health, and independence of the working population. Were I asked how I would propose to relieve such a family, I would say, show them how they may live comfortably within their incomes; let them be taught and trained to habits of industry, frugality, sobriety, cleanliness, &c., and with this 12s. or 14s. they may live in health and happiness as others in similar circumstances have lived and are now living. The man who maintains himself and his family in comfort on 12s. or 14s. of weekly income, possesses what he well deserves, happiness at home, and he stands forth in his neighbourhood a noble example of honest independence. I am persuaded that the filth, fever, and destitution in many families is occasioned, not by their small incomes, but by a misapplication or a prodigal waste of a part, in some cases a great part, of their otherwise sufficient wages. Frequently cases are found where, with a want of skill and economy, there is combined the intemperate use of intoxicating liquors, and here the misery may be said to be complete.'

The false opinions as to destitution being the general cause of fever, and as to its propagation, have had extensively the disastrous effect of preventing efforts being made for the removal of the circumstances which are proved to be followed by a diminution of the pestilence.

The opinion of the majority of the medical officers of the unions in England on this topic, acting in districts in every condition, might be expressed in the terms used by *Dr. Davidson*:

'It has already been shown that filth and deficient ventilation tend much to spread the contagion of typhus, being almost constant concomitants; and that while it generally affects the whole members, or the large proportion of a family among the lower orders, it rarely spreads in this manner among the better classes of society, who attend more to cleanliness and ventilation. And the evil will continue to assail us so long as our cities contain so many narrow and filthy lanes, so long as the houses situated there are little better than dens or hovels, so long as dunghills and other nuisances are allowed to accumulate in their vicinity, so long as these hovels are crowded with inmates, and so long as there is so much poverty and destitution. Why, then, should we not have a legislative enactment that would level these hovels to the ground—that would regulate the width of every street—that would regulate the ventilation of every dwelling-house—that would prevent the lodging-houses of the poor from being crowded with human beings, and that would provide for their destitution? It may be said that this would interfere too much with the liberty of the subject, and no doubt it would be vehemently opposed by many interested persons. In place, however, of being an infringement on the liberty of the subject, it might rather be designated an attempt to prevent the improper liberties of the subject; for what right, moral or constitutional, has any man to form streets, construct houses, and crowd them with human beings, so as to deteriorate health and shorten life, because he finds it profitable to do so? As well ought the law to tolerate the sale of unwholesome food because it might be profitable to the retailer of it.'

COMPARATIVE CHANCES OF LIFE IN DIFFERENT CLASSES OF THE COMMUNITY

It is proper to observe, that so far as I was informed upon the evidence received in the Factory Inquiry, and more recently on the cases of children of migrant families, that opinion is erroneous which ascribes greater sickness and mortality to the children employed in factories than amongst the children who remain in such homes as these towns afford to the labouring classes. However defective the ventilation of many of the factories may yet be, they are all of them drier and more equably warm than the residence of the parent; and we had proof that weakly children have been put into the better-managed factories as healthier places for them than their own home. It is an appalling fact that, of all who are born of the labouring classes in Manchester, more than 57 per cent die before they attain five years of age; that is, before they can be engaged in factory labour, or in any other labour whatsoever.

Of 4,629 deaths of persons of the labouring classes who died in the year 1840 in Manchester, the numbers who died were at the several periods as follows:

Under 5 years of age .... 2,649 or 1 in 1^{7}/10
Above 5 and under 10 .... 215 or 1 in 22
Above 10 and under 15 .... 107 or 1 in 43
Above 15 and under 20 .... 135 or 1 in 34

At seven, eight, or nine years of age the children of the working classes begin to enter into employment in the cotton and other factories. It appears that at the period between 5 and 10 years of age the proportions of deaths which occur amongst the labouring classes, as indicated by these returns, are not so great as the proportions of deaths which occur amongst the children of the middle classes who are not so engaged. Allowing for the circumstances that some of the weakest of the labourers' children will have been swept away in the first stage, the effect of employment is not shown to be injurious in any increase of the proportion who die in the second stage.

In a return obtained from a district differently situated (Bethnal Green, where the manufactory is chiefly domestic) it appears that of 1,268 deaths amongst the labouring classes in the year 1839, no less than 783, or 1 in $1^4/_7$, died at their own residences under 5 years of age. One in 15 of the deaths occurred between 5 and 10, the age when employment commences. The proportion of deaths which occurred between 10 and 15, the period at which full employment usually takes place, is 1 in 60 only.

In that district the average age of deaths in the year 1839 was as follows, in the several classes, from a population of 62,018:

BETHNAL GREEN

No. of Deaths		Average Age of Deceased
101	Gentlemen and persons engaged in professions, and their families	45 years
237	Tradesmen and their families	26
1,258	Mechanics, servants, and labourers, and their families.	16

The mean chances of life amongst the several classes in Leeds appear from the returns to the Registrar-general generally to correspond with the anticipations raised by the descriptions given of the condition of the labouring population.

LEEDS BOROUGH

No. of Deaths		Average Age of Deceased
79	Gentlemen and persons engaged in professions, and their families	44 years
824	Tradesmen, farmers, and their families	27
3,395	Operatives, labourers, and their families	19

But in Liverpool (which is a commercial and not a manufacturing town) where, however, the condition of the dwellings are reported to be the worst, where, according to the report of Dr. Duncan, 40,000 of the population live in cellars, where 1 in 25 of the population are annually attacked with fever,—there the mean chances of life appear from the returns to the Registrar-general to be still lower than in Manchester, Leeds, or amongst the silk weavers in Bethnal Green. During the year 1840, the deaths, distinguishable in classes, were as follows:

LIVERPOOL, 1840

No. of Deaths		*Average Age of Deceased*
137	Gentry and professional persons, &c.	35 years
1,738	Tradesmen and their families	22
5,597	Labourers, mechanics, and servants, &c.	15

Of the deaths which occurred amongst the labouring classes, it appears that no less than 62 per cent. of the total number were deaths under five years of age. Even amongst those entered as shopkeepers and tradesmen, no less than 50 per cent. died before they attained that period. The proportion of mortality for Birmingham, where there are many insalubrious manufactories, but where the drainage of the town and the general condition of the inhabitants is comparatively good, was, in 1838, 1 in 40: whilst in Liverpool it was 1 in 31.

By the inspection of a map of Leeds, which Mr. Baker has prepared at my request, to show the localities of epidemic diseases, it will be perceived that they similarly fall on the uncleansed and close streets and wards occupied by the labouring classes; and that the track of the cholera is nearly identical with the tract of fever.

The Effects of Preventive Measures
Employers' Influence on the Health of Workpeople by the Promotion of Personal Cleanliness

I proceed to another instance of the power of the employers to protect the health, as well as the morals of their workpeople, by influencing their habits of personal cleanliness.

But I shall first submit a few instances of the extent and prevalence of personal uncleanliness amongst whole classes of workpeople.

Mr. John Kennedy, in the course of the examinations of some colliers in Lancashire, asked one of them:

> 'How often do the drawers (those employed in drawing coals) wash their bodies?—None of the drawers ever wash their bodies. I never wash my body; I let my shirt rub the dirt off; my shirt will show that. I wash my neck and ears, and face, of course.
>
> 'Do you think it usual for the young women (engaged in the colliery) to do the same as you do?—I do not think it is usual for the lasses to wash their bodies; my sisters never wash themselves, and seeing is believing; they wash their faces, necks, and ears.
>
> 'When a collier is in full dress, he has white stockings, and very tall shirt necks, very stiffly starched, and ruffles?—That is very sure, sir; but they never wash their bodies underneath; I know that; and their legs and bodies are as black as your hat.'

One labourer remembered that a particular event took place at Easter, 'because it was then he washed his feet.' The effects of these habits are seen at the workhouse on almost every one of the paupers admitted. When it is necessary to wash them on their admission, they usually manifest an extreme repugnance to the process. Their common feeling was expressed by one of them when he declared that he considered it 'equal to robbing him of a great coat which he had had for some years.' The filthy condition in which they are found on admission into the hospitals is frequently sufficient to account for the state of disease in which they appear, and the act of cleansing them is itself the most efficient cure. The out-door service of the union medical officers amidst such a population is often most painful and disgusting: *e.g.*—

Mr. J. F. Handley, medical officer of the Chipping Norton union, states in his report:

> 'When the small-pox was prevalent in this district, I attended a man, woman, and five children, all lying ill with the confluent species of that disorder, in one bed-room, and having only two beds amongst them. The walls of the cottage were black, the sheets were black, and the patients themselves were blacker still; two of the children were absolutely sticking together. It was indeed a gloomy scene. I have relished many a biscuit and glass of wine in Mr. Grainger's dissecting-room when ten dead bodies were lying on the tables under dissection, but was entirely deprived of appetite during my attendance upon these cases. The smell on entering the apartments was exceedingly nauseous, and the room would not admit of free ventilation.'

Such conditions of the population, of habitual personal and domestic filth, are not necessary to any occupation; they are not the necessary consequence of poverty, and are the type of neglect and indolence; this is proved by the example of men engaged in the same occupations with improved habits. The medical officers of the Merthyr Tydvill union, in their returns, represent the health of the colliery population to be very good, a circumstance which is ascribed to their habitual cleanliness.

Mr. J. L. Roberts, surgeon, states:

> 'The colliers in our district invariably, on their return from the pits in the evening to their houses, strip to the skin, and wash themselves perfectly clean in a tub of lukewarm water, and wipe with towels until the cuticle is dry. The miners are not so particular. I firmly believe that the health of other workmen employed generally about the ironworks is not so permanently good as the colliers; they, generally speaking, not undergoing complete ablution as the colliers do. Generally, the colliers are quite free from any cutaneous disease, or at least not so much affected with psora, &c., as the generality of their fellow-workmen. Cutaneous diseases are frequent amongst children from want of cleanliness.'

In the places of work where there is the greatest need for cleanliness, in every place where there is a steam-engine, hot water, which is commonly allowed to run waste, is already provided in abundance for warm or tepid baths, not only for the workpeople, but, where there are numerous engines, for the whole population. If the same hot water arose at the same heat and abundance from any natural spring, baths would be erected, and medical treatises would be written in commendation of its medicinal virtues, which, the better opinion appears now to be, are ascribable, in the majority of instances, simply to the hot water, and to its application in cases where it had not before been used. Hot or tepid baths are deemed of more importance for the labouring classes in winter than are cold baths in summer, and they might be generally provided for the working classes in the manufacturing districts at a cost utterly inconsiderable.

A few years since a gentleman, observing some ditches in London, in the neighbourhood of the City-road, smoking with clean hot water running away from the steam-engine of a manufactory, directed attention to the waste, and suggested the expediency of using that water to supply public warm or tepid baths. After a time the suggestion was acted upon as a private speculation, and large swimming-baths were constructed; one, with superior accommodation and decorations at 1s.; another, with less costly fittings-up, at 6d. the bath. These were luxurious tepid baths, kept at a heat of 84°. The example appears to have been followed in Westminster by the establishment of similar tepid swimming-baths, where only 3d. is charged to persons of the working-class. As many as 2,000 and 3,000 of this class have resorted to these baths in one day, and the bath at the lowest charge is stated to make the best return for the capital invested in it. Similar establishments are, we believe, in progress in other parts of the metropolis.

RECAPITULATION OF CONCLUSIONS

First, as to the extent and operation of the evils which are the subject of the inquiry:—

That the various forms of epidemic, endemic, and other disease caused, or aggravated, or propagated chiefly amongst the labouring classes by atmospheric impurities produced by decomposing animal and vegetable substances, by damp and filth, and close and overcrowded dwellings prevail amongst the population in every part of the kingdom, whether dwelling in separate houses, in rural villages, in small towns, in the larger towns—as they have been found to prevail in the lowest districts of the metropolis.

That such disease, wherever its attacks are frequent, is always found in connexion with the physical circumstances above specified, and that where those circumstances are removed by drainage, proper cleansing, better ventilation, and other means of diminishing atmospheric impurity, the frequency and intensity of such disease is abated; and where the removal of the noxious agencies appears to be complete, such disease almost entirely disappears.

That high prosperity in respect to employment and wages, and various and abundant food, have afforded to the labouring classes no exemptions from attacks of epidemic disease, which have been as frequent and as fatal in periods of commercial and manufacturing prosperity as in any others.

That the formation of all habits of cleanliness is obstructed by defective supplies of water.

That the annual loss of life from filth and bad ventilation are greater than the loss from death or wounds in any wars in which the country has been engaged in modern times.

That these adverse circumstances tend to produce an adult population short-lived, improvident, reckless, and intemperate, and with habitual avidity for sensual gratifications.

That these habits lead to the abandonment of all the conveniences and decencies of life, and especially lead to the overcrowding of their homes, which is destructive to the morality as well as the health of large classes of both sexes.

That defective town cleansing fosters habits of the most abject degradation and tends to the demoralization of large numbers of human beings, who subsist by means of what they find amidst the noxious filth accumulated in neglected streets and byeplaces.

That the expenses of local public works are in generally unequally and unfairly assessed, oppressively and uneconomically collected, by separate collections, wastefully expended in separate and inefficient operations by unskilled and practically irresponsible officers.

That the existing law for the protection of the public health and the constitutional machinery for reclaiming its execution, such as the Courts Leet, have fallen into desuetude, and are in the state indicated by the prevalence of the evils they were intended to prevent.

Secondly. As to the means by which the present sanitary condition of the labouring classes may be improved:—

The primary and most important measures, and at the same time the most practicable, and within the recognized province of public administration, are drainage, the removal of all refuse of habitations, streets, and roads, and the improvement of the supplies of water.

That the chief obstacles to the immediate removal of decomposing refuse of towns and habitations have been the expense and annoyance of the hand labour and cartage requisite for the purpose.

That this expense may be reduced to one-twentieth or to one-thirtieth, or rendered inconsiderable, by the use of water and self-acting means of removal by improved and cheaper sewers and drains.

That appropriate scientific arrangements for public drainage would afford important facilities for private land-drainage, which is important for the health as well as sustenance of the labouring classes.

That the expense of public drainage, of supplies of water laid on in houses, and of means of improved cleansing would be a pecuniary gain, by diminishing the existing charges attendant on sickness and premature mortality.

That for the protection of the labouring classes and of the ratepayers against inefficiency and waste in all new structural arrangements for the protection of the public health, and to ensure public confidence that the expenditure will be beneficial, securities should be taken that all new local public works are devised and conducted by responsible officers qualified by the possession of the science and skill of civil engineers.

That for the prevention of the disease occasioned by defective ventilation, and other causes of impurity in places of work and other places where large numbers are assembled, and for the general promotion of the means necessary to prevent disease, that it would be good economy to appoint a district medical officer independent of private practice, and with the securities of special qualifications and responsibilities to initiate sanitary measures and reclaim the execution of the law.

And that the removal of noxious physical circumstances, and the promotion of civic, household, and personal cleanliness, are necessary to the improvement of the moral condition of the population; for that sound morality and refinement in manners and health are not long found co-existant with filthy habits amongst any class of the community.

> I have the honour to be,
> Gentlemen,
> Your obedient servant,
> EDWIN CHADWICK.

IGNAZ SEMMELWEIS (1818–1865)

The Etiology, Concept, and Prophylaxis of Childbed Fever

In 1846, when Ignaz Semmelweis became an assistant in Vienna's Lying-In Hospital, the fame of Viennese medicine was established throughout Europe. A persistent thorn in the hospital's side, however, was the staggering mortality rate from childbed, or puerperal, fever at the very clinic it used to train medical students. Almost one in every three pregnant women who entered this notorious clinic died, as opposed to only three in every one hundred women who were treated at the second clinic, which trained midwives. Semmelweis set out to explain this discrepancy. Rejecting the widely held notion that puerperal fever was a peculiar kind of epidemic disease, he discovered that it was instead a specific form of blood poisoning. This finding did not in itself elicit the censure of his colleagues: It was Semmelweis's explanation of how the disease was transmitted that they condemned. At the time, students and physicians routinely went straight from dissecting putrid corpses to examining pregnant women without so much as washing their hands. Semmelweis argued that this practice carried lethal matter from hand to womb and insisted that students and physicians disinfect with chlorine before handling patients: "Murder must cease," he declared. Despite an immediate and dramatic drop in mortality after his recommendations were implemented, his colleagues scorned them as utter nonsense and discontinued the new measures. Ostracized and embittered, Semmelweis returned to his native Budapest in 1851, where, after a decades-long struggle to win acceptance for his revolutionary discoveries regarding antisepsis and the nature of infection, he died from the very disease that would bring him undying fame.

Medicine's highest duty is saving threatened human life, and obstetrics is the branch of medicine in which this duty is most obviously fulfilled. Frequently it is necessary to deliver a child in transverse lie. Mother and child will probably die if the birth is left to nature, while the obstetrician's timely helping hand, almost painlessly and taking only a few minutes, can save both.

I was already familiar with this prerogative of obstetrics from the theoretical lectures on the specialty. I found it perfectly confirmed as I had the opportunity to learn the practical aspects of obstetrics in the large Viennese maternity hospital. But unfortunately the number of cases in which the obstetrician achieves such blessings vanishes in comparison with the number of victims to whom his help is of no avail.

From *The Etiology, Concept, and Prophylaxis of Childbed Fever*, ed. and trans. K. Codell Carter (Madison: University of Wisconsin Press, 1983).

This dark side of obstetrics is childbed fever. Each year I saw ten or fifteen crises in which the salvation of mother and child could be achieved. I also saw many hundreds of maternity patients treated unsuccessfully for childbed fever. Not only was therapy unsuccessful, the etiology seemed deficient. The accepted etiology of childbed fever, on the basis of which I saw so many hundreds of maternity patients treated unsuccessfully, cannot contain the actual causal factor of the disease.

The large gratis Viennese maternity hospital is divided into two clinics; one is called the first, the other the second. By Imperial Decree of 10 October 1840, Court Commission for Education Decree of 17 October 1840, and Administrative Ordinance of 27 October 1840, all male students were assigned to the first clinic and all female students to the second. Before this time student obstetricians and midwives received training in equal numbers in both clinics.

TABLE 1

	First Clinic			Second Clinic		
	Births	*Deaths*	*Rate*	*Births*	*Deaths*	*Rate*
1841	3,036	237	7.7	2,442	86	3.5
1842	3,287	518	15.8	2,659	202	7.5
1843	3,060	274	8.9	2,739	164	5.9
1844	3,157	260	8.2	2,956	68	2.3
1845	3,492	241	6.8	3,241	66	2.03
1846	4,010	459	11.4	3,754	105	2.7
Total	20,042	1,989		17,791	691	
Avg.			9.92			3.38

From the time the first clinic began training only obstetricians until June 1847, the mortality rate in the first clinic was consistently greater than in the second clinic, where only midwives were trained. Indeed, in the year 1846, the mortality rate in the first clinic was five times as great as in the second, and through a six-year period it was, on the average, three times as great. This is shown in Table 1.

It has not been questioned and has been expressed thousands of times that the horrible ravages of childbed fever are caused by epidemic influences. By epidemic influences one understands atmospheric-cosmic-terrestrial changes, as yet not precisely defined, that often extend over whole countrysides, and by which childbed fever is generated in persons predisposed by the puerperal state. But if the atmospheric-cosmic-terrestrial conditions of Vienna cause puerperal fever in predisposed persons, how is it that for many years these conditions have affected persons in the first clinic while sparing similarly predisposed persons in the second? To me there appears no doubt that if the ravages of childbed fever in the first clinic are caused by epidemic influences, the same conditions must operate with minimal variation in the second clinic.

These considerations alone forced me to the unshakable conviction that epidemic influences were not responsible for the horrible devastations of the maternity patients in the first clinic.

Once I had come to this conviction, other supporting considerations occurred to me. If the atmospheric influences of Vienna occasion an epidemic in the maternity hospital, then necessarily there must be an epidemic among maternity patients throughout Vienna because the entire population is subject to the same influences. But in fact, while the puerperal disease rages most furiously in the maternity hospital, it is only infrequently observed either in Vienna at large or in the surrounding countryside. During a cholera epidemic, people in general are affected, not just those in a particular hospital. A common and successful expedient for halting an epidemic of childbed fever is to close the maternity hospitals. Hospitals are closed not to force maternity patients to die somewhere else, but because of the belief that if patients deliver in the hospital they are subject to epidemic influences, whereas if they deliver elsewhere they will remain healthy. However, this proves one is not dealing with a disease dependent on atmospheric influences, because these influences would extend beyond the hospital into every part of the city. This proves that the disease is endemic—a disease due to causes limited by the boundaries of the hospital.

With a few exceptions, maternity hospitals that are not teaching institutions or that train only midwives are more favorable than institutions that train obstetricians. Table 1 shows the different mortality rates of two divisions of one institution; a similar difference occurred in the two divisions of the maternity hospital at Strasbourg. Later we will speak more of these circumstances.

As explained before, these considerations strengthened my conviction that the great mortality of the first clinic was not due to epidemic influences but rather to harmful endemic factors (i.e., to a cause manifested so horribly only within the first clinic). Because of the bad reputation of the first clinic, everyone sought admission to the second clinic. For this reason, the second clinic was often unable to resume admissions at the specified time because it was impossible to accommodate new arrivals. Or if the second clinic began to admit, within a few hours it was necessary to resume admitting patients to the first clinic because the passageway was crowded with such a great number of persons awaiting admission to the second clinic. In a short time all the free places were taken. In the five years I was associated with the first clinic, not once did overcrowding make it necessary to reopen admission to the second clinic. This was true even though once each week the first clinic admitted continuously for a period of forty-eight hours. In spite of this overcrowding, the mortality rate in the second clinic was strikingly smaller.

It has been proposed that the evil reputation of the institution, with its great annual contingent of deaths, so frightens the newly admitted patients that they become ill and die. The patients really do fear the first clinic. Frequently one must witness moving scenes in which patients, kneeling and wringing their hands, beg to be released in order to seek admission to the second clinic. Such persons have usually been admitted because they are ignorant of the reputation of the first clinic, but they soon become suspicious because of the large number of doctors present. One sees maternity patients with abnormally high pulse rates, bloated stomachs, and dry tongues (in other words, very ill with puerperal fever), still insisting only hours before death that they are perfectly healthy, because they know that treatment by the physicians is the forerunner of death. Nevertheless, I could not convince myself that fear was the cause of the high mortality rate in the first clinic. As a physician, I could not understand how fear, a psychological condition, could bring about such physical changes as occur in childbed fever. Moreover, it would have required a long period of time with consistently unequal mortality rates for ordinary people, who did not have access to hospital reports, to become aware that one clinic had a much greater mortality rate than the other. Fear could not account for the initial difference.

Even religious practices did not escape attention. The hospital chapel was so located that when the priest was summoned to administer last rites in the second clinic, he could go directly to the room set aside for ill patients. On the other hand, when he was summoned to the first clinic he had to pass through five other rooms because the room containing ill patients was sixth in line from the chapel. According to accepted Catholic practice, when visiting the sick to administer last rites, the priest generally arrived in ornate vestments and was preceded by a sacristan who rang a bell. This was supposed to occur only once in twenty-four hours. Yet twenty-four hours is a long time for someone suffering from childbed fever. Many who appeared tolerably healthy at the time of the priest's visit, and who therefore did not require last rites, were so ill a few hours later that the priest had to be summoned again. One can imagine the impression that was created on the other patients when the priest came several times a day, each time accompanied by the clearly audible bell. Even to me it was very demoralizing to hear the bell hurry past my door. I groaned within for the victim who had fallen to an unknown cause. The bell was a painful admonition to seek this unknown cause with all my powers. It had been proposed that even this difference in the two clinics explained the different mortality rates. During my first period of service, I appealed to the compassion of the servant of God and arranged for him to come by a less direct route, without bells, and without passing through the other clinic rooms. Thus, no one outside the room containing the ill patients knew of the priest's presence. The two clinics were made identical in this respect as well, but the mortality rate was unaffected.

It had also been suggested that the mortality rate in the first clinic resulted from the offense to modesty incurred through the presence of males at delivery. As those familiar with the Viennese maternity hospital realize, patients are troubled by fear but not by offended modesty. Moreover, it is not clear how this offended modesty would bring about the exudative mortal processes of the disease.

Based on experience of over fifteen years in three different institutions, all of which were severely afflicted with childbed fever, I regard the disease, without a single exception, as a resorption fever dependent on the resorption of decaying animal-organic matter. Resorption first causes disintegration of the blood. This is followed by exudation. In the overwhelming majority of cases the decaying animal-organic matter is conveyed to the individual from external sources. These are the cases represented as epidemics of childbed fever; these are the cases that can be prevented. Occasionally, decaying animal-organic matter is generated within the attacked organism. This is self-infection and cannot always be prevented.

The source of decaying animal-organic matter can be a corpse of any age, of either sex, regardless of the preceding disease, regardless whether the corpse is a pregnant woman or not. Only the degree of decomposition of the corpse should be taken into consideration. These assorted corpses are the ones which people who practiced in the first clinic examined. The source of decaying animal-organic matter can be a diseased person of any age, of either sex, regardless whether the individual suffers from childbed fever; only whether the decaying animal-organic matter is a result of the disease comes into question. In the first clinic in October 1847 childbed fever was caused by a discharging medullary carcinoma of the uterus, and in November 1847 by the exhalations of a carious knee. In the maternity ward of the St. Rochus Hospital childbed fever was caused by the ichorous products of various surgical disorders. The source of the decaying animal-organic matter is every physiological animal-organic structure that, having been withdrawn from the vital order, has reached a specific degree of decay. Not the nature of the structure but only the degree of decomposition comes into question. In the obstetrical clinic at Pest during the school years 1856–57 and 1857–58 childbed fever was caused by physiological blood and normal lochial discharge that adhered to the bed linen and began to decay.

Decaying animal-organic matter is carried by examining fingers, operating hands, instruments, bed linen, the atmosphere, sponges, basins, hands of midwives and attendants. In other words, anything that is contaminated by decaying animal-organic matter and that comes into contact with the genitals of patients.

The decaying animal-organic matter is resorbed at the inner surface of the uterus from the external orifice upward. As a result of pregnancy, this surface is denuded of its mucous membrane and is therefore unusually resorbant.

In rare cases, decaying animal-organic matter originates inside the affected person. This occurs when organic matter that should be discharged during delivery begins to decay before being discharged. In being resorbed, it causes childbed fever by self-infection. The organic matter can be lochia, decidual remnants, clotted blood that is retained in the uterus, etc. Alternatively, the decaying animal-organic matter can be a product of pathological processes. For example, as a result of a difficult operation with forceps, portions of the genitals may be crushed and become gangrenous. Upon resorption, the gangrenous particles cause childbed fever by self-infection.

Suppose we explain childbed fever as a fever of resorption in which the introduction of decaying animal-organic matter leads to disintegration of the blood and to exudation. Then childbed fever is not a disease unique to and appearing only in the newly delivered, because as a result of resorption the disease may arise during pregnancy or when giving birth. The disease can be conveyed to infants, whether male or female. In consequence of resorption of decaying matter it can also be found among anatomists, surgeons, in operative cases in surgical wards, etc. Kolletschka also had this disease. Thus childbed fever is not a species of disease; rather it is a type of pyemia.

Various concepts are associated with the expression 'pyemia' and it is necessary, therefore, to explain that I understand this term as referring to disintegration of the blood through decaying animal-organic matter. One type of pyemia I call childbed fever, because in pyemia of maternity patients one finds phenomena in the genital region that are not found in other people. Anatomists and surgeons who die of pyemia do not have endometritis [serious infection of the mucous membrane of the uterus], etc.

Childbed fever is not a contagious disease. A contagious disease is one that produces the contagion by which the disease is spread. This contagion brings about only the same disease in other individuals. Smallpox is a contagious disease because smallpox generates the contagion that causes smallpox in others. Childbed fever is different. This fever can be caused in healthy patients through other diseases.

The only cause of childbed fever is decaying animal-organic matter that is either introduced to the individual from external sources or generated internally. Thus, the prophylaxis of childbed fever involves preventing the introduction of external decaying matter, preventing the internal generation of decaying matter, and removing as quickly as possible any existing decaying matter or preventing its resorption.

Decaying matter is usually spread in manual examinations. Given a large number of students, it is safer to avoid contamination than to clean what has once been contaminated. I therefore appeal to all governments to proclaim laws forbidding those engaged in maternity hospitals from activities likely to contaminate their hands. The imperative necessity of such laws is made clear by my experience in the first clinic; in spite of all my exertions, I did not succeed in limiting childbed fever to cases of self-infection. Bear in mind that the semester for practical obstetrics does not begin on a fixed day when all can simultaneously be made aware of their responsibilities. Rather, a few students join and leave each day. Because one cannot repeat the same things every day, it can easily happen that many are first warned after they have been there several days. Consider that the forty-two students in the first clinic spend the largest part of their day in the morgue performing pathological and forensic autopsies, in the divisions of the general hospital, in various operations, and in other courses. In all these activities, their hands become not only contaminated but actually saturated with decaying matter. Moreover, although it is difficult to believe, these students will not take the time necessary for chlorine washings to disinfect their hands completely.

This pernicious behavior—whereby many human lives are prematurely destroyed, whereby additional generations of misled physicians are sent out into practice, and whereby cases of infection outside the maternity hospitals are then used as evidence that childbed fever is epidemic—can only be ended by such laws. If, in consequence of the law, students in maternity hospitals have clean hands, then the most ardent lecture on epidemic influences will no longer cause epidemics. Without this law, such lectures make students careless, and childbed fever is increased by hands contaminated with decaying matter. I therefore implore all governments to proclaim such laws in order that the childbearing sex will not be further decimated, in order that life yet unborn will not be infected with seeds of death by those very persons who are called to protect life. Such a law would not hinder other aspects of medical education, because practical obstetrics is a relatively short course. Moreover, the law would significantly promote the teaching of practical obstetrics, because the most informative cases would no longer occur while students are occupied in other activities.

In order to disinfect the hands completely it is necessary to oil them before they are contaminated so that the decaying matter cannot penetrate the pores. Thereafter the hands must be washed with soap and then exposed to the operation of a chemical agent to destroy the decaying matter. I employ chloride of lime and wash as long as is necessary to make the hands slippery. Hands treated in this way are completely disinfected. Decaying matter is carried not only by the examining finger but also by everything contaminated that can come into contact with the genitals. These items must, therefore, either be disinfected or no longer used.

It is easy to explain why the relative mortality in smaller maternity hospitals is greater than in large ones. In small hospitals the teaching material is restricted and every patient must be used. If they are examined with contaminated hands, a high percentage of the patients will become infected. In Vienna there is such an excess of teaching material that hundreds of individuals are not used for teaching and thus are not infected.

In order that these measures will be observed everywhere, medical personnel must be made to swear in the oath and in the official instructions given when they receive their diplomas that they will conscientiously discharge all that is required by these prophylactic measures. Instead of losing 1 patient for every 3 or 4 that are admitted, those who observe these measures may lose as few as 1 in 400—certainly less than 1 in 100.

JOSEPH LISTER (1827-1912)

"On the Antiseptic Principle in the Practice of Surgery"

In Joseph Lister's day, fear, physical agony, and massive infection made surgery the treatment of last resort. It was solving the last difficulty that Lister would make his life's work. Lister was no doubt introduced to the most important scientific instrument of the nineteenth century while still a child, for his father spent his leisure time absorbed in his microscope. Coming from an English Quaker family, Lister was educated in London and Scotland, becoming house physician at the Edinburgh Hospital in 1854 and professor of surgery at Glasgow University in 1861. A large part of his practice involved treating broken limbs, and Lister began to note a signal fact: Although it was commonly believed that all contused wounds produced pus, compound fractures suppurated, while simple ones did not. Open wounds, therefore, differed from closed ones, and, arguing on the basis of Pasteur's recent discoveries, Lister speculated that exposed wounds were more likely to putrefy because they came in contact with airborne bacteria. An obvious solution was to destroy these microbes, and after experimenting with a number of techniques, Lister found that using carbolic spray during surgery and applying thick layers of bandages soaked in carbolic solution over the wound nearly eliminated infection. Because it was linked to Pasteur's germ theory, still widely regarded with skepticism, "listerism" and its antiseptic surgical dressing were not widely adopted until the Franco-German War provided a vast field for their application. Surgeons reported remarkable success with Lister's technique, and it soon became world famous. The step from antisepsis to asepsis still remained to be taken, however, for physicians had yet to realize that their hands and instruments presented far graver danger to a wound than did the air around it.

In the course of an extended investigation into the nature of inflammation, and the healthy and morbid conditions of the blood in relation to it, I arrived, several years ago, at the conclusion that the essential cause of suppuration in wounds is decomposition, brought about by the influence of the atmosphere upon blood or serum retained within them, and, in the case of contused wounds, upon portions of tissue destroyed by the violence of injury.

To prevent the occurrence of suppuration, with all its attendant risks, was an object manifestly desirable; but till lately apparently unattainable, since it seemed hopeless to attempt to exclude the oxygen, which was universally regarded as the agent by which putrefaction was effected. But when it had been shown by the researches

From *Medical Classics*, Vol. 1 (Baltimore: Williams & Wilkins, 1936–37).

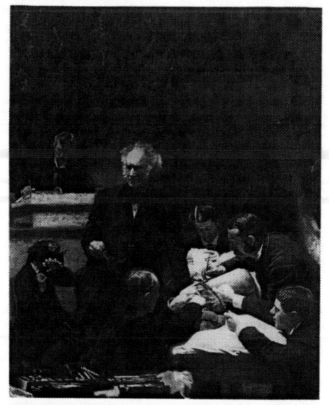

18. Thomas Eakins, The Gross Clinic. *Jefferson Medical College of Thomas Jefferson University, Philadelphia. Although Eakins highlights the use of anesthesia in this painting, he also exposes the absence of antisepsis. The doctors' black frock coats and naked hands signal an era in which hospital wards reeked with the stench of gangrene, and surgeons went directly from the dissecting room to the operating table, sporting their needles and thread in the lapels of their coats. As Dr. Lawrence Tait observed in the 1860s, "The only correct garb of the surgeon was a frock coat (the oldest and shabbiest in his wardrobe) which was kept in the surgeon's room and never renewed or cleaned during his twenty years of operating work"* (Logan Clendening, Behind the Doctor *[London: William Heinemann, 1933], p. 386). The horror that still clung to surgery is captured in the figure to Dr. Gross's right; her averted face and agonized gesture serve as poignant counterpoints to the clinical composure and avid attention of the surgeons.*

of Pasteur that the septic property of the atmosphere depended, not on the oxygen or any gaseous constituent, but on minute organisms suspended in it, which owed their energy to their vitality, it occurred to me that decomposition in the injured part might be avoided without excluding the air, by applying as a dressing some material capable of destroying the life of the floating particles.

Upon this principle I have based a practice of which I will now attempt to give a short account.

The material which I have employed is carbolic or phenic acid, a volatile organic compound which appears to exercise a peculiarly destructive influence upon low forms of life, and hence is the most powerful antiseptic with which we are at present acquainted.

The first class of cases to which I applied it was that of compound fractures, in which the effects of decomposition in the injured part were especially striking and pernicious. The results might have been such as to establish conclusively the great principle, that *all the local inflammatory mischief and general febrile disturbance which follow severe injuries are due to the irritating and poisoning influence of decomposing blood or sloughs.* For these evils are entirely avoided by the antiseptic treatment, so that limbs which otherwise would be unhesitatingly condemned to amputation may be retained with confidence of the best results.

In conducting the treatment, the first object must be the destruction of any septic germs which may have been introduced into the wound, either at the moment of the accident or during the time which has since elapsed. This is done by introducing the acid of full strength into all accessible recesses of the wound by means of a piece of rag held in dressing forceps and dipped in the liquid.

The next object to be kept in view is to guard effectually against the spreading of decomposition into the wound along the stream of blood and serum which oozes out during the first few days after the accident, when the acid originally applied has been washed out, or dissipated by absorption and evaporation. This part of the treatment has been greatly improved during the last few weeks. The method which I have hitherto published consisted in the application of a piece of lint dipped in the acid, overlapping the sound skin to some extent, and covered with a tin cap, which was daily raised in order to touch the surface of the lint with the antiseptic. This method certainly succeeded well with wounds of moderate size; and, indeed, I may say that in all the many cases of this kind which have been so treated by myself or my house-surgeons, not a single failure has occurred. When, however, the wound is very large, the flow of blood and serum is so profuse, especially during the first twenty-four hours, that the antiseptic application cannot prevent the spread of decomposition into the interior unless it overlaps the sound skin for a very considerable distance, and this was inadmissible by the method described above, on account of the extensive sloughing of the surface of the cutis which it would involve. This difficulty has, however, been overcome by employing a paste composed of common whitening (carbonate of lime) mixed with a solution of one part of carbolic acid in four parts of boiled linseed oil, so as to form a firm putty. This application contains the acid in too dilute a form to excoriate the skin, which it may be made to cover to any extent that may be thought desirable, while its substance serves as a reservoir of the antiseptic material. So long as any discharge continues, the paste should be changed daily; and, in order to prevent the chance of mischief occurring during the process, a piece of rag dipped in the solution of carbolic acid in oil is put on next the skin, and maintained there permanently, care being taken to avoid raising it along with the putty. This rag is always kept in an antiseptic condition from contact with the paste above it, and destroys any germs that may fall upon it during the short time that should alone be allowed to pass in the changing of the dressing. And here I would desire earnestly to enforce the necessity of persevering with the antiseptic application, in spite of the appearance of suppuration, so long as other symptoms are favourable. The surgeon is extremely apt to suppose that any suppuration is an indication that the antiseptic treatment has failed, . . .

Another instructive experiment is to dress a granulating sore with some of the putty above described, overlapping the sound skin extensively, when we find in the course of twenty-four hours that pus has been produced by the sore, although the application has been perfectly antiseptic; and, indeed, the larger the amount of carbolic acid in the paste the greater is the quantity of pus formed, provided we avoid such a proportion as would act as a caustic. The carbolic acid, though it prevents decomposition, induces suppuration—obviously by acting as a chemical stimulus; and we may safely infer that putrescent organic materials (which we know to be chemically acrid) operate in the same way.

I left behind me in Glasgow a boy, thirteen years of age, who between three and four weeks previously met with a most severe injury to the left arm, which he got entangled in a machine at a fair. There was a wound six inches long and three inches broad, and the skin was very extensively undetermined beyond its limits, while the soft parts generally were so much lacerated that a pair of dressing forceps introduced at the wound, and pushed directly inwards, appeared beneath the skin at the opposite aspect of the limb. From this wound several tags of muscle were hanging, and among them there was one consisting of about three inches of the triceps in almost its entire thickness; while the lower fragment of the bone, which was broken high up, was protruding four and a half inches, stripped of muscle, the skin being tucked in under it. Without the assistance of the antiseptic treatment, I should certainly have thought of nothing else but amputation at the shoulder-joint; but as the radial pulse could be felt, and the fingers had sensation, I did not hesitate to try to save the limb, and adopted the plan of treatment above described, wrapping the arm from the shoulder to below the elbow in the antiseptic application, the whole interior of the wound, together with the protruding bone, having previously been freely treated with strong carbolic acid. About the tenth day the discharge, which up to that time had been only sanious and serous, showed a slight admixture of slimy pus, and this increased till, a few days before I left, it amounted to about three drachms in twenty-four hours. But the boy continued, as he had been after the second day, free from unfavourable symptoms, with pulse, tongue, appetite, and sleep natural, and strength increasing, while the limb remained, as it had been from the first, free from swelling, redness, or pain. I therefore persevered with the antiseptic dressing, and before I left, the discharge was already somewhat less, while the bone was becoming firm. I think it likely that in that boy's case I should have found merely a superficial sore had I taken off all the dressings at the end of three weeks, though, considering the extent of the injury, I thought it prudent to let the month expire before disturbing the rag next to the skin. But I feel sure that if I had resorted to ordinary dressing when the pus first appeared, the progress of the case would have been exceedingly different.

The next class of cases to which I have applied the antiseptic treatment is that of abscesses. Here, also, the results have been extremely satisfactory, and in beautiful harmony with the pathological principles indicated above.

Ordinary contused wounds are of course amenable to the same treatment as compound fractures, which are a complicated variety of them. I will content myself with mentioning a single instance of this class of cases. In April last a volunteer was discharging a rifle, when it burst, and blew back the thumb with its metacarpal bone, so that it could be bent back as on a hinge at the trapezial joint, which had evidently been opened, while all the soft parts between the metacarpal bones of the thumb and forefinger were torn through. I need not insist before my present audience on the ugly character of such an injury. My house-surgeon, Mr. Hector Cameron, applied carbolic acid to the whole raw surface, and completed the dressing as if for compound fracture. The hand remained free from pain, redness, or swelling, and, with the exception of a shallow groove, all the wound consolidated without a drop of matter, so that if it had been a clean cut, it would have been regarded as a good example of primary union. The small granulating surface soon healed, and at present a linear cicatrix alone tells of the injury he sustained, while his thumb has all its movements and his hand a firm grasp.

If the severest form of contused and lacerated wounds heal thus kindly under the antiseptic treatment, it is obvious that its application to simple incised wounds must be merely a matter of detail. I have devoted a good deal of attention to this class, but I have not as yet pleased myself altogether with any of the methods I have employed. I am, however, prepared to go so far as to say that a solution of carbolic acid in twenty parts of water, while a mild and cleanly application, may be relied on for destroying any septic germs that may fall upon the wound during the performance of an operation; and also that for preventing the subsequent introduction of others, the paste above described, applied as for compound fractures, gives excellent results. Thus I have had a case of strangulated inguinal hernia, in which it was necessary to take away half a pound of thickened omentum, heal without any deep-seated suppuration or any tenderness of the sac or any fever; and amputations, including one immediately below the knee, have remained absolutely free from constitutional symptoms.

There is, however, one point more that I cannot but advert to—namely, the influence of this mode of treatment upon the general healthiness of a hospital. Previously to its introduction, the two large wards in which most of my cases of accident and of operation are treated were amongst the unhealthiest in the whole surgical division of the Glasgow Royal Infirmary, in consequence, apparently, of these wards being unfavourably placed with reference to the supply of fresh air; and I have felt ashamed, when recording the results of my practice, to have so often to allude to hospital gangrene or pyaemia. It was interesting, though melancholy, to observe that, whenever all, or nearly all, the beds contained cases with open sores, these grievous complications were pretty sure to show themselves; so that I came to welcome simple fractures, though in themselves of little interest either for myself or the students, because their presence diminished the proportion of open sores among the patients.

But since the antiseptic treatment has been brought into full operation, and wounds and abscesses no longer poison the atmosphere with putrid exhalations, my wards, though in other respects under precisely the same circumstances as before, have completely changed their character; so that during the last nine months not a single instance of pyaemia, hospital gangrene, or erysipelas has occurred in them.

As there appears to be no doubt regarding the cause of this change, the importance of the fact can hardly be exaggerated.

LOUIS PASTEUR (1822–1895)

"On the Extension of the Germ Theory to the Etiology of Certain Common Diseases"

Although Louis Pasteur was a chemist by profession, his discoveries in agriculture, alcoholic fermentation, and silk production had incalculable and far-reaching effects on the theory and practice of medicine. After studying at the École Normale in Paris and teaching in Dijon and Strasbourg, Pasteur was appointed dean of the faculty of natural science at Lille, where the major industry was the manufacture of alcohol. Having grown up in Burgundy, Pasteur was all too familiar with farmers' complaints about wine "falling sick," butter turning rancid, and milk growing sour. At Lille, he became convinced that all these transmutations had a common cause: minuscule living creatures, or "germs." Pasteur's next challenge was to explain where the microorganisms responsible for spoiling wine came from. In a series of epoch-making experiments that demolished the idea of spontaneous generation, Pasteur found that if substances were heated and sealed off from the air, no contamination resulted; only with exposure to the air did decomposition set in. With this experiment, the process of "pasteurization" was invented. Pasteur could now direct his attention to epidemic diseases, and he did so with overwhelming success. In addition to rescuing the French silk industry by eradicating the microbe that was decimating silkworms, he also saved farmers from catastrophic losses by developing vaccines for chicken cholera, splenic fever, and swine fever. Having achieved miraculous effects in the field of agriculture, in 1880, Pasteur broadened the scope of his enterprise and published the momentous essay that extended his "germ theory" to the diseases of humankind.

When I began the studies now occupying my attention, I was attempting to extend the germ theory to certain common diseases. I do not know when I can return to that work. Therefore in my desire to see it carried on by others, I take the liberty of presenting it to the public in its present condition.

I. Furuncles. In May, 1879, one of the workers in my laboratory had a number of furuncles, appearing at short intervals, sometimes on one part of the body and sometimes on another. Constantly impressed with the thought of the immense part played by microscopic organisms in Nature, I queried whether the pus in the furuncles might not contain one of these organisms whose presence, development, and chance trans-

From *The Harvard Classics: Scientific Papers,* ed. Charles W. Eliot (1897; reprint, New York: P. F. Collier & Son, 1910).

portation here and there in the tissues after entrance would produce a local inflammation, and pus formation, and might explain the recurrence of the illness during a longer or shorter time. It was easy enough to subject this thought to the test of experiment.

First observation.—On June second, a puncture was made at the base of the small cone of pus at the apex of a furuncle on the nape of the neck. The fluid obtained was at once sowed in the presence of pure air—of course with the precautions necessary to exclude any foreign germs, either at the moment of puncture, at the moment of sowing in the culture fluid, or during the stay in the oven, which was kept at the constant temperature of about 35° C. The next day, the culture fluid had become cloudy and contained a single organism, consisting of small spherical points arranged in pairs, sometimes in fours, but often in irregular masses. Two fluids were preferred in these experiments—chicken and yeast bouillon. According as one or the other was used, appearances varied a little. These should be described. With the yeast water, the pairs of minute granules are distributed throughout the liquid, which is uniformly clouded. But with the chicken bouillon, the granules are collected in little masses which line the walls and bottom of the flasks while the body of the fluid remains clear, unless it be shaken: in this case it becomes uniformly clouded by the breaking up of the small masses from the walls of the flasks.

Second observation.—On the tenth of June a new furuncle made its appearance on the right thigh of the same person. Pus could not yet be seen under the skin, but this was already thickened and red over a surface the size of a franc. The inflamed part was washed with alcohol, and dried with blotting paper passed through the flame of an alcohol lamp. A puncture at the thickened portion enabled us to secure a small amount of lymph mixed with blood, which was sowed at the same time as some blood taken from the finger of the hand. The following days, the blood from the finger remained absolutely sterile: but that obtained from the center of the forming furuncle gave an abundant growth of the same small organism as before.

Third observation.—The fourteenth of June, a new furuncle appeared on the neck of the same person. The same examination, the same result, that is to say the development of the microscopic organism previously described and complete sterility of the blood of the general circulation, taken this time at the base of the furuncle outside of the inflamed area.

At the time of making these observations I spoke of them to Dr. Maurice Reynaud, who was good enough to send me a patient who had had furuncles for more than three months. On June thirteenth I made cultures of the pus from a furuncle of this man. The next day there was a general cloudiness of the culture fluids, consisting entirely of the preceding parasite, and of this alone.

Fourth observation.—June fourteenth, the same individual showed me a newly forming furuncle in the left axilla: there was wide-spread thickening and redness of the skin, but no pus was yet apparent. An incision at the center of the thickening showed a small quantity of pus mixed with blood. Sowing, rapid growth for twenty-four hours and the appearance of the same organism. Blood from the arm at a distance from the furuncle remained completely sterile.

June 17, the examination of a fresh furuncle on the same individual gave the same result, the development of a pure culture of the same organism.

Fifth observation.—July twenty-first, Dr. Maurice Reynaud informed me that there was a woman at the Lariboisière hospital with multiple furuncles. As a matter of fact her back was covered with them, some in active suppuration, others in the ulcerating stage. I took pus from all of these furuncles that had not opened. After a few hours, this pus gave an abundant growth in cultures. The same organism, without admixture, was found. Blood from the inflamed base of the furuncle remained sterile.

In brief, it appears certain that every furuncle contains an aerobic microscopic parasite, to which is due the local inflammation and the pus formation that follows.

II. On Osteomyelitis. On the fourteenth of February, at the request of Dr. Lannelongue I went to the Sainte-Eugènie hospital, where this skillful surgeon was to operate on a little girl of about twelve years of age. The right knee was much swollen, as well as the whole leg below the calf and a part of the thigh above the knee. There was no external opening. Under chloroform, Dr. Lannelongue made a long incision below the knee which let out a large amount of pus; the tibia was found denuded for a long distance. Three places in the bone were trephined. From each of these, quantities of pus flowed. Pus from inside and outside the bone was collected with all possible precautions and was carefully examined and cultivated later. The direct microscopic study of the pus, both internal and external, was of extreme interest. It was seen that both contained large numbers of the organism similar to that of furuncles, arranged in pairs, in fours and in packets, some with sharp clear contour, others only faintly visible and with very pale outlines. The external pus contained many pus corpuscles, the internal had none at all. It was like a fatty paste of the furuncular organism. Also, it may be noted, that growth of the small organism had begun in less than six hours after the cultures were started. Thus I saw, that it corresponded exactly with the organism of furuncles. The diameter of the individuals was found to be one one-thousandth of a millimeter. If I ventured to express myself so I might say that in this case at least the osteomyelitis was really a furuncle of the bone marrow. It is undoubtedly easy to induce osteomyelitis artificially in living animals.

III. On puerperal fever.—First observation. On the twelfth of March, 1878, Dr. Hervieux was good enough to admit me to his service in the Maternity to visit a woman delivered some days before and seriously ill with puerperal fever. The lochia were extremely fetid. I found them full of micro-organisms of many kinds. A small amount of blood was obtained from a puncture on the index finger of the left hand, (the finger being first properly washed and dried with a *sterile* towel,) and then sowed in chicken bouillon. The culture remained sterile during the following days.

The thirteenth, more blood was taken from a puncture in the finger and this time growth occurred. As death took place on the sixteenth of March at six in the morning, it seems that the blood contained a microscopic parasite at least three days before.

The fifteenth of March, eighteen hours before death, blood from a needle-prick in the left foot was used. This culture also was fertile.

The first culture, of March thirteenth, contained only the organism of furuncles; the next one, that of the fifteenth, contained an organism resembling that of furunculosis, but which always differed enough to make it easy usually to distinguish it. In this way; whilst the parasite of furuncles is arranged in pairs, very rarely in chains of three or four elements, the new one, that of the culture of the fifteenth, occurs in long chains, the number of cells in each being indefinite. The chains are flexible and often appear as little tangled packets like tangled strings of pearls.

Interpretation of the disease and of the death.—After confinement, the pus that always naturally forms in the injured parts of the uterus instead of remaining pure becomes contaminated with microscopic organisms from outside, notably the organism in long chains and the pyogenic vibrio. These organisms pass into the peritoneal cavity through the tubes or by other channels, and some of them into the blood, probably by the lymphatics. The resorption of the pus, always extremely easy and prompt when it is pure, becomes impossible through the presence of the parasites, whose entrance must be prevented by all possible means from the moment of confinement.

On May twenty-eighth, a rabbit was inoculated under the skin of the abdomen with five drops of the preceding culture of the pyogenic vibrio. The days following an enormous abscess formed which opened spontaneously on the fourth of June. An abundantly cheesy pus came from it. About the abscess there was extensive induration. On the eighth of June, the opening of the abscess was larger, the suppuration active. Near its border was another abscess, evidently joined with the first, for upon pressing it with the finger, pus flowed freely from the opening in the first abscess. During the whole of the month of June, the rabbit was sick and the abscesses suppurated, but less and less. In July they closed; the animal was well. There could only be felt some nodules under the skin of the abdomen.

What disturbances might not such an organism carry into the body of a parturient woman, after passing into the peritoneum, the lymphatics or the blood through the maternal placenta! Its presence is much more dangerous than that of the parasite arranged in chains. Furthermore, its development is always threatening, because, as said in the work already quoted (April, 1878) this organism can be easily recovered from many ordinary waters.

I may add that the organism in long chains, and that arranged in pairs are also extremely widespread, and that one of their habitats is the mucous surfaces of the genital tract.

Apparently there is no puerperal parasite, properly speaking. I have not encountered true septicemia in my experiments: but it ought to be among the puerperal affections.

Seventh observation.—On June eighteenth, M. Doléris informed me that a woman had been confined at the Cochin Hospital five days before and that fears were entertained as to the results of an operation that had been performed, it having been necessary to do an embryotomy. The lochia were sowed on the 18th; there was not the slightest trace of growth the next day nor the day after. Without the least knowledge of this woman since the eighteenth, on the twentieth I ventured to assert that she would get well. I sent to inquire about her. This is the text of the report: *"The woman is doing extremely well; she goes out tomorrow."*

Interpretation of the facts.—The pus naturally formed on the surface of the injured parts did not become contaminated with organisms brought from without. *Natura medicatrix* carried it off, that is to say the vitality of the mucous surfaces prevented the development of foreign germs. The pus was easily resorbed, and recovery took place.

I beg the Academy to permit me, in closing, to submit certain definite views, which I am strongly inclined to consider as legitimate conclusions from the facts I have had the honor to communicate to it.

Under the expression *puerperal fever* are grouped very different diseases, but all appearing to be the result of the growth of common organisms which by their presence infect the pus naturally formed on injured surfaces, which spread by one means or another, by the blood or the lymphatics, to one or another part of the body, and there induce morbid changes varying with the condition of the parts, the nature of the parasite, and the general constitution of the subject.

Whatever this constitution, does it not seem that by taking measures opposing the production of these common parasitic organisms recovery would usually occur, except perhaps when the body contains, before confinement, microscopic organisms, in contaminated internal or external abscesses, as was seen in one striking example (fifth observation). The antiseptic method I believe likely to be sovereign in the vast majority of cases. It seems to me that *immediately after confinement* the application of antiseptics should be begun. Carbolic acid can render great service, but there is another antiseptic, the use of which I am strongly inclined to advise, this is boric acid in concentrated solution, that is, four per cent. at the ordinary temperature. This acid, whose singular influence on cell life has been shown by M. Dumas, is so slightly acid that it is alkaline to certain test papers, as was long ago shown by M. Chevreul, besides this it has no odor like carbolic acid, which odor often disturbs the sick. Lastly, its lack of hurtful effects on mucous membranes, notably of the bladder, has been and is daily demonstrated in the hospitals of Paris.

Would it not be of great service to place a warm concentrated solution of boric acid, and compresses, at the bedside of each patient; which she could renew frequently after saturating with the solution, and this also after confinement? It would also be acting the part of prudence to place the compresses, before using, in a hot air oven at 150° C., more than enough to kill the germs of the common organisms.

Was I justified in calling this communication *"On the extension of the germ theory to the etiology of certain common diseases"*? I have detailed the facts as they have appeared to me and I have mentioned interpretations of them: but I do not conceal from myself that, in medical territory, it is difficult to support one's self wholly on subjective foundations. I do not forget that Medicine and Veterinary practice are foreign to me. I desire judgment and criticism upon all my contributions. Little tolerant of frivolous or prejudiced contradiction, contemptuous of that ignorant criticism which doubts on principle, I welcome with open arms the militant attack which has a method in doubting and whose rule of conduct has the motto "More light."

PART 6

The Healer

"The Hippocratic Oath"

The one work universally associated with Hippocrates was in all likelihood written by neither him nor his disciples. Many of its ethical precepts, in fact, are at odds with key passages found throughout the Hippocratic corpus. Scholars believe, instead, that the Oath is the product of an esoteric sect of Pythagoreans, who wished to reform the practice of medicine and sanctify the soul of the physician in accordance with their own religious values. Although its formal qualities identify the Oath as a typical guild document of the classical era, its dictates do not accord with either the medical practices or social mores of Greco-Roman culture. Many Hippocratic treatises, for example, promoted surgery as a highly valuable medical intervention and went to great lengths to describe its various procedures and techniques. By the same token, there were generally no injunctions against physicians' assisting with abortions or suicides. Such practices were commonly accepted in Greco-Roman society, and neither religious doctrine nor legal stricture typically condemned them.

I swear by Apollo Physician and Asclepius and Hygieia and Panaceia and all the gods and goddesses, making them my witnesses, that I will fulfill according to my ability and judgment this oath and this covenant:

To hold him who has taught me this art as equal to my parents and to live my life in partnership with him, and if he is in need of money to give him a share of mine, and to regard his offspring as equal to my brothers in male lineage and to teach them this art—if they desire to learn it—without fee and covenant; to give a share of precepts and oral instruction and all the other learning to my sons and to the sons of him who has instructed me and to pupils who have signed the covenant and have taken an oath according to the medical law, but to no one else.

I will apply dietetic measures for the benefit of the sick according to my ability and judgment; I will keep them from harm and injustice.

I will neither give a deadly drug to anybody if asked for it, nor will I make a suggestion to this effect. Similarly I will not give to a woman an abortive remedy. In purity and holiness I will guard my life and my art.

I will not use the knife, not even on sufferers from stone, but will withdraw in favor of such men as are engaged in this work.

Whatever houses I may visit, I will come for the benefit of the sick, remaining free of all intentional injustice, of all mischief and in particular of sexual relations with both female and male persons, be they free or slaves.

From *The Hippocratic Oath: Text, Translation, and Interpretation,* by Ludwig Edelstein, Supplements to the *Bulletin of the History of Medicine,* no. 1 (Baltimore: Johns Hopkins University Press, 1943).

What I may see or hear in the course of the treatment or even outside of the treatment in regard to the life of men, which on no account one must spread abroad, I will keep to myself holding such things shameful to be spoken about.

If I fulfill this oath and do not violate it, may it be granted to me to enjoy life and art, being honored with fame among all men for all time to come; if I transgress it and swear falsely, may the opposite of all this be my lot.

The Bible (A.D. 1st Century)

The word *gospel* is a translation into Middle English of the Greek *evangelion,* which means "goods news." The gospel that the four evangelists—Matthew, Mark, Luke, and John—propagated was the new dispensation and law as exemplified in the life, death, and resurrection of Jesus Christ. If what Christians call the Old Testament is the story of a people, the New Testament is the story of an individual, the son of God, through whom the Word—the disembodied voice of Yahweh—takes on human form and flesh. Mark's Gospel (ca. 60–70) is generally regarded to be the earliest, with Matthew and Luke, whose accounts are indebted to his, coming a decade or so later, and John, whose narrative is largely independent, later still. In Mark, we see a Jesus who is the subverter of both secular and religious authority, a hero of the common people who freely mixes with children, women, laborers, beggars, the poor, the sick, and the outcast. Expanding on the theme of Jesus' charismatic mission and appeal, Matthew focuses on His *exousia*—or "power"—which is demonstrated by His ability to expound the law, absolve sins, and perform miracles. Matthew stresses that Jesus' authority is totally unlike that of the magician or scribe, for it encompasses the power of the healer, who can cast out "unclean spirits" and "heal all manner of sickness and all manner of disease." In John, the reach of Jesus' authority as healer extends its dominion over death itself, heralding a new order in which death is no more and the dead body can be summoned back to life from the very depths of the grave.

MATTHEW

8.1 When he came down from the mountain, great crowds followed him; 2 and behold, a leper came to him and knelt before him, saying, "Lord, if you will, you can make me clean." 3 And he stretched out his hand and touched him, saying, "I will; be clean." And immediately his leprosy was cleansed. 4 And Jesus said to him, "See that you say nothing to any one; but go, show yourself to the priest, and offer the gift that Moses commanded, for a proof to the people."

5 As he entered Caper'na-um, a centurion came forward to him, beseeching him 6 and saying, "Lord, my servant is lying paralyzed at home, in terrible distress." 7 And he said to him, "I will come and heal him." 8 But the centurion answered him, "Lord, I am not worthy to have you come under my roof; but only say the word, and my servant will be healed."

From *The Oxford Annotated Bible with Apocrypha* (Revised Standard Version), ed. Herbert G. May and Bruce M. Metzger (New York: Oxford University Press, 1965). Copyright 1946 by the Division of Christian Education of the National Council of Churches of Christ in the U.S.A.

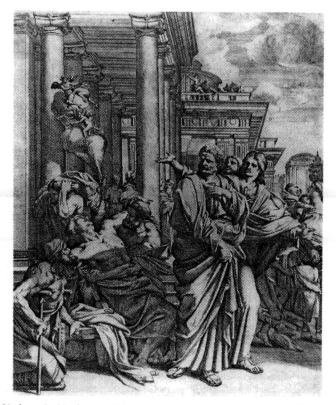

19. Rémy Vuibert, In Umbra tua Viuemus in Gentibus *(Cure of One Possessed by the Devil), 1639. Clements C. Fry Print Collection at Harvey Cushing/John Hay Whitney Medical Library-Historical Library, Yale University. The New Testament repeatedly links Jesus' authority to heal with the practice of exorcism. Here, a muscular and magisterial Christ casts out demons with a mere glance as onlookers wildly gesticulate in amazement. The similarity between the possessed man in Vuibert's print and that of the collapsing epileptic in Picart's engraving (fig. 12, marked A) is unmistakable.*

13 And to the centurion Jesus said, "Go; be it done for you as you have believed." And the servant was healed at that very moment.

14 And when Jesus entered Peter's house, he saw his mother-in-law lying sick with a fever; 15 he touched her hand, and the fever left her, and she rose and served him. 16 That evening they brought to him many who were possessed with demons; and he cast out the spirits with a word, and healed all who were sick. 17 This was to fulfil what was spoken by the prophet Isaiah, "He took our infirmities and bore our diseases."

MARK

5.1 They came to the other side of the sea, to the country of the Ger'asenes. 2 And when he had come out of the boat, there met him out of the tombs a man with an unclean spirit, 3 who lived among the tombs; and no one could bind him any more, even with a chain; 4 for he had often been bound with fetters and chains, but the chains he wrenched apart, and the fetters he broke in pieces; and no one had the strength to subdue him. 5 Night and day among the tombs and on the mountains he was always crying out, and bruising himself with stones. 6 And when he saw Jesus from afar, he ran and worshiped him; 7 and crying out with a loud voice, he said, "What have you to do with me, Jesus, Son of the Most High God? I adjure you by God, do not torment me." 8 For he had said to him, "Come out of the man, you unclean spirit!" 9 And Jesus asked him, "What is your name?" He replied, "My name is Legion; for we are many." 10 And he begged him eagerly not to send them out of the country. 11 Now a great herd of swine was feeding there on the hillside; 12 and they begged him, "Send us to the swine, let us enter them." 13 So he gave them leave. And the unclean spirits came out, and entered the swine; and the herd, numbering about two thousand, rushed down the steep bank into the sea, and were drowned in the sea.

14 The herdsmen fled, and told it in the city and in the country. And people came to see what it was that had happened. 15 And they came to Jesus, and saw the demoniac sitting there, clothed and in his right mind, the man who had had the legion; and they were afraid.

21 And when Jesus had crossed again in the boat to the other side, a great crowd gathered about him; and he was beside the sea. 22 Then came one of the rulers of the synagogue, Ja'irus by name; and seeing him, he fell at his feet, 23 and besought him, saying, "My little daughter is at the point of death. Come and lay your hands on her, so that she may be made well, and live." 24 And he went with him.

And a great crowd followed him and thronged about him. 25 And there was a woman who had had a flow of blood for twelve years, 26 and who had suffered much under many physicians, and had spent all that she had, and was no better but rather grew worse. 27 She had heard the reports about Jesus, and came up behind him in the crowd and touched his garment. 28 For she said, "If I touch even his garments, I shall be made well." 29 And immediately the hemorrhage ceased; and she felt in her body that she was healed of her disease. 30 And Jesus, perceiving in himself that power had gone forth from him, immediately turned about in the crowd, and said, "Who touched my garments?" 31 And his disciples said to him, "You see the crowd pressing around you, and yet you say, 'Who touched me?'" 32 And he looked around to see who had done it. 33 But the woman, knowing what had been done to her, came in fear and trembling and fell down before him, and told him the whole truth. 34 And he said to her, "Daughter, your faith has made you well; go in peace, and be healed of your disease."

35 While he was still speaking, there came from the ruler's house some who said, "Your daughter is dead. Why trouble the Teacher any further?" 36 But ignoring what they said, Jesus said to the ruler of the synagogue, "Do not fear, only believe." 37 And he allowed no one to follow him except Peter and James and John the brother of James. 38 When they came to the house of the ruler of the synagogue, he saw a

tumult, and people weeping and wailing loudly. 39 And when he had entered, he said to them, "Why do you make a tumult and weep? The child is not dead but sleeping." 40 And they laughed at him. But he put them all outside, and took the child's father and mother and those who were with him, and went in where the child was. 41 Taking her by the hand he said to her, "Tal'itha cu'mi"; which means, "Little girl, I say to you, arise." 42 And immediately the girl got up and walked; for she was twelve years old. And immediately they were overcome with amazement. 43 And he strictly charged them that no one should know this, and told them to give her something to eat.

JOHN

11.1 Now a certain man was ill, Laz'arus of Bethany, the village of Mary and her sister Martha.

3 So the sisters sent to him, saying, "Lord, he whom you love is ill."

5 Now Jesus loved Martha and her sister and Laz'arus. 6 So when he heard that he was ill, he stayed two days longer in the place where he was. 7 Then after this he said to the disciples, "Let us go into Judea again."

17 Now when Jesus came, he found that Laz'arus had already been in the tomb four days.

21 Martha said to Jesus, "Lord, if you had been here, my brother would not have died. 22 And even now I know that whatever you ask from God, God will give you." 23 Jesus said to her, "Your brother will rise again." 24 Martha said to him, "I know that he will rise again in the resurrection at the last day." 25 Jesus said to her, "I am the resurrection and the life; he who believes in me, though he die, yet shall he live, 26 and whoever lives and believes in me shall never die. Do you believe this?" 27 She said to him "Yes, Lord; I believe that you are the Christ, the Son of God, he who is coming into the world."

32 Then Mary, when she came where Jesus was and saw him, fell at his feet, saying to him, "Lord, if you had been here, my brother would not have died." 33 When Jesus saw her weeping, and the Jews who came with her also weeping, he was deeply moved in spirit and troubled; 34 and he said, "Where have you laid him?" They said to him, "Lord, come and see." 35 Jesus wept. 36 So the Jews said, "See how he loved him!" 37 But some of them said, "Could not he who opened the eyes of the blind man have kept this man from dying?"

38 Then Jesus, deeply moved again, came to the tomb; it was a cave, and a stone lay upon it. 39 Jesus said, "Take away the stone." Martha, the sister of the dead man, said to him, "Lord, by this time there will be an odor, for he has been dead four days." 40 Jesus said to her, "Did I not tell you that if you would believe you would see the glory of God?" 41 So they took away the stone. And Jesus lifted up his eyes and said, "Father, I thank thee that thou hast heard me. 42 I knew that thou hearest me always, but I have said this on account of the people standing by, that they may believe that thou didst send me." 43 When he had said this, he cried with a loud voice, "Laz'arus, come out." 44 The dead man came out, his hands and feet bound with bandages, and his face wrapped with a cloth. Jesus said to them, "Unbind him, and let him go."

ASAF JUDAEUS (A.D. 7TH CENTURY)

"Admonition"

Considered to be the earliest medical writer in Hebrew, Asaf most probably lived in seventh-century Mesopotamia. Author of several works on medicine and cosmography, Asaf is also known for having written an ethical admonition that incorporated the precepts and the phraseology of the Torah. During the ceremony in which he and his colleague John formally administered their words of caution, pupils were required to respond by promising to abide by their teachers' directives "with pure heart, with whole soul, and with all our strength." The overriding conviction embodied in the admonition is that the power to heal comes exclusively from the one true God and that to believe otherwise—to place one's faith in magic or witchcraft—is to commit an act of idolatry. In keeping with this fundamental premise, only the virtuous could heal. Asaf's directives, therefore, served to safeguard the physician's therapeutic efficacy by admonishing him to lead a religious and morally exemplary life.

Beware of causing death to anyone by administering the juices of poisonous roots. Do not administer to an adulterous wife an abortifacient drug. Let not the beauty of woman arouse in thee the passion of adultery. Divulge not any secret entrusted to thee and do no act of injury or of harm for any price. Do not close thy heart to mercy toward the poor and the needy. Say not of the good that it is evil, nor of the evil that it is good. Walk not in the path of sorcerers who raise enmity in marital couples through incantation, magic and witchcraft. Do not covet any possession as a reward for having aided in an act of infamy. In thy treatment do not apply the arts of the idolater, and place no trust in idols, for they are naught and are of no avail. On the contrary, ye must despise their servants; dead spirits are their idols without ability to help their lifeless images; how much can they avail the living human beings? Put thy trust in the Eternal, the God of Truth; He kills and He likewise brings to life; He punishes and He heals the wound; He gives to man understanding to be of help; He punishes in righteousness and justice, but He restores in love and in mercy; He makes plants of healing to grow up and He implants into the perfect heart the ability to heal, in order to make known His great grace and His wondrous works before great multitudes, so that all living may understand that He is the Creator and beside Him there is none who can help. The nations place their trust in idols which cannot help them in the hour of need, nor save them in their distress; thus their hope and their longings lead unto death. It is proper, therefore, that ye separate yourselves from them, that ye keep yourselves far removed from their idols and that ye call upon the

---

From *The Jews and Medicine: Essays,* by Harry Friedenwald, Vol. 1 (Hoboken, N.J.: KTAV Publishing House, 1967).

name of the Eternal, the living God, the God of the spirits of all flesh, in Whose hand lies the power over the souls of all living and the spirits of all mankind, to kill or to bring to life; no one can escape from His might. Keep Him in mind at all times, seek Him in truth, rectitude, and perfection; then will all the works of your hands succeed. He will help you to be of aid to others and ye will be praised highly by all mankind; the people will forsake their idols for the service of the Eternal, for they will recognize that they had placed their trust in nought, that they had wearied themselves in vain in the service of gods which cannot be of help. Therefore be ye strong and not indolent, for great reward awaits your work. God will be with you, if ye are with Him. If ye keep the covenant of your oath and if ye follow our instructions, then ye will be honored as saints in the eyes of all mankind who will say: "Happy the nation whose God is the Lord; the people whom He has chosen for His own inheritance" (Ps., 33:12).

"On the Precautions That Physicians Must Observe"

Not only a physician, Arnald of Villanova was also an astrologer, alchemist, diplomat, and reformer, whose advice was sought by kings and popes. More than one hundred treatises on subjects ranging from medicine to theology have been attributed to him. Arnald translated the works of Arabic physicians into Latin, hoping to systematize all medical knowledge on the basis of Galen's theories. Although *De Cautelis Medicorum* was published under Arnald's name, Part III was taken from the *Codex Salernitanus* of Breslau, whereas Part I is most likely his own work. Whatever its origins, the treatise gives us a window onto a battle of wits in which patients maneuvered to protect themselves from quacks, and physicians countered with stratagems devised to "prove" their competence. The choice of weapon in this contest was the flask of urine, whose physical properties were believed to hold vital clues to the patient's condition and prognosis. More gamesmanship than medical craft, the analysis of a patient's urine sorely tested not only what was thought to be a physician's diagnostic acumen but also the quality of his bedside manner.

I

We must consider the precautions with regard to urines, by which we can protect ourselves against people who wish to deceive us. The very first shall consist in finding out whether the urine be of man or of another animal or another fluid; and if it is human urine it is diagnosed in four ways.

The second precaution is with regard to the individual who brings the urine. You must look at him sharply and keep your eyes straight on him or on his face; and if he wishes to deceive you he will start laughing or the color of his face will change, and then you must curse him forever and in all eternity.

The third precaution is also with regard to the individual who brings the urine, whether man or woman, for you must see whether he or she is pale, and after you have ascertained that this is the individual's urine, say to him: "Verily, this urine resembles you," and talk about the pallor, because immediately you will hear all about his illness. It commonly happens with poor people and those of moderate means that they go to the doctor when they are afflicted very seriously.

From "Bedside Manners in the Middle Ages: The Treatise *De Cautelis Medicorum* Attributed to Arnald of Villanova," trans. Henry Sigerist, *Quarterly Bulletin, Northwestern University Medical School* 20 (1946): 135–143. Manuscript from the collection of the Galter Health Sciences Library, Northwestern University, Chicago. Reprinted in *Henry E. Sigerist on the History of Medicine*, ed. Felix Marti-Ibañez (New York: MD Publications, 1960).

Tabule

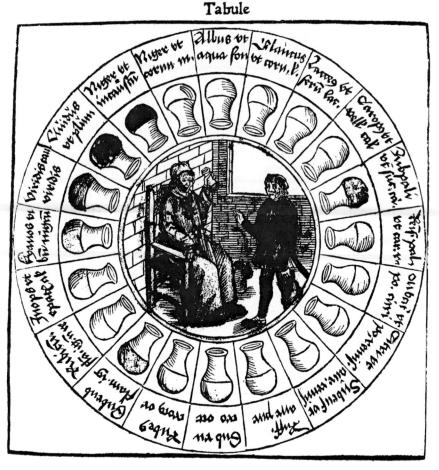

20. Woodcut of urine flasks from Ulrich Binder, Epiphaniae Medicorum, *1506. Wellcome Institute Library, London. This sixteenth-century uroscopy wheel was a common pictorial device designed to aid doctors in diagnosing their patients' ailments. They would compare the color, odor, and texture of their patients' urine with those indicated on the chart. Physicians were also known to taste the urine—a practice that enabled them to diagnose patients with diabetes, whose urine was noticeably sweet.*

The fourth precaution is with regard to sex. An old woman wants to have your opinion. You inquire whose urine it is, and the old woman will say to you: "Don't you know it?" Then look at her in a certain way from the corner of your eye, and ask: "What relation is it of yours?" And if she is not too crooked, she will say that the patient is a male or female relation, or something from which you can distinguish the sex. Should she say: "We are not related," then ask what the patient used to do when he was in good health, and from the patient's doing you can recognize or deduce the sex.

The fifth precaution is that you must ask if the patient is old. If the messenger says yes, you must say that he greatly suffers from the stomach, and that he spits a lot, and in the morning more than at any other time, for old people have by nature a cold stomach.

The sixth precaution: whether this illness has lasted for a long time or not. If the messenger says that it has, you must say that the patient is altogether irritable and that one can help him, or some such talk. If he says no, you must say that the patient is altogether oppressed because in the beginnings of diseases there is much matter that oppresses the organ.

There is a seventh precaution, and it is a very general one; you may not find out anything about the case, then say that he has an obstruction in the liver. He may say: "No, sir, on the contrary he has pains in the head, or in the legs or in other organs." You must say that this comes from the liver or from the stomach; and particularly use the word, obstruction, because they do not understand what it means, and it helps greatly that a term is not understood by the people.

The eighth precaution is with regard to conception. An old woman consults you because the patient cannot become pregnant. Perhaps you do not know the cause but say that she cannot hold her husband's sperm which she could have done very well if she had been well disposed.

The eleventh precaution is taken with regard to white or yellow wine. If you have any doubts in this respect, be cautious and put the lid of the urinal down and pour out a little of the content in such a way that the wine in being poured out touches your finger. Then you must give her the urinal and act as if you were going to blow your nose whereby you put the finger that has been dipped in, on or next to your nose; then you will smell the odor of wine, whereupon you must take the urinal again and say to her: "Get away and be ashamed of yourself!"

The thirteenth precaution: whenever the old woman asks what disease the patient has, you must say: "You would not understand me if I told you, and it would be better for you to ask what he should do." And then she will see that you have judgment in the matter and will keep quiet. But perhaps she will say: "Sir, he is very hot; therefore he seems to have a fever."—"Thus it seems to you and other lay people who do not know how to distinguish between fever and other diseases."

The fourteenth precaution: when you have been called to a patient, feel the pulse before you examine the urine and make them talk so that the condition of the animal virtue becomes apparent to you. After having recognized these factors you will be able to evaluate the urine better and with more certainty and you may proceed thus.

The fifteenth precaution is: should the patient be in a bad condition so that you think that he may die the following day, do not go to him but send your servant to bring you the urine, or tell them to bring it to-morrow in the early morning because you wish that they prepare for the meal and that after you have seen the urine you will tell what they shall administer. And so from the report of the person who brings the urine you will be able to form an opinion about the patient, whether he is in good or bad condition.

The sixteenth precaution is that when you come to a patient you should always do something new lest they say that you cannot do anything without the books.

The seventeenth precaution is that if by hard luck you come to the home of the patient and find him dead and somebody perhaps says: "Sir, what have you come for?" You shall say that you have not come for that, and say that you well knew that he was going to die that night but that you wanted to know at what hour he had died.

III

Physician! When you shall be called to a sick man, in the name of God seek the assistance of the Angel who has attended the action of the mind and from inside shall attend departures of the body. You must know from the beginning how long the sick has been laboring, and in what way the illness has befallen him, and by inquiring about the symptoms, if it can be done, ascertain what the disease is. This is necessary because after having seen the faeces and urine and the condition of the pulse you may not be able to diagnose the disease, but if you can announce the symptoms the patient will have confidence in you as in the author of his health and therefore one must devote greatest pains to knowing the symptoms.

Therefore, when you come to a house, inquire before you go to the sick whether he has confessed, and if he has not, he should confess immediately or promise you that he will confess immediately, and this must not be neglected because many illnesses originate on account of sin and are cured by the Supreme Physician after having been purified from squalor by the tears of contrition, according to what is said in the Gospel: "Go, and sin no more, lest something worse happens to you."

Entering the sickroom do not appear very haughty or overzealous, and return, with the simple gesture, the greetings of those who rise to greet you. After they have seated themselves you finally sit down facing the sick; ask him how he feels and reach out for his arm, and all that we shall say is necessary so that through your entire behavior you obtain the favor of the people who are around the sick. And because the trip to the patient has sharpened your sensitivity, and the sick rejoices at your coming or because he has already become stingy and has various thoughts about the fee, therefore by your fault as well as his the pulse is affected, is different and impetuous from the motion of the spirits.

Let me give you one more warning: do not look at a maid or a daughter or a wife with an improper or covetous eye and do not let yourself be entangled in woman affairs—for there are medical operations that excite the helper's mind; otherwise your judgment is affected, you become harmful to the patient, and people will expect less from you. And so, be pleasant in your speech, diligent and careful in your medical dealings, eager to help. And adhere to this without fallacy.

When you have been invited for dinner you should not throw yourself upon the party and at the table should not occupy the place of honor although it is customary to assign the place of honor to the priest and the physician. Then you should not disdain certain drinks, nor find fault with certain dishes, nor be disgusted perhaps because you are hardly accustomed to appease your hunger with millet bread in peasant fashion. If you act thus your mind will feel at ease. And while the attention is concentrated on the variety of dishes, inquire explicitly from some of the attendants about the patient or about his condition. If you do this the sick will have great confidence in you, because he sees that you cannot forget him in the midst of delicacies. When you leave the table and come to the sick, you must tell him that you have been served well, at which the patient greatly rejoices because he was very anxious to have you well served.

If it is the time and place to feed the sick you will feed him. It is necessary, however, that you set the time for the patient's meals, namely in intermittent fevers when the sick have a real remission; in continuous fevers when there happens to be a quiet moment because a decline of their fever does not occur before the crisis.

You shall feed the sick according to the season of the year and according to the change of seasons and of the disease; and quantity and quality of food must be varied according to the diseases, for you shall give the patient ampler food in intermittent than in continuous fever, and colder food in a continuous than in intermittent fever, more food in winter and spring, less in summer and autumn because they stand it very badly.

Remember, furthermore, that in the beginning of the disease the physician endeavors to oppose it with digestive remedies, for he is the helper of nature and must aid it. Nature namely proceeds to making the crisis, to the triumph over the disease; she wishes to reduce the forces of the disease by changing the condition and quality of the matter and by dispersing it among the organs so that the parts be separated from each other and she may reach her end and more easily than expected with complete results in one weak expulsion. In the same way, the physician in order to drive out the matter that must be driven out, must be prepared to treat the digested matters, according to the aphorism in the first book of Hippocrates. Consideration of the cause of the disease determines the choice of remedies that digest the humors; for if the patient suffers from cholera you will give vinegar syrup; if he suffers from a cold humor you will give oxymel, and everything else as I have said in another chapter. Oh physician, thanks be given to God.

HEINRICH KRAMER (ca. 1430–1505)
AND JAMES SPRENGER (ca. 1436–1495)

Malleus Maleficarum

Appointed by Pope Innocent III as Inquisitors of Northern Germany, Heinrich Kramer and James Sprenger were two Dominican monks who undertook the defense of the Catholic Church against the assaults of witchcraft and sorcery. Born in Lower Alsace, Kramer quickly rose to prominence in the Dominican order, becoming both Prior and Master of Sacred Theology at a young age. A staunch defender of papal supremacy in all matters of the faith, Kramer drew enormous crowds by his legendary preaching. In 1484, together with Sprenger, he was delegated by the Pope to seek out and prosecute witches and sorcerers. Another prominent Dominican, Sprenger was born in Basle, where he zealously restored the "Primitive and Strict Obedience" in his own religious order. In 1480, he was elected Dean of the Faculty of Theology at the University of Cologne. *Malleus Maleficarum,* the treatise he coauthored with Kramer, dominated European jurisprudence in matters of witchcraft, devil worship, and exorcism well into the eighteenth century, definitively signaling the "decline of magic" and its systematic appropriation by the Church. In giving their instructions for performing an exorcism, Kramer and Sprenger made certain to Christianize every aspect of a ritual still tied to the use of pagan incantation and heathen amulets.

CHAPTER VI

Prescribed Remedies; to wit, the Lawful Exorcisms of the Church, for all Sorts of Infirmities and Ills due to Witchcraft; and the Method of Exorcising those who are Bewitched.

It has already been stated that witches can afflict men with every kind of physical infirmity; therefore it can be taken as a general rule that the various verbal or practical remedies which can be applied in the case of those infirmities which we have just been discussing are equally applicable to all other infirmities, such as epilepsy or leprosy, for example. And as lawful exorcisms are reckoned among the verbal remedies and have been most often considered by us, they may be taken as a general type of such remedies. . . .

In the first place, that is said to be lawful in the Christian religion which is not superstitious; and that is said to be superstitious which is over and above the prescribed form of religion. See *Colossians* ii: Which things indeed have a show of wis-

From *Malleus Maleficarum,* ed. and trans. Montague Summers (1928; reprint, New York: Dover, 1971).

dom in superstition: on which the gloss says: Superstition is undisciplined religion, that is, religion observed with defective methods in evil circumstances.

. . . [W]hen a work is done by virtue of the Christian religion, as when someone wishes to heal the sick by means of prayer and benediction and sacred words (which is the matter we are considering), such a person must observe seven conditions by which such benedictions are rendered lawful. And even if he uses adjurations, through the virtue of the Divine Name, and by the virtue of the works of Christ, His Birth, Passion and Precious Death, by which the devil was conquered and cast out; such benedictions and charms and exorcisms shall be called lawful, and they who practise them are exorcists or lawful enchanters. See S. Isidore, *Etym.* VIII, Enchanters are they whose art and skill lies in the use of words.

And the first of these conditions, as we learn from S. Thomas, is that there must be nothing in the words which hints at any expressed or tacit invocation of devils. If such were expressed, it would be obviously unlawful. If it were tacit, it might be considered in the light of intention, or in that of fact: in that of intention, when the operator has no care whether it is God or the devil who is helping him, so long as he attains his desired result; in that of fact, when a person has no natural aptitude for such work, but creates some artificial means. And of such not only must physicians and astronomers be the judges, but especially Theologians. For in this way do necromancers work, making images and rings and stones by artificial means; which have no natural virtue to effect the results which they very often expect: therefore the devil must be concerned in their works.

Secondly, the benedictions or charms must contain no unknown names; for according to S. John Chrysostom such are to be regarded with fear, lest they should conceal some matter of superstition.

Thirdly, there must be nothing in the words that is untrue; for if there is, the effect of them cannot be from God, Who is not a witness to a lie. But some old women in their incantations use some such jingling doggerel as the following:

> Blessed MARY went a-walking
> Over Jordan river.
> Stephen met her, and fell a-talking, etc.

Fourthly, there must be no vanities, or written characters beyond the sign of the Cross. Therefore the charms which soldiers are wont to carry are condemned.

Fifthly, no faith must be placed in the method of writing or reading or binding the charm about a person, or in any such vanity, which has nothing to do with the reverence of God, without which a charm is altogether superstitious.

Sixthly, in the citing and uttering of Divine words and of Holy Scripture attention must only be paid to the sacred words themselves and their meaning, and to the reverence of God; whether the effect be looked for from the Divine virtue, or from the relics of Saints, which are a secondary power, since their virtue springs originally from God.

Seventhly, the looked-for effect must be left to the Divine Will; for He knows whether it is best for a man to be healed or to be plagued, or to die. This condition was set down by S. Thomas.

So we may conclude that if none of these conditions be broken, the incantation will be lawful. And S. Thomas writes in this connexion on the last chapter of *S. Mark*: And these signs shall follow them that believe; in my name shall they cast out devils; they shall take up serpents.

For in man himself lies the cause by reason of which the devil receives his power in other matters which are brought about by man, namely, sin, either original or actual. This then is the significance of the words that are used in exorcism, as when it is said, "Depart, O Satan, from him"; and likewise of the things that are then done.

In conclusion, and for the sake of clearness, we may recommend this form of exorcism for a person who is bewitched. Let him first make a good confession (according to the often-quoted Canon: If by sortilege, etc.). Then let a diligent search be made in all corners and in the beds and mattresses and under the threshold of the door, in case some instrument of witchcraft may be found. The bodies of animals bewitched to death are at once to be burned. And it is expedient that all bed-clothes and garments should be renewed, and even that he should change his house and dwelling. But in case nothing is found, then he who is to be exorcised should if possible go into the church in the morning, especially on the Holier Days, such as the Feasts of Our Lady, or on some Vigil; and the better if the priest also has confessed and is in a state of grace, for then the stronger will he be. And let him who is to be exorcised hold in his hand a Holy Candle as well as he can, either sitting or kneeling; and let those who are present offer up devout prayers for his deliverance. And let him begin the Litany at "Our help is in the Name of the Lord," and let one be appointed to make the responses: let him sprinkle him with Holy Water, and place a stole round his neck, and recite the Psalm "Haste thee, O God, to deliver me"; and let him continue the Litany for the Sick, saying at the Invocation of the Saints, "Pray for him and be favourable; deliver him, O Lord," continuing thus to the end. But where the prayers are to be said, then in the place of the prayers let him begin the exorcism, and continue in the way we have declared, or in any other better way, as seems good to him. And this sort of exorcism may be continued at least three times a week, that so through many intercessions the grace of health may be obtained.

Finally, he must receive the Sacrament of the Eucharist; although some think that this should be done before the exorcism. And at his confession the confessor must inquire whether he is under any bond of excommunication, and if he is, whether he has rashly omitted to obtain absolution from his Judge; for then, although he may at his discretion absolve him, yet when he has regained his health, he must seek absolution also from the Judge who excommunicated him.

It should further be noted that, when the exorcist is not ordained to the Order of Exorcist, then he may proceed with prayers; and if he can read the Scriptures, let him read the beginnings of the four Gospels of the Evangelists, and the Gospel beginning, "There was an Angel sent"; and the Passion of our Lord; all of which have great power to expel the works of the devil. Also let the Gospel of S. John, "In the beginning was the Word," be written and hung round the sick man's neck, and so let the grace of healing be looked for from God.

Our second main consideration is what is to be done when no healing grace results from exorcisms. Now this may happen for six reasons; and there is a seventh about which we suspend any definite judgement. For when a person is not healed, it is due either to want of faith in the bystanders or in those who present the sick man, or to the sins of them who suffer from the bewitchment, or to a neglect of the due and fitting remedies, or to some flaw in the faith of the exorcist, or to the lack of a greater trust in the powers of another exorcist, or to the need of purgation and for the increased merit of the bewitched person.

Concerning the first four of these the Gospel teaches us in the incident of the only son of his father, who was a lunatic, and of the disciples of Christ being there present (*S. Matthew* xvii. and *S. Mark* ix.). For in the first place He said that the multitude were without faith; whereupon the father prayed Him, saying: Lord, I believe: help Thou mine unbelief. And JESUS said to the multitude: O faithless and perverse generation, how long shall I be with you?

"The Vices and Virtues of Physicians"

Abolitionist, social reformer, and signer of the Declaration of Independence, Benjamin Rush attacked the leading medical theories of his day and advanced a new and simplified system of nosology based on the idea that all forms of illness are produced by specific irritants. Sound therapy consisted in removing the aggravating agent either through bleeding or purgation; not surprisingly, the lancet and a dose of calomel were Rush's trusted and indispensable therapeutic aides. Rush's ideas were often considered radical, and his repeated claims that Philadelphia's frequent epidemics of yellow fever were brought on by the filth of its own streets—and not imported from elsewhere—earned him public censure, involving him at one point in a lawsuit and at another in a challenge to a duel. Rush received his B.A. from Princeton in 1760 and his M.D. in 1768 from the University of Edinburgh. A year later he was appointed Professor of Chemistry at the College of Philadelphia, completing the faculty of the first medical school in the colonies. During the course of his forty-four-year career, Rush privately instructed more than two thousand students in addition to his official teaching responsibilities. In 1783, Rush became physician to the Pennsylvania Hospital, where he introduced new methods in the treatment of the insane, serving in this post until his death.

The vices of physicians may be divided into three heads.

I. As they relate to the Supreme Being.
II. To their patients, and
III. To their professional brethren.

1st. Under the first head I shall begin by lamenting, that men whose educations necessarily open to them the wisdom and goodness of the Creator, and whose duties lead them constantly to behold his power over human life, and all its comforts, should be so very prone to forget him. This they evidence by their neglect of that worship, which is paid to him in different forms, under true, or false names, in every country. If it be a fact, that physicians are more inclined to infidelity, than any other body of men, it must be ascribed chiefly to this cause.

Our business leads us daily into the abodes of pain and misery. It obliges us likewise, frequently to witness the fears with which our friends leave the world, and the anguish which follows, in their surviving relatives. A pious word, dropped from the lips of a physician in such circumstances of his patients, often does more good than

From *Selected Writings of Benjamin Rush,* ed. Dagobert D. Runes (New York: Philosophical Library, 1947).

a long, and perhaps an ingenious discourse from another person, inasmuch as it falls upon the heart, in the moment of its deepest depression from grief.

2d. An undue confidence in medicine, to the exclusion of a Divine and Superintending Power over the health and lives of men, is another vice among physicians. A Dr. ——, in New York prescribed on an evening, for a sick man. The next day he called and asked him how he was, "Much better (said he) thank God." "Thank God! (said the doctor) thank me, it was I who cured you."

3d. Drunkenness is a medical vice, which offends not only God, but man. It is generally induced by fatigue, and exposure to great heat and cold. But a habit of drinking intemperately is often incurred by a social spirit, leading physicians to accept of offers of wine, or spirits and water, in every house they enter, in the former part of the day. Good men have often been seduced and ruined by this complaisant practice.

4th. The members of our profession have sometimes been charged with an irreverent, and profane use of the name of the Supreme Being, . . .

II. In speaking of the vices of physicians as far as they relate to their patients, I pass over numerous acts of imposture. They are all more or less contrary to good morals. I shall at present only mention the more obvious and positive vices which belong to this head. They are

1st. Falsehood. This vice discovers itself chiefly in the deceptions which are practised by physicians with respect to the cause, nature, and probable issue of diseases. What oceans of falsehoods have issued from the members of our profession, upon the cause of pestilential epidemics, in all ages and countries! How many false names have been given to them to conceal their existence! In England the plague of 1664, was called, for several months, by the less alarming name of a spotted fever.

Equally criminal is the practice among physicians of encouraging patients to expect a recovery, in diseases which have arrived at their incurable stage. The mischief done by falsehood in this case, is the more to be deplored, as it often prevents the dying from settling their worldly affairs, and employing their last hours in preparing for their future state.

2d. Inhumanity is a vice which sometimes appears in the conduct of physicians to their patients. It discovers itself in the want of prompt and punctual attendance upon the sick, and in a careless or unfeeling manner in sick rooms.

3d. Avarice, in all its forms of meanness, oppression, and cruelty, is a frequent vice among physicians. It discovers itself,

1st. In a denial of services to the poor. I once heard a physician's eminence estimated by the fewness of his bad debts, and by his doing no business, for which he was not paid. We had a trader in medicine of this kind in Philadelphia, many years ago, who constantly refused to attend poor people, and when called upon to visit them, drove them from his door by a name so impious, that I shall not mention it. This sordid conduct is sometimes aggravated by being exercised towards old patients, who have been unfortunate in business, in the evening of their lives. We owe much to the families, who employ us in the infancy of our knowledge and experience. It is an act, therefore, of ingratitude, as well as avarice, to neglect them under the pressure of age and poverty, as well as sickness, or to consign them over to young physicians or quacks, who are ignorant of their constitutions and habits, and strangers to the respect they commanded in their better days.

3d. To undertake the charge of sick people, and to neglect them afterwards, is a vice of a malignant dye in a physician. Many lives have been lost, by the want of punctual and regular attention to the varying symptoms of diseases; but still more have been sacrificed by the criminal preference, which has been given by physicians to ease, convivial company, or public amusements and pursuits, to the care of their patients. The most important contract that can be made, is that which takes place between a sick man and his doctor. The subject of it is human life. The breach of this contract, by willful negligence, when followed by death, is murder; and it is because our penal laws are imperfect, that the punishment of that crime is not inflicted upon physicians who are guilty of it.

5th. The last vice I shall mention under this head, is, obstinacy in adhering to old and unsuccessful modes of practice, in diseases which have yielded to new remedies.

III. Agreeably to our order, I should proceed next to mention the vices of physicians towards their professional brethren, but for obvious reasons, I shall pass over this disagreeable part of our subject in silence, and hasten, with pleasure, to speak of the VIRTUES of physicians.

1. Piety towards God has, in many instances, characterized some of the first physicians in ancient and modern times. Hippocrates did homage to the gods of Greece, and Galen vanquished atheism for a while, in Rome, by proving the existence of a god, from the curious structure of the human body.

2. Humanity has been a conspicuous virtue among physicians in all ages and countries. It manifests itself,

1st. In their sacrifices and sufferings, in order to acquire a knowledge of all the different branches of medicine. For this, they spend months, and years, in dissecting dead bodies, or in the smoke of laboratories; or in visiting foreign, and sometimes uncivilized countries; or in making painful and expensive experiments upon living animals. Many physicians have contracted diseases, and some have perished in these loathsome and dangerous enterprizes, all of which are intended for the benefit of their fellow-creatures.

2d. No sooner do they enter upon the duties of their profession, than they are called upon to exhibit their humanity by sympathy, with pain and distress in persons of all ranks. It is this heaven-born principle, which produces such acts of self-denial of company, pleasure, and sleep, in physicians.

. . . [Galen] has left the following remark upon record, in speaking of the education of a young man, intended for the study of medicine. "Does he suffer" says the venerable man, "with the sufferings of others? Does he naturally feel the tenderest commiseration for the woes incident to his fellow mortals? you may reasonably infer that he will be passionately devoted to an art, that will instruct him in what manner to afford them relief." This noble sympathy, in physicians, in sometimes so powerful, as to predominate over the fear of death; hence we observe them to expose, and frequently to sacrifice their lives, in contending with mortal epidemics.

3d. Humanity in physicians manifests itself in gratuitous services to the poor. The greatest part of the business of Dr. Sydenham, seems to have been confined to poor people. It is true, he now and then speaks of a noble lady, and of a learned prelate, in the history of cases, but these were accidental patients.

Public dispensaries were projected, and are still conducted, chiefly by physicians. These excellent institutions mark an aera in the history of human beneficence. They yearly save many thousand lives.

4th. Humanity in physicians discovers itself in *pecuniary* contributions, as well as in advice, for the relief of the poor. I have read an account of a physician in England, who gave all the fees he received on a Sunday, to charitable purposes.

Dr. Fothergill once heard of the death of a citizen of London, who had left his family in indigent circumstances. As soon as he was interred, the doctor called upon his widow, and informed her, that he had, some years before, received thirty guineas for as many visits he had paid her husband in the days of his prosperity. "I have since heard," said the doctor "of his reverse of fortune. Take this purse. It contains all that I received from him. It will do thy family more good, than it will do me."

Similar anecdotes of his liberality might be multiplied without end. It is said, he gave away one half of all the income of his extensive and lucrative business, amounting, in the course of life, to one hundred thousand pounds.

III. Physicians have been distinguished in many instances, for their patriotism. By this virtue, I mean a disposition to promote all the objects of utility, convenience, and pleasure, and to remove all the evils of the country to which we belong. It embraces all the interests and wants of every class of citizens, and manifests itself in a great variety of forms. I shall briefly enumerate them.

1st. It appears in acts of liberality to promote science, and particularly medicine. The British Museum was the gift of a physician to the British nation. Dr. Radcliff founded a library at Oxford, and bequeathed three hundred pounds to be applied to the maintenance of a constant succession of students of medicine, who should spend three years in foreign countries, in search of medical knowledge.

2d. Patriotism in physicians has discovered itself in attempts and plans to obviate the prevailing diseases of their native country. Hippocrates was once invited by the kings of Illyria and Peonia, to come to the relief of their subjects, who were afflicted by the plague.

A physician delivered Calcutta from an epidemic malignant fever, by pointing out a new and effectual mode of conveying off its filth. The city of Frankfort, in Germany, was saved from an occasional pestilence, by a physician tracing its origin to a number of offensive privies.

3d. Physicians have contributed largely to the prosperity of their respective countries, by recommending and patronizing plans for promoting agriculture, commerce, morals and literature. Dr. Fothergill's garden at Upton, was a kind of hotbed of useful plants, for the whole nation. His active mind was always busy in devising public improvements that were calculated to increase the wealth, the knowledge, the happiness and even the elegance of his country.

If you feel, gentlemen, in hearing these details of the exploits of the illustrious worthies of our profession, as I do in relating them, you will not regret the day, you devoted yourselves to the study of medicine.

ELIZABETH BLACKWELL (1821–1910)

The Influence of Women in the Profession of Medicine

The first woman to receive a medical degree, Elizabeth Blackwell came from an English family of reformers and abolitionists who settled in New York in 1832. Here they opened a progressive school for children, carried on their work against slavery, and led the movement for women's higher education. Blackwell decided to become a physician while tending a sick friend but, upon writing to several physicians about her intentions, was told there was no way to realize them. Undeterred, Blackwell obtained private instruction in anatomy and applied to medical colleges in Philadelphia and New York state, finally gaining admission to Geneva Medical School, where she graduated in 1849. A scandalous and unheard-of entity at the time, a woman physician was barred from practice in any existing institution, so Blackwell started a dispensary of her own. In 1857, together with her sister Emily, also a physician, and Dr. Marie Zakrezewska, she founded the New York Infirmary for Women and Children. Intent on furthering the cause of women physicians in England, Blackwell settled there in 1869, and after working in London for several years, she returned to Hastings, New York, where she died at the age of eighty-nine.

In the short time that we meet together to-day I will ask you to let me dwell upon the way in which the most beneficial influence of women in the medical profession may be exercised. I wish also to point out certain dangers, as well as advantages, with which medical study is now surrounded.

The avenues by which all may enter into the profession are now so much more widely thrown open that there is little difficulty in the way of any man or woman who may wish to acquire a legal right to practise medicine. The democratic principle is everywhere steadily gaining ground, and the individual allowed to try his strength in the great battle of life. Large numbers of women are taking advantage of this wider individual liberty to enter the medical profession. In Great Britain our seventy-three registered lady-doctors are few compared with the 3,000 in the United States, yet the nine students who are now connected with our London school, with, in addition, the Edinburgh classes, the Dublin students, and the latest fact that the Glasgow Medical College has just opened its doors to women, clearly indicate that the movement has taken sturdy root in our country, . . .

It is quite certain that the wide adoption of the medical profession by women cannot continue to be an insignificant matter; it must exercise an appreciable effect on future society for good or evil.

From *The Influence of Women in the Profession of Medicine: Address Given at the Opening of the Winter Session of the London School of Medicine for Women* (Baltimore, 1890).

Now, there is no career nobler than that of the physician. The progress and welfare of society is more intimately bound up with the prevailing tone and influence of the medical profession than with the status of any other class of men. This exceptional influence is not only due to the great importance of dealing with the issues of life and death in health and disease, but it is still more owing to the fact that the body and the mind are so inseparably blended in the human constitution, that we cannot deal with one portion of this compound nature without in more or less degree affecting the other. Our ministrations to body and soul cannot be separated by a sharply-defined line. The arbitrary distinction between the physician of the body and the physician of the soul—doctor and priest—tends to disappear as science advances. Every branch of medicine involves moral considerations, both as regards the practitioner and the patient. Even the amputation of a limb, the care of a case of fever, the birth of a child, all contain a moral element which is evident to the clear understanding, and which cannot be neglected without injury to the doctor, to the individual, and to society.

If, then, we recognise that, although just reward for honest labour is fair, we must not enter upon medicine as a trade for getting money, but from a higher motive this motive, as it influences conduct, becomes on that account a moral motive or an ideal which should guide our future practical life as physicians. Now, this ideal necessitates a distinct conception of what is right or wrong for us, in medicine, both as human beings and as women. Simply sensuous life, without an ideal or without higher principles of action than the limited needs of every day, tends to degrade the individual and all who surround him.

What we need is a clear idea of what is really right or wrong, with the reasons on which the judgment is based, instead of a confused notion or a vague and ever-shifting standard.

No women student of medicine can safely ignore this subject. It is a vital one for us, and only a true answer to it will make our entrance into the profession a marked advance in social progress.

I do not attempt to disguise the difficulty of laying down the law of right and wrong in medicine; not only because medicine, as every other part of social life, is subject to the growth of evolution, but because in a state of society that has not yet succeeded in moulding itself on the fundamental principles of Christianity, we are involved in faulty social conditions which prevent us from embodying our moral perceptions in every phase of practical life.

You will see in the course of your medical studies—particularly if you study abroad—much to shock your enlightened intellect and revolt your moral sense. In practice also you will be subjected to strong temptations of the most varied character. But just for the reason that as women we ought to see more clearly the broken bridge or approaching danger, in the onward rush of the male intellect, I now dwell on our special responsibility, and shall endeavour to give the reasons for it.

My object is not to limit, but to enlarge our work in medicine, when I seek to define our ideal. It is true that the great object of this human life of ours is essentially one for every human being, man or woman, barbarous or civilized. It is to become a nobler creature, and to help all others to a higher human status during this brief span of earthly life. But as variety in unity is a law of creation, so there are infinite methods of progress, producing harmony instead of monotony, when the individual or classes of individuals are true to the guiding principles of their own nature.

For the ideal of every creature must be found in the relation of its own nature to the universe around it. Right and wrong are based upon the sound understanding of this positive foundation. It is this fact of variety in unity, in the progress of the race, which justifies the hope that the entrance of women into the medical profession will advance that profession.

In order to carry out this noble aspiration, we must understand what the special contribution is, that women may make to medicine, what the aspect of morality which they are called upon to emphasize.

It is not blind imitation of men, nor thoughtless acceptance of whatever may be taught by them that is required, for this would be to endorse the widespread error that the race is men. Our duty is loyalty to right and opposition to wrong, in accordance with the essential principles of our own nature.

Now, the great essential fact of woman's nature is the spiritual power of maternity.

We should do miserable injustice to this great fact if, looking at it with semiblind eyes, we only see the shallow material aspect of this remarkable speciality. It is the great spiritual life underlying the physical which gives us our true womanly ideal.

What are the spiritual principles necessarily involved in this special creation of one-half the race—principles which lie within the material facts of gestation and the care of infancy and childhood, which constitute the distinctive material domain of women?

They are the subordination of self to the welfare of others; the recognition of the claim which helplessness and ignorance make upon the stronger and more intelligent; the joy of creation and bestowal of life; the pity and sympathy which tend to make every woman the born foe of cruelty and injustice; and hope—*i.e.,* the realization of the unseen—which foresees the adult in the infant, the future in the present.

All these are great moral tendencies, and they are necessarily involved in the mighty potentiality of maternity. They lay upon women the weighty responsibility of becoming more and more the moral guides in life's journey. Women are called upon very specially to judge all practical action as right or wrong, and to exercise influence for this high morality in whatever direction it can be most powerfully exerted.

We see the indication of this providential inherited impulse to moral action, in the great and increasing devotion of women to the relief of social suffering and their sturdy opposition to wrong-doing, which form a distinguishing characteristic of our age. These spiritual mothers of the race are often more truly incarnations of the grand maternal life, than those who are technically mothers in the lower physical sense.

With sound intellectual growth the range of moral influence increases. But such sound growth can only take place under the guidance of moral principle; for moral perception becomes reason as the intellectual faculties grow, and reason is the true light for all. It is in this high moral life, enlarged by intelligence, that the ideal of womanhood lies. It is through the moral, guiding the intellectual, that the beneficial influence of woman in any new sphere of activity will be felt.

Thus, from their inherited tendencies, as well as from the existent individuality of their nature, women must seek a high moral standard as their ideal, and acknowledge the supremacy of right over every sphere of intellectual activity. The highest type of moral excellence which we can find in the age in which we live, the beneficence which it exerts, the means by which it has been attained, form so many landmarks to guide us in our search for the right.

It is a noteworthy feature of the present day that some of our best men, witnessing the failure of so many panaceas for the intolerable evils that afflict society, are longing for that untried force—the action and co-operation of good women. 'Our only hope is in women!' is a cry that may sometimes be heard from the enlightened male conscience. But still more significant is the awakening of an increasing number of women themselves.

There is no line of practical work outside domestic life, so eminently suited to these noble aspirations as the legitimate study and practice of medicine. The legitimate study requires the preservation in full force of those beneficent moral qualities—tenderness, sympathy, guardianship—which form an indispensable spiritual element of maternity; whilst, at the same time, the progress of the race demands that the intellectual horizon be enlarged, and the understanding strengthened by the observation and reasoning which will give increased efficiency to those moral qualities.

The true physician must possess the essential qualities of maternity. The sick are as helpless in his hands as the infant. They depend absolutely upon the insight and judgment, the honesty and hopefulness, of the doctor.

The fact also that every human being we are called on to treat, is, like the infant and the child, soul as well as body, must never be forgotten. Successful treatment requires the insight which comes from recognition of these facts and the sympathy that they demand. In the infinite variety of human ailments the physician will find that she must often be the confessor of her patient, and the consulting-room should have the sacredness of the Confessional, and she must always be the counsellor and guide.

In those two departments of medicine which seem to me peculiarly valuable to women physicians, which I shall refer to later—viz., midwifery and preventive medicine—it would be hard to say whether the moral or intellectual qualities of the physician were called most largely into play, so inseparably are they blended. What patience and hopefulness also are demanded in the lingering trial of chronic illness! What discrimination and union of gentleness and firmness these cases require! Then think of the children in our families! To the girls and boys, the young women and men, who grow up under our ministrations, what an inspirer of nobleness and purity, what a guardian from temptation the true physician can be!

Again, in the treatment of the poor, an immense demand is made upon our pity, patience, and courage. These poor victims of our social stupidity are often extremely trying. The faulty arrangements which compel us to see thirty, fifty even, in an hour exhaust the nervous system of the doctor. It requires faith and courage to recognise the real human soul under the terrible mask of squalor and disease in these crowded masses of poverty, and to resist the temptation to regard them as 'clinical material.'

The attitude of the student and doctor to the sick poor is a real test of the true physician.

It is not a brilliant theorizer that the sick person requires, but the experience gained by careful observation and sound common-sense, united to the kindly feeling and cheerfulness which make the very sight of the doctor a cordial to the sick. If these necessary results of intellectual training can be secured in harmony with the moral structure of womanhood, then a step of real social progress is made by our study of medicine.

The more thoroughly the human organization is investigated, the more wonderful will the unapproachable mechanism for the use of human life be seen to be. We shall never regret any amount of time and care spent in acquiring the most intimate knowledge of human anatomy. For even if we never perform a surgical operation, the thorough knowledge of the human framework with whose aberrations we have to deal, gives a firm foundation for practice that nothing else can supply.

We are happy in drawing into our schools a large number of capable women—women who may not only be a gain as physicians, but who may exert a most beneficial influence on the profession itself, if they bring into it fresh and independent life.

It is much to be regretted that our students are now compelled to go abroad for the completion of their medical education, for methods of study injurious to morality are exaggerated abroad. The abuse of the poor as subjects of experimental investigation, in whose treatment all decent reserves of modesty are so often stripped away; the contempt felt for the mass of women where chastity is not recognised as an obligatory male virtue; the atrocious cruelty of their experiments on animals—all these results of active intellect, unguided by large morality, as seen in full force abroad, make me deplore the necessity which drives so many of our best but inexperienced students away, in search of more efficient training than they can obtain at home.

The two special dangers against which I would warn our students are:

First, the blind acceptance of what is called 'authority' in medicine.

Second, the narrow and superficial materialism which prevails so widely amongst scientific men.

Our women students especially need caution as to the blind acceptance of authority. Young women come into such a new and stimulating intellectual atmosphere when entering upon medical study, that they breathe it with keen delight; they are inclined to accept with enthusiasm the brilliant theory or statement which the active intellect of a clever teacher lays before them. They are accustomed to accept the government and instruction of men as final, and it hardly occurs to them to question it. It is not the custom to realize the positive fact, that methods and conclusions formed by one-half of the race only, must necessarily require revision as the other half of humanity rises into conscious responsibility.

It is a difficult lesson also, fully to recognise the limitations of the human intellect, which recognition, nevertheless, is necessary before we can grasp this important and positive fact in human experience—viz., that the Moral must guide the Intellectual, or there is no halting-place in the rapid incline to error.

. . . [T]he worship of the intellect, or so-called knowledge, as an end in itself, entirely regardless of the character of the means by which we seek to gain it, is the most dangerous error that science can make.

The second danger against which the student of medicine must guard is the materialism which seems to arise from undue absorption in the physical aspect of nature, and which spreads like a blight in our profession.

The basis of materialism is the assertion that only sense is real.

Our medical studies necessarily begin with minute and prolonged study of what we term 'dead matter.' If this study be carried on without reverence, it appears to blind the student to any reality except the material under his scalpel or in his crucible—*i.e.,* the facts that the senses reveal. Proceeding logically from this false premise, that only sense is real, mind is looked upon as an outcome of the brain, and life as the result of organization of matter, which is destroyed when the organization of the material body is broken up.

Love, Hope, Reverence, are realities of a different order from the senses, but they are positive and constant facts, always active, always working out mighty changes in human life.

A thoughtful writer has characterized Materialism as an attempt to explain the Universe in terms of mass and motion rather than in terms of Intelligence, Love, and Will, and it is a true criticism.

The tendency of unprejudiced science in our day is to show the unsatisfactory character of the terms 'matter' and 'spirit.' For the exaltation of what we term 'matter' tends constantly to lose itself in what we call 'spirit.'

Reality always transcends sense. As the vibrations of ether are only known as light and colour, and the vibrations of the atmosphere are translated into sound, so in the careful observation of our own mental states, in the experiences of dream-land, in the study of clairvoyants and somnambulists and the revelations of hypnotism, we gain an insight into states of consciousness independent of the senses—states where the old distinctions between matter and spirit seem to become quite inapplicable.

Í must not now dwell longer on this new and valuable department of medical investigation—psycho-physiology. But it is an inspiring thought that true science supports the noblest intuitions of humanity, and its tendency is to furnish proof suited to our age of these intuitions. I have specially dwelt on this subject now, because the discouragement which results from the false reasoning of materialism, injuring hope, aspiration, and our sense of justice, is especially antagonistic to women, whose distinctive work is joyful creation.

"My Most Humiliating Jim Crow Experience"

It is only within this generation that Hurston's work as novelist, anthropologist, and folklorist has been accorded a place within America's cultural and academic heritage. Raised in rural Florida, Zora Neale Hurston eventually made her way to New York City, where she graduated from Barnard College in 1927, after studying anthropology under Franz Boas and Margaret Mead. Determined to preserve the traditions of her native region, Hurston spent five years in the field, combing the South for African-American folktales, sermons, songs, rituals, and hoodoo practices. The culmination of this work, *Mules and Men* (1935), was the first book of its kind by an African-American, and it has since become a classic text in cultural studies. The forms and rhythms of vernacular expression that Hurston gleaned from her odyssey across the South pervade her novels and short stories and pointed the way to new stylistic directions in American fiction. Hurston also published her autobiography, *Dust Tracks on the Road* (1942), more than fifty short stories and essays, and four novels, including the celebrated *Their Eyes Were Watching God* (1937), in which she describes the psychological development and liberation of a woman who discovers the power of the cultural traditions that sustain her.

My most humiliating Jim Crow experience came in New York instead of the South as one would have expected. It was in 1931 when Mrs. R. Osgood Mason was financing my researches in anthropology. I returned to New York from the Bahama Islands ill with some disturbances of the digestive tract.

Godmother (Mrs. Mason liked for me to call her Godmother) became concerned about my condition and suggested a certain white specialist at her expense. His office was in Brooklyn.

Mr. Paul Chapin called up and made the appointment for me. The doctor told the wealthy and prominent Paul Chapin that I would get the best of care.

So two days later I journeyed to Brooklyn to submit myself to the care of the great specialist.

His reception room was more than swanky, with a magnificent hammered copper door and other decor on the same plane as the door.

But his receptionist was obviously embarrassed when I showed up. I mentioned

From *I Love Myself When I Am Laughing . . . and Then Again When I Am Looking Mean and Impressive: A Zora Neale Hurston Reader,* ed. Alice Walker (Old Westbury, N.Y.: The Feminist Press, 1979). Reprinted by permission of Lucy A. Hurston.

the appointment and got inside the door. She went into the private office and stayed a few minutes, then the doctor appeared in the door all in white, looking very important, and also very unhappy from behind his rotund stomach.

He did not approach me at all, but told one of his nurses to take me into a private examination room.

The room was private all right, but I would not rate it highly as an examination room. Under any other circumstances, I would have sworn it was a closet where the soiled towels and uniforms were tossed until called for by the laundry. But I will say this for it, there was a chair in there wedged in between the wall and the pile of soiled linen.

The nurse took me in there, closed the door quickly and disappeared. The doctor came in immediately and began in a desultory manner to ask me about my symptoms. It was evident he meant to get me off the premises as quickly as possible. Being the sort of objective person I am, I did not get up and sweep out angrily as I was first disposed to do. I stayed to see just what would happen, and further to torture him more. He went through some motions, stuck a tube down my throat to extract some bile from my gall bladder, wrote a prescription and asked for twenty dollars as fee.

I got up, set my hat at a reckless angle and walked out, telling him that I would send him a check, which I never did. I went away feeling the pathos of Anglo-Saxon civilization.

And I still mean pathos, for I know that anything with such a false foundation cannot last. Whom the gods would destroy, they first made mad.

Balm in Gilead:
Journey of a Healer

Professor of Education at Harvard University, Sara Lawrence Lightfoot is the author of several books, including *Worlds Apart: Relationships between Families and Schools* and *The Good High School: Portraits of Character and Culture*. In 1984, she received the MacArthur Foundation Award, which allowed her time to write *Balm in Gilead: Journey of a Healer* (1988), a biographical study of her mother's life and work. Pediatrician, psychoanalyst, mother of three, and author of *Mental Health Teams in the Schools* (1971) and *Young Inner City Families* (1975), Dr. Margaret Cornelia Morgan Lawrence was born in New York City in 1914 but spent her childhood in Virginia and Mississippi. The death of her eleven-month-old brother soon after she was born had a devastating impact on her family, and by the time Margaret Morgan was ten, she had decided to become a doctor so she could "save babies." At the age of fourteen, she moved to New York to pursue her goal, doing brilliantly in her studies and eventually earning her medical degree from the Columbia University College of Physicians & Surgeons in 1940. That same year, her husband, Charles Lawrence, whom she had married in 1938, entered the doctoral program in sociology at Columbia University while she began her pediatric internship at Harlem Hospital. Dedicated to community service, Margaret Lawrence also enrolled at Columbia's School of Public Health, where Benjamin Spock's interdisciplinary approach to teaching childcare would soon push her work in new directions. In 1943, the Lawrence family moved to Nashville, where Charles joined the sociology faculty at Fisk University and Margaret started teaching at Meharry Medical College while practicing at a pediatric clinic. During the next three years, Margaret Morgan Lawrence came to realize that much of her work revolved around "the unravelling of family stories," and she became increasingly drawn to the psychological and cultural dimensions of doctoring. Returning to New York City with her family in 1947, she began her residency in psychiatry at the New York State Psychiatric Institute and started her studies at Columbia's Psychoanalytic Center, completing her training at the age of thirty-seven. In 1963, Lawrence became head of the Developmental Psychiatry Service at Harlem Hospital, where she practiced for more than twenty years, developing an interdisciplinary approach to psychotherapy and conducting pioneering work in the city's day care centers and community mental health clinics.

From *Balm in Gilead: Journey of a Healer,* Radcliffe Biography Series (Reading, Mass.: Addison-Wesley, 1988). Copyright 1988 by Sara Lawrence Lightfoot. Reprinted by permission of Addison-Wesley Publishing Company, Inc.

How can I bear my sorrow?
I am sick at heart . . .
I am wounded at the sight of my people's wound,
I go like a mourner, overcome with horror.

Is there no balm in Gilead,
   no physician there?
Why has no skin grown over their wound?
                    JEREMIAH (8:18–8:22)

It is rare, I think, for parents to let their children—of any age—grow up and become peers. My parents, Margaret and Charles Lawrence, encouraged their three children's autonomy and equality, making it possible for each of us to feel both closer to and more separate from them as we grew older. That combination of intimacy and identity made this book possible. I thank my parents for their enthusiastic participation in this project—their eagerness to tell their stories, their courage in revisiting old haunts and uncovering family secrets. But mostly I feel indebted to them for the strength of our relationships, which allowed me to mix the roles of daughter, inquirer, and narrator, and to blend the passion of a family member with the skepticism of a social scientist.

The consultation room, where we meet for our interviews, is . . . full of treasures that reflect Margaret's history and passions. Family photographs are carefully arranged to allow everyone's face to be seen. There are African Mkonda statues, a redwood image made by a sculptor friend of "Mother and Child," a calendar picturing beautiful brown Indian women with babies on their backs, a miniature porcelain black infant, and a handwoven hanging from West Africa that covers an entire wall. Because this is where Margaret sees her adult patients, there are the more typical doctor's office furnishings: a medical degree from the College of Physicians and Surgeons, Columbia University, 1940; a Master of Science in Public Health degree from the Columbia School of Public Health, 1943; diplomas from the American Board of Pediatrics, 1948, and the New York Psychiatric Institute, 1950; and a Certificate in Psychoanalysis from the Columbia Psychoanalytic Clinic for Training and Research, 1951.

The worst traumas of her professional training are perhaps those that made Margaret feel forced into a childlike dependence. . . . [One] such moment came in Margaret's senior year at Cornell. She had concluded her career there with a flourish. As she moved closer to medical school, the momentum and energy of her academic pursuits increased, her grades soared, and she knew with increasing certainty that her dream would be realized. In the beginning of her senior year, she took the medical aptitude exams required of prospective medical students. Margaret remembers that "it didn't so much depend on past knowledge, but on aptitude, on figuring things out." For the first time since she had come north, the girl from Vicksburg managed to do very well on a standardized test. When the dean of the medical school told her she had done "very well" on the examination, she was overjoyed and newly confident. This was another sign that "medicine was right for me."

When the same dean called Margaret into his office toward the end of her senior year, she assumed that this would be the ritualized visit offered to all incoming medical students. She expected that he would offer acknowledgment of her fine work in college and congratulations for her successful admission to medical school. "I took it that everyone was having these conversations with the dean." As she sat in the chair facing the dean, Margaret's mind savored all the anticipated events. "I recall happily considering medical school, looking forward to my graduation, planning for my parents' arrival, working on renting an apartment for them to stay in . . ." Her pleasant reveries were interrupted by the dean's voice, which seemed to be cautious and apologetic even before Margaret could hear the words. Then the message—with all its horror—began to penetrate, and Margaret grew blank and silent. "The dean said there had been a number of meetings of the Admissions Committee about me, that my application had been carefully considered, that I was a very good student and a promising physician, but that I would *not* be admitted. He said he was sorry."

This was impossible. Margaret couldn't believe what she heard. Still stunned, she heard his explanation for the rejection. "You know," he said, without a hint of emotion in his voice, "twenty-five years ago there was a Negro man admitted to Cornell Medical School and it didn't work out. . . . He got tuberculosis." Each of the dean's words was like a knife. There was nothing to say. "I cannot remember my response . . . I *must* have said something. . . ." She left the office in a daze, devastated by the death of a dream she had pursued with all her energy since she was a young girl.

Margaret's pain cut right to her soul. "My experience was one of depersonalization. . . . It was as if I was lost in a strange world . . . I walked around like this for days and days . . . I remember one brief conversation with my comparative anatomy professor . . . but there was nobody who could really be with me where I was." The reliving of this tale nearly fifty years later brings back the pain and tears as Margaret speaks of a "lost identity." "Who am I?" she wondered.

Somehow out of the depths of despair, Margaret was able to reach out. After days of aimless wondering, she managed to make a telephone call to Madeline Ramée, an administrator with the National Council of the Episcopal Church, a group that had awarded Margaret a scholarship for her undergraduate education.

Miss Ramée received Margaret's painful news with a welcome equanimity. She did not share Margaret's panic but moved quickly to think about alternatives. "She wrote back and said, 'Hold on! . . . We have contacts at Columbia Medical School. Make your application.'" By now, it was very late in the spring, well past the usual application deadlines, but Margaret moved quickly and Miss Ramée pursued her contacts. Before she knew it, Margaret was on her way to New York to be interviewed by Columbia's Admissions Committee. The stonefaced, gray men sat in a line before her and asked lots of questions, one of which Margaret remembers: "Suppose in your clinical years you go on the ward and a white patient refuses to have you as a doctor. What would you do?" Margaret's response was straightforward and seemed to satisfy the concerns of the committee. "I would come back to my clinical supervisor and I'd ask for another patient." She was admitted. "So that was that," says Margaret of the smooth conclusion to her terrifying experience. "I had fallen apart . . . but I came back." When Margaret Morgan was admitted to Columbia Medical School in the fall of 1936, she was the third black medical student and the second black woman to attend, although she was the only black there during her four years of school. She was also one of ten woman students out of a class of one hundred and four.

The only other time in her life that Margaret experienced the same sense of "acute depersonalization"—"floating through space somewhere"—was at the end of her psychoanalytic training sixteen years later. When she had arrived at the Columbia Psychoanalytic Center in 1946, she was the first and only black trainee. The center was dominated by Dr. Sandor Rado, its founder and director. Rado had been a close associate of Freud's and was a major figure in the interpretation of Freudian theory and practice in this country. A short Jewish man of Hungarian background, he was opinionated, outspoken, and uncompromising in his power. The trainees both revered and feared him, treasuring every pearl of wisdom that came out of his mouth.

At the conclusion of her training, now thirty-seven and the mother of three children, ages six, seven, and eight, Margaret took the oral examinations required for the final certificate of graduation and was eager to push on with her life. This had been a costly and consuming process, in terms of both time and psychic energy, and she could almost taste the feeling of relief and liberation she would feel when it was all over. On the eve of her departure, having successfully passed the oral examination, Margaret was called into Dr. Rado's office. Just as in the conference with the dean of the Cornell Medical School, she arrived with the expectation of a ritualized, appreciative encounter. After all, she had thrived in her training analysis, successfully completed the required course work, learned a great deal in supervision, and passed the final examination. But, as she was now more sophisticated and skeptical, it occurred to her that the Rado meeting might not be merely ritual or congratulations. She was not, however, prepared for what she heard: "The committee has decided that before awarding you a certificate, you should have a consultation with Dr. Abram Kardiner to see if you need further analysis." This time the blow did not leave Margaret speechless. She was fighting angry and "by now I was free enough to say my piece." "Why?" she inquired. "I won't tell you," Rado shot back. "You'll have to go to Kardiner. That was the committee's decision." "Why can't you tell me?" said Margaret, her voice steady but her insides ravaged. Dr. Rado, unaccustomed to any questioning of his authority, rose from his chair, his body rigid with anger. Margaret looked into his red and contorted face as their confrontation escalated. "You will have to go," he finally threatened, to which she replied, "I refuse to have this consultation." Then there was silence as the two adversaries tried to figure out how to extract themselves from the deadlock. Margaret, her mind racing furiously, offered a compromise. "David Levy has been my supervisor, and Gene Milch, my analyst; I would be willing to talk to one of them but not to Kardiner." But after she offered this suggestion, she asked once again, "Why can't you tell me?" And Rado kept turning away, refusing to answer, as if he were harboring some terrible, unspeakable truth. Finally he spoke the words that ended the session, words that felt unsatisfactory to both of them. Both of their faces showed defeat. "You see Levy, but if that is not satisfactory, you will have to see Kardiner."

"This was on Friday afternoon," recalls Margaret as if it were yesterday. "I made an appointment to see David Levy on the following Monday morning . . . that was a weekend of *suffering."* Once again, the pain was so deep that Margaret "lost her identity." Again the question from the depths of her soul: "Who am I?" This time the loss seemed more severe because she would be taking her family down with her. Charles and the children had been part of this quest.

"This was the longest weekend I have ever lived. Margaret felt like a puppet in the hands of these powerful men. Her fate hung on their impulses, their needs, their fears and apprehensions. The drama was further complicated by the nature of the man whom Rado had wanted to pull into the act, Abram Kardiner. Kardiner, an analyst and professor at the institute, was also the author of *Mark of Oppression,* a popular and controversial book about the Negro psyche. A few years before, when he had been gathering data for the book, he had asked Margaret to be a research assistant. He had wanted her to go into the field and spend several months interviewing Negroes in the Deep South. Margaret had declined his offer. "I said I couldn't do it because I had three children and a husband, and I was in the midst of psychiatric and psychoanalytic training." She was also suspicious of his perspective and his methods, and worried that in his research Negroes might be portrayed as powerless and inarticulate. But she did not mention these apprehensions. It was enough to offer him the facts of her already overcrowded life. Kardiner was furious that this black trainee—the only one he had available to him—would dare to refuse his offer. He needed her to make his work legitimate, and she had the nerve to decline the chance to work with him.

On the Monday following the agonizing, long weekend, Margaret arrived at David Levy's office. This was a friendly place and she trusted him. Levy had been her supervisor and they had developed a satisfying, caring relationship. She repeated her conversation with Sandor Rado, trying to remain distant and cool, and trying to pull herself out of her weekend daze. Levy had already heard a short version of the confrontation from Milch, who had called him with the news the night before. He then revealed the terrible, hidden secret that Rado had refused to let Margaret hear. His voice sought clarification but had no edge of condemnation. "Someone told Rado that you had said that you didn't want to work with Negro patients. . . . Is that true?" Margaret couldn't believe her ears. Nothing could be further from the truth. She shot back, "Absolutely not!" Levy's reply was both relieving and deeply troubling. Almost casually, he said, "Well, just forget it then. I'll take care of it."

So easily remedied. Just a phone call from this powerful person would remove the nightmare. "What extraordinary power. . . . In the meantime, I had been devastated for two days, thinking my life was in ruins. The whole thing seemed so unreal. Where did this idea come from? Where did Rado get this accusation which he couldn't tell me? How could they accuse me of rejecting my identification as a Negro? *That* was a lie. That I had never done! Those people who were supposed to be experts on motivation telling me I didn't want to be a Negro." Margaret is raging as she speaks.

How could this rumor have gotten started? Why wasn't it stopped by those mentors who knew her well? Was there anything she had done—some slight slip of the tongue, some almost imperceptible gesture, some challenging question she asked—that might have given them the impression that she was forsaking her people? Were they trying to put a barrier in her path, forcing her to jump extra hoops in order to test her mettle? When she declined Kardiner's offer to work on his research, did he misinterpret her response as a decision not to work with Negro patients? But she had not wanted to work for *him*! Even today, for Margaret it remains a murky mystery. The whole scene still seems "unreal," impossible to comprehend, and she shakes with the memory. Then her voice grows calm as she puts it back in the past where it won't hurt so much. "David Levy was powerful enough to say, 'Let's drop it' . . . then life went on after that . . . with just enough scar to remember."

PART 7

The Experimenter

EDWARD JENNER (1749–1823)

"An Inquiry into the Causes and Effects of the Variolae Vaccinae, or Cow-Pox"

In Edward Jenner's day, smallpox was one of the most feared diseases in the world, leaving its victims, if not dead, then horribly scarred for life with pockmarks. Although many European countries, as well as Africa, China, India, and Turkey, had developed various methods of immunization, then called "variolation," none of these was free of risk. In England, Lady Wortley Montagu worked to introduce the Turkish practice of inoculating the young with a needle prick under the skin, the means by which she had had her own children immunized. Her persuasive powers even convinced the Princess of Wales to follow suit with the royal offspring, but only after the procedure was performed safely and successfully on seven criminals and seven orphans. Despite the tremendous benefits of variolation, the process—which depended on the transmission of a deadly disease from one human to another—carried the risk of communicating an unmitigated form of smallpox or even some other disease, such as syphilis. A safer and more effective method of prevention was needed, and it was precisely this that Edward Jenner, a young English physician from Gloucestershire, set out to find. A former pupil of John Hunter, Jenner had a keen interest in natural science, and he soon noticed something that linked two different diseases: Cowherds and milkmaids sometimes developed pustules similar to those found on cows suffering from cowpox. Furthermore, after they were inoculated with smallpox, they showed no signs of the disease. These facts seemed to confirm the widespread belief among dairy farmers that contracting cowpox gave immunity against smallpox, and Jenner set out to lend scientific validity to humble folklore. In a series of experiments that began on May 14, 1796, Jenner began to inoculate his neighbors and relatives with pus taken from cowpox pustules, and then with matter containing the smallpox virus. In case after case, no symptoms of smallpox developed. When his results were first published in 1798, they were greeted with ridicule: The idea that virulent matter taken from animals could protect humans from their own diseases was completely foreign to medical thinking. Within a few years, however, Jenner's discovery earned not only general acceptance but the sum of ten thousand pounds, conferred on him by the British Parliament as a token of the nation's profound gratitude.

The deviation of man from the state in which he was originally placed by nature seems to have proved to him a prolific source of diseases. From the love of splendour,

From *The Harvard Classics: Scientific Papers,* ed. Charles W. Eliot (1897; reprint, New York: P. F. Collier & Son, 1910).

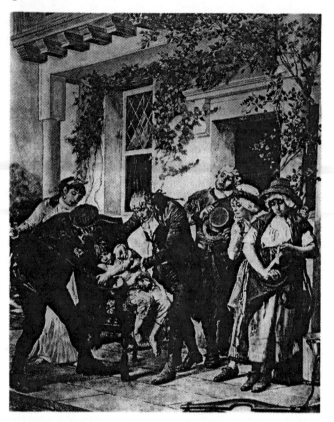

21. *Watercolor by William Thompson (after a painting by Gaston Melingue) depicting Edward Jenner inoculating a child. Wellcome Institute Library, London. On May 14, 1796, Edward Jenner inoculated the eight-year-old James Phipps with matter taken from pustules on the hand of a dairymaid, Sarah Nelmes, who had contracted cowpox. The painting depicts Jenner making an incision with his lancet in the arm of Phipps, who is portrayed as the feisty, if somewhat reluctant, hero of the scene. Nelmes stands binding her sores in the foreground, with her milk pail and yoke beside her. Thompson's tableau of human experimentation has a distinctly pastoral quality to it, helping to domesticate, and thus legitimate, the search for new medical knowledge.*

from the indulgences of luxury, and from his fondness for amusement he has familiarised himself with a great number of animals, which may not originally have been intended for his associates.

The wolf, disarmed of ferocity, is now pillowed in the lady's lap. The cat, the little tiger of our island, whose natural home is the forest, is equally domesticated and caressed. The cow, the hog, the sheep, and the horse, are all, for a variety of purposes, brought under his care and dominion.

There is a disease to which the horse, from his state of domestication, is frequently subject. The farriers have called it the grease. It is an inflammation and swelling in the heel, from which issues matter possessing properties of a very peculiar kind, which seems capable of generating a disease in the human body (after it has undergone the modification which I shall presently speak of), which bears so strong a resemblance to the smallpox that I think it highly probable it may be the source of the disease.

In this dairy country a great number of cows are kept, and the office of milking is performed indiscriminately by men and maid servants. One of the former having been appointed to apply dressings to the heels of a horse affected with the grease, and not paying due attention to cleanliness, incautiously bears his part in milking the cows, with some particles of the infectious matter adhering to his fingers. When this is the case, it commonly happens that a disease is communicated to the cows, and from the cows to the dairymaids, which spreads throughout the farm until most of the cattle and domestics feel its unpleasant consequences. This disease has obtained the name of the cow-pox. It appears on the nipples of the cows in the form of irregular pustules. At their first appearance they are commonly of a palish blue, or rather of a colour somewhat approaching to livid, and are surrounded by an erysipelatous inflammation. These pustules, unless a timely remedy be applied, frequently degenerate into phagedenic ulcers, which prove extremely troublesome. The animals become indisposed, and the secretion of milk is much lessened. Inflamed spots now begin to appear on different parts of the hands of the domestics employed in milking, and sometimes on the wrists, which quickly run on to suppuration, first assuming the appearance of the small vesications produced by a burn. Most commonly they appear about the joints of the fingers and at their extremities; but whatever parts are affected, if the situation will admit, these superficial suppurations put on a circular form, with their edges more elevated than their centre, and of a colour distantly approaching to blue. Absorption takes place, and tumours appear in each axilla. The system becomes affected—the pulse is quickened; and shiverings, succeeded by heat, with general lassitude and pains about the loins and limbs, with vomiting, come on. The head is painful, and the patient is now and then even affected with delirium. These symptoms, varying in their degrees of violence, generally continue from one day to three or four, leaving ulcerated sores about the hands, which, from the sensibility of the parts, are very troublesome, and commonly heal slowly, frequently becoming phagedenic, like those from whence they sprung. The lips, nostrils, eyelids, and other parts of the body are sometimes affected with sores; but these evidently arise from their being heedlessly rubbed or scratched with the patient's infected fingers. No eruptions on the skin have followed the decline of the feverish symptoms in any instance that has come under my inspection, one only excepted, and in this case a very few appeared on the arms: they were very minute, of a vivid red colour, and soon died away without advancing to maturation; so that I cannot determine whether they had any connection with the preceding symptoms.

Thus the disease makes its progress from the horse to the nipple of the cow, and from the cow to the human subject.

Morbid matter of various kinds, when absorbed into the system, may produce effects in some degree similar; but what renders the cow-pox virus so extremely singular is that the person who has been thus affected is forever after secure from the infection of the smallpox; neither exposure to the variolous effluvia, nor the insertion of the matter into the skin, producing this distemper.

In support of so extraordinary a fact, I shall lay before my reader a great number of instances.

CASE I.—Joseph Merret, now an under gardener to the Earl of Berkeley, lived as a servant with a farmer near this place in the year 1770, and occasionally assisted in milking his master's cows. Several horses belonging to the farm began to have sore heels, which Merret frequently attended. The cows soon became affected with the cow-pox, and soon after several sores appeared on his hands. Swellings and stiffness in each axilla followed, and he was so much indisposed for several days as to be incapable of pursuing his ordinary employment. Previously to the appearance of the distemper among the cows there was no fresh cow brought into the farm, nor any servant employed who was affected with the cow-pox.

In April, 1795, a general inoculation taking place here, Merret was inoculated with his family; so that a period of twenty-five years had elapsed from his having the cow-pox to this time. However, though the variolous matter was repeatedly inserted into his arm, I found it impracticable to infect him with it; an efflorescence only, taking on an erysipelatous look about the centre, appearing on the skin near the punctured parts. During the whole time that his family had the smallpox, one of whom had it very full, he remained in the house with them, but received no injury from exposure to the contagion.

It is necessary to observe that the utmost care was taken to ascertain, with the most scrupulous precision, that no one whose case is here adduced had gone through the smallpox previous to these attempts to produce that disease.

Had those experiments been conducted in a large city, or in a populous neighbourhood, some doubts might have been entertained; but here, where population is thin, and where such an event as a person's having had the smallpox is always faithfully recorded, no risk of inaccuracy in this particular can arise.

CASE II.—Sarah Portlock, of this place, was infected with the cow-pox when a servant at a farmer's in the neighbourhood, twenty-seven years ago.

In the year 1792, conceiving herself, from this circumstance, secure from the infection of the smallpox, she nursed one of her own children who had accidentally caught the disease, but no indisposition ensued. During the time she remained in the infected room, variolous matter was inserted into both her arms, but without any further effect than in the preceding case.

CASE V.—Mrs. H——, a respectable gentlewoman of this town, had the cow-pox when very young. She received the infection in rather an uncommon manner: it was given by means of her handling some of the same utensils which were in use among the servants of the family, who had the disease from milking infected cows. Her hands had many of the cow-pox sores upon them, and they were communicated to her nose, which became inflamed and very much swollen. Soon after this event Mrs. H—— was exposed to the contagion of the smallpox, where it was scarcely possible for her to have escaped, had she been susceptible of it, as she regularly attended a relative who had the disease in so violent a degree that it proved fatal to him.

In the year 1778 the smallpox prevailed very much at Berkeley, and Mrs. H——, not feeling perfectly satisfied respecting her safety (no indisposition having followed her exposure to the smallpox), I inoculated her with active variolous matter. The same appearance followed as in the preceding cases—an efflorescence on the arm without any effect on the constitution.

C ASE VI.—It is a fact so well known among our dairy farmers that those who have had the smallpox either escape the cow-pox or are disposed to have it slightly, that as soon as the complaint shews itself among the cattle, assistants are procured, if possible, who are thus rendered less susceptible of it, otherwise the business of the farm could scarcely go forward.

In the month of May, 1796, the cow-pox broke out at Mr. Baker's, a farmer who lives near this place. The disease was communicated by means of a cow which was purchased in an infected state at a neighbouring fair, and not one of the farmer's cows (consisting of thirty) which were at that time milked escaped the contagion. The family consisted of a man servant, two dairymaids, and a servant boy, who, with the farmer himself, were twice a day employed in milking the cattle. The whole of this family, except Sarah Wynne, one of the dairymaids, had gone through the smallpox. The consequence was that the farmer and the servant boy escaped the infection of the cow-pox entirely, and the servant man and one of the maid servants had each of them nothing more than a sore on one of their fingers, which produced no disorder in the system. But the other dairymaid, Sarah Wynne, who never had the smallpox, did not escape in so easy a manner. She caught the complaint from the cows, and was affected with the symptoms described . . . in so violent a degree that she was confined to her bed, and rendered incapable for several days of pursuing her ordinary vocations in the farm.

March 28, 1797, I inoculated this girl and carefully rubbed the variolous matter into two slight incisions made upon the left arm. A little inflammation appeared in the usual manner around the parts where the matter was inserted, but so early as the fifth day it vanished entirely without producing any effect on the system.

C ASE IX.—Although the cow-pox shields the constitution from the smallpox, and the smallpox proves a protection against its own future poison, yet it appears that the human body is again and again susceptible of the infectious matter of the cow-pox, as the following history will demonstrate.

William Smith, of Pyrton in this parish, contracted this disease when he lived with a neighbouring farmer in the year 1780. One of the horses belonging to the farm had sore heels, and it fell to his lot to attend him. By these means the infection was carried to the cows, and from the cows it was communicated to Smith. On one of his hands were several ulcerated sores, and he was affected with such symptoms as have been before described.

In the year 1791 the cow-pox broke out at another farm where he then lived as a servant, and he became affected with it a second time; and in the year 1794 he was so unfortunate as to catch it again. The disease was equally as severe the second and third time as it was on the first.

In the spring of the year 1795 he was twice inoculated, but no affection of the system could be produced from the variolous matter; and he has since associated with those who had the smallpox in its most contagious state without feeling any effect from it.

CASE XII.—The paupers of the village of Tortworth, in this county, were inoculated by Mr. Henry Jenner, Surgeon, of Berkeley, in the year 1795. Among them, eight patients presented themselves who had at different periods of their lives had the cow-pox. One of them, Hester Walkley, I attended with that disease when she lived in the service of a farmer in the same village in the year 1782; but neither this woman, nor any other of the patients who had gone through the cow-pox, received the variolous infection either from the arm or from mixing in the society of the other patients who were inoculated at the same time. This state of security proved a fortunate circumstance, as many of the poor women were at the same time in a state of pregnancy.

CASE XVI.—Sarah Nelmes, a dairymaid at a farmer's near this place, was infected with the cow-pox from her master's cows in May, 1796. She received the infection on a part of her hand which had been previously in a slight degree injured by a scratch from a thorn. A large pustulous sore and the usual symptoms accompanying the disease were produced in consequence. The pustule was so expressive of the true character of the cow-pox, as it commonly appears upon the hand, that I have given a representation of it in the annexed plate. The two small pustules on the wrists arose also from the application of the virus to some minute abrasions of the cuticle, but the livid tint, if they ever had any, was not conspicuous at the time I saw the patient. The pustule on the forefinger shews the disease in an earlier stage. It did not actually appear on the hand of this young woman, but was taken from that of another, and is annexed for the purpose of representing the malady after it has newly appeared.

CASE XVII.—The more accurately to observe the progress of the infection I selected a healthy boy, about eight years old, for the purpose of inoculation for the cow-pox. The matter was taken from a sore on the hand of a dairymaid, who was infected by her master's cows, and it was inserted, on the 14th of May, 1796, into the arm of the boy by means of two superficial incisions, barely penetrating the cutis, each about half an inch long.

On the seventh day he complained of uneasiness in the axilla, and on the ninth he became a little chilly, lost his appetite, and had a slight headache. During the whole of this day he was perceptibly indisposed, and spent the night with some degree of restlessness, but on the day following he was perfectly well.

The appearance of the incisions in their progress to a state of maturation were much the same as when produced in a similar manner by variolous matter. The only difference which I perceived was in the state of the limpid fluid arising from the action of the virus, which assumed rather a darker hue, and in that of the efflorescence spreading round the incisions, which had more of an erysipelatous look than we commonly perceive when variolous matter has been made use of in the same manner; but the whole died away (leaving on the inoculated parts scabs and subsequent eschars) without giving me or my patient the least trouble.

In order to ascertain whether the boy, after feeling so slight an affection of the system from the cow-pox virus, was secure from the contagion of the smallpox, he was inoculated the 1st of July following with variolous matter, immediately taken from a pustule. Several slight punctures and incisions were made on both his arms, and the matter was carefully inserted, but no disease followed. The same appearances were observable on the arms as we commonly see when a patient has had variolous matter applied, after having either the cow-pox or smallpox. Several months afterwards he was again inoculated with variolous matter, but no sensible effect was produced on the constitution.

Here my researches were interrupted till the spring of the year 1798, when, from the wetness of the early part of the season, many of the farmers' horses in this neighbourhood were affected with sore heels, in consequence of which the cow-pox broke out among several of our dairies, which afforded me an opportunity of making further observations upon this curious disease.

A mare, the property of a person who keeps a dairy in a neighbouring parish, began to have sore heels the latter end of the month of February, 1798, which were occasionally washed by the servant men of the farm, Thomas Virgoe, William Wherret, and William Haynes, who in consequence became affected with sores in their hands, followed by inflamed lymphatic glands in the arms and axillae, shiverings succeeded by heat, lassitude, and general pains in the limbs. A single paroxysm terminated the disease; for within twenty-four hours they were free from general indisposition, nothing remaining but the sores on their hands.

CASE XVIII.—John Baker, a child of five years old, was inoculated March 16, 1798, with matter taken from a pustule on the hand of Thomas Virgoe, one of the servants who had been infected from the mare's heels. He became ill on the sixth day with symptoms similar to those excited by cow-pox matter. On the eighth day he was free from indisposition.

There was some variation in the appearance of the pustule on the arm. Although it somewhat resembled a smallpox pustule, yet its similitude was not so conspicuous as when excited by matter from the nipple of the cow, or when the matter has passed from thence through the medium of the human subject.

This experiment was made to ascertain the progress and subsequent effects of the disease when thus propagated. We have seen that the virus from the horse, when it proves infectious to the human subject, is not to be relied upon as rendering the system secure from variolous infection, but that the matter produced by it upon the nipple of the cow is perfectly so. Whether its passing from the horse through the human constitution, as in the present instance, will produce a similar effect, remains to be decided. This would now have been effected, but the boy was rendered unfit for inoculation from having felt the effects of a contagious fever in a workhouse soon after this experiment was made.

CASE XIX.—William Summers, a child of five years and a half old, was inoculated the same day with Baker, with matter taken from the nipples of one of the infected cows, at the farm alluded to.

CASE XX.—From William Summers the disease was transferred to William Pead, a boy of eight years old, who was inoculated March 28th.

CASE XXI.—April 5th: Several children and adults were inoculated from the arm of William Pead. The greater part of them sickened on the sixth day, and were well on the seventh, but in three of the number a secondary indisposition arose in consequence of an extensive erysipelatous inflammation which appeared on the inoculated arms. One of these patients was an infant of half a year old. Hannah Excell, an healthy girl of seven years old, and one of the patients above mentioned, received the infection from the insertion of the virus under the cuticle of the arm in three distinct points.

CASE XXII.—From the arm of this girl matter was taken and inserted April 12th into the arms of John Macklove, one year and a half old, Robert F. Jenner, eleven months old, Mary Pead, five years old, and Mary James, six years old.

Among these, Robert F. Jenner did not receive the infection. The arms of the other three inflamed properly and began to affect the system in the usual manner; but being under some apprehensions from the preceding cases that a troublesome erysipelas might arise, I determined on making an experiment with the view of cutting off its source. Accordingly, after the patients had felt an indisposition of about twelve hours, I applied in two of these cases out of the three, on the vesicle formed by the virus, a little mild caustic, composed of equal parts of quick-lime and soap, and suffered it to remain on the part six hours. It seemed to give the children but little uneasiness, and effectually answered my intention in preventing the appearance of erysipelas. Indeed, it seemed to do more, for in half an hour after its application the indisposition of the children ceased. These precautions were perhaps unnecessary, as the arm of the third child, Mary Pead, which was suffered to take its common course, scabbed quickly, without any erysipelas.

CASE XXIII.—After the many fruitless attempts to give the smallpox to those who had had the cow-pox, it did not appear necessary, nor was it convenient to me, to inoculate the whole of those who had been the subjects of these late trials; yet I thought it right to see the effects of variolous matter on some of them, particularly William Summers, the first of these patients who had been infected with matter taken from the cow. He was, therefore, inoculated with variolous matter from a fresh pustule; but, as in the preceding cases, the system did not feel the effects of it in the smallest degree. I had an opportunity also of having this boy and William Pead inoculated by my nephew, Mr. Henry Jenner, whose report to me is as follows: "I have inoculated Pead and Barge, two of the boys whom you lately infected with the cowpox. On the second day the incisions were inflamed and there was a pale inflammatory stain around them. On the third day these appearances were still increasing and their arms itched considerably. On the fourth day the inflammation was evidently subsiding, and on the sixth day it was scarcely perceptible. No symptom of indisposition followed.

"To convince myself that the variolous matter made use of was in a perfect state I at the same time inoculated a patient with some of it who never had gone through the cow-pox, and it produced the smallpox in the usual regular manner."

These experiments afforded me much satisfaction; they proved that the matter, in passing from one human subject to another, through five gradations, lost none of its original properties, J. Barge being the fifth who received the infection successively from William Summers, the boy to whom it was communicated from the cow.

I shall now conclude this inquiry with some general observations on the subject, and on some others which are interwoven with it.

Although I presume it may be unnecessary to produce further testimony in support of my assertion "that the cow-pox protects the human constitution from the infection of the smallpox," yet it affords me considerable satisfaction to say that Lord Somerville, the President of the Board of Agriculture, to whom this paper was shewn by Sir Joseph Banks, has found upon inquiry that the statements were confirmed by the concurring testimony of Mr. Dolland, a surgeon, who resides in a dairy country remote from this, in which these observations were made. With respect to the opinion adduced "that the source of the infection is a peculiar morbid matter arising in the horse," although I have not been able to prove it from actual experiments conducted immediately under my own eye, yet the evidence I have adduced appears sufficient to establish it.

It is curious also to observe that the virus, which with respect to its effects is undetermined and uncertain previously to its passing from the horse through the medium of the cow, should then not only become more active, but should invariably and completely possess those specific properties which induce in the human constitution symptoms similar to those of the variolous fever, and effect in it that peculiar change which for ever renders it unsusceptible of the variolous contagion.

In some of the preceding cases I have noticed the attention that was paid to the state of the variolous matter previous to the experiment of inserting it into the arms of those who had gone through the cow-pox. This I conceived to be of great importance in conducting these experiments, and, were it always properly attended to by those who inoculate for the smallpox, it might prevent much subsequent mischief and confusion. With the view of enforcing so necessary a precaution I shall take the liberty of digressing so far as to point out some unpleasant facts relative to mismangement in this particular, which have fallen under my own observation.

A medical gentleman (now no more), who for many years inoculated in this neighborhood, frequently preserved the variolous matter intended for his use on a piece of lint or cotton, which, in its fluid state, was put into a vial, corked, and conveyed into a warm pocket; a situation certainly favourable for speedily producing putrefaction in it. In this state (not unfrequently after it had been taken several days from the pustules) it was inserted into the arms of his patients, and brought on inflammation of the incised parts, swellings of the axillary glands, fever, and sometimes eruptions. But what was this disease? Certainly not the smallpox; for the matter having from putrefaction lost or suffered a derangement in its specific properties, was no longer capable of producing that malady, those who had been inoculated in this manner being as much subject to the contagion of the smallpox as if they had never been under the influence of this artificial disease; and many, unfortunately, fell victims to it, who thought themselves in perfect security. The same unfortunate circumstance of giving a disease, supposed to be the smallpox, with inefficacious variolous matter, having occurred under the direction of some other practitioners within my knowledge, and probably from the same incautious method of securing the variolous matter, I avail myself of this opportunity of mentioning what I conceive to be of great importance; and, as a further cautionary hint, I shall again digress so far as to add another observation on the subject of inoculation.

Whether it be yet ascertained by experiment that the quantity of variolous matter inserted into the skin makes any difference with respect to the subsequent mildness or violence of the disease, I know not; but I have the strongest reason for supposing that if either the punctures or incisions be made so deep as to go *through* it and wound the adipose membrane, that the risk of bringing on a violent disease is greatly increased. I have known an inoculator whose practice was "to cut deep enough (to use his own expression) to see a bit of fat," and there to lodge the matter. The great number of bad cases, independent of inflammations and abscesses on the arms, and the fatality which attended this practice, was almost inconceivable; and I cannot account for it on any other principle than that of the matter being placed in this situation instead of the skin.

It was the practice of another, whom I well remember, to pinch up a small portion of the skin on the arms of his patients and to pass through it a needle, with a thread attached to it previously dipped in variolous matter. The thread was lodged in the perforated part, and consequently left in contact with the cellular membrane. This practice was attended with the same ill success as the former. Although it is very improbable that any one would now inoculate in this rude way by design, yet these observations may tend to place a double guard over the lancet, when infants, whose skins are comparatively so very thin, fall under the care of the inoculator.

At what period the cow-pox was first noticed here is not upon record. Our oldest farmers were not unacquainted with it in their earliest days, when it appeared among their farms without any deviation from the phaenomena which it now exhibits. Its connection with the smallpox seems to have been unknown to them. Probably the general introduction of inoculation first occasioned the discovery.

Its rise in this country may not have been of very remote date, as the practice of milking cows might formerly have been in the hands of women only; which I believe is the case now in some other dairy countries, and, consequently, that the cows might not in former times have been exposed to the contagious matter brought by the men servants from the heels of horses. Indeed, a knowledge of the source of the infection is new in the minds of most of the farmers in this neighbourhood, but it has at length produced good consequences; and it seems probable, from the precautions they are now disposed to adopt, that the appearance of the cow-pox here may either be entirely extinguished or become extremely rare.

Should it be asked whether this investigation is a matter of mere curiosity, or whether it tends to any beneficial purpose, I should answer that, notwithstanding the happy effects of inoculation, with all the improvements which the practice has received since its first introduction into this country, it not very unfrequently produces deformity of the skin, and sometimes, under the best management, proves fatal.

These circumstances must naturally create in every instance some degree of painful solicitude for its consequences. But as I have never known fatal effects arise from the cow-pox, even when impressed in the most unfavourable manner, producing extensive inflammations and suppurations on the hands; and as it clearly appears that this disease leaves the constitution in a state of perfect security from the infection of the smallpox, may we not infer that a mode of inoculation may be introduced preferable to that at present adopted, especially among those families which, from previous circumstances, we may judge to be predisposed to have the disease unfavourably? It is an excess in the number of pustules which we chiefly dread in the smallpox; but in the cow-pox no pustules appear, nor does it seem possible for the contagious matter to produce the disease from effluvia, or by any other means than contact, and that probably not simply between the virus and the cuticle; so that a single individual in a family might at any time receive it without the risk of infecting the rest or of spreading a distemper that fills a country with terror.

R.T.H. LAËNNEC (1781–1826)

A Treatise on the Diseases of the Chest and on Mediate Auscultation

In 1804, René Théophile Hyacinthe Laënnec received his degree from the École de Santé of Paris, which excelled in the young field of pathological anatomy, the science that was to become the foundation of a new paradigm of disease. Challenging the age-old conception that diseases resulted from the body's general state of imbalance or irritation, physicians began to assert that illness could be caused by pathological processes in specific anatomical sites, or "seats." Although the practice of postmortem examination had suggested this idea, it remained to be demonstrated on the living body. Following in the steps of Leopold Auenbrugger, who had invented the technique of percussion to identify signs of morbidity in the thoracic region, Laënnec decided to concentrate on sounds that this region produced on its own. He suspected that the noises emitted by the heart and lungs held vital clues to any anatomical changes occurring within them and, therefore, to the patient's general state of health. The procedure of laying one's ear directly on the patient's chest, however, soon revealed its distinct disadvantages, bringing physician and patient into closer contact than either may have wanted. Moreover, as intimate as this method of auscultation was, it still did not permit the physician to hear the interior of the body clearly and distinctly. A way of amplifying the sounds had to be found, and inspiration was to come from an unexpected quarter. One day, Laënnec happened upon some children playing a game; they were tapping messages to one another at either end of a long beam. Immediately upon arriving at his clinic, Laënnec proceeded to fashion and use the first stethoscope: He rolled up a piece of paper, placed one end on a patient's chest, the other to his ear, and listened. A flutist in his leisure time, Laënnec had a gifted ear for sound, and in time, he became a virtuoso on various prototypes of the modern stethoscope, recording his observations on thoracic activity in astonishing detail and precision. The work that resulted, *A Treatise on the Diseases of the Chest and on Mediate Auscultation* (1818), not only established new disease categories but signaled the beginning of a new era of medical instrumentation that made the inner workings of the living, breathing body "visible" in unprecedented ways. After serving as physician in chief to the Hôpital Necker for close to a decade, Laënnec fell ill and died from pulmonary consumption, a disease whose signs he had come to know so very intimately.

From *Epoch-Making Contributions to Medicine, Surgery, and the Allied Sciences*, comp. C.N.B. Camac (Philadelphia: W. B. Saunders, 1909).

Of all the diseases which are essentially local, those of the thoracic organs are unquestionably the most frequent; while in point of danger they can only be compared with organic affections of the brain. The heart, lungs, and brain constitute, according to the happy expression of Bordeu, *the tripod of life*; and none of these organs can sustain any considerable or extensive morbid change without the greatest danger. The delicacy of their organization and their incessant motion account for the frequency and severity of their diseases. In no other texture of the animal system is idiopathic and primary inflammation so frequent a source of severe disorder and death as in the lungs; and no other is so liable to become the seat of *accidental productions* of every kind, more especially of tubercles, the most common of all. It may even be asserted that in maladies of every sort, whatever be their seat, death scarcely ever occurs without the chest becoming affected in one way or another; and that, in most cases, life does not seem in peril until the supervention of a congested state of the lungs, serous effusion into the pleura, or a great disorder of the circulation. The brain in general becomes affected only subsequently to these changes; and frequently remains undisturbed even to the last moment of life.

However dangerous diseases of the chest may be, they are, nevertheless, more frequently curable than any other severe internal affection. For this double reason medical men in all ages have been desirous of obtaining a correct diagnosis of them.

Diseases of the brain, not in themselves numerous, are distinguished, for the most part, by constant and striking symptoms; the soft and yielding walls of the abdomen allow us to examine, through the medium of touch, the organs of that cavity, and thus to judge, in some measure, of their size, position, and degree of sensibility, and also of the extraneous substances that may be formed in them. On the other hand, the diseases of the thoracic viscera are very numerous and diversified, and yet have almost all the same class of symptoms. Of these, the most common and prominent are cough, dyspnoea, and, in some expectoration. These, of course, vary in different diseases; but their variations are by no means of that determinate kind which can enable us to consider them as certain indications of known variations in the diseases. The consequence is that the most skilful physician who trusts to the pulse and general symptoms is often deceived in regard to the most common and best known complaints of this cavity. Nay, I will go so far as to assert, and without fear of contradiction from those who have been long accustomed to the examination of dead bodies, that, before the discovery of Auenbrugger, one-half of the acute cases of peripneumony and pleurisy, and almost all the chronic pleurisies, were mistaken by practitioners; and that, in such instances as the superior tact of a physician enabled him to suspect the true nature of the disease, his conviction was rarely sufficiently strong to prompt and justify the application of very powerful remedies. The percussion of the chest, according to the method of the ingenious observer just mentioned, is one of the most valuable discoveries ever made in medicine. By means of it several diseases which had hitherto been cognisable by general and equivocal signs only, are brought within the immediate sphere of our perceptions, and their diagnosis, consequently, rendered both more easy and more certain. It is not to be concealed, however, that this mode of exploration is very incomplete. Confined, in a great measure, to the indication of *fulness* or *emptiness,* it is only applicable to a limited number of organic lesions; it does not enable us to discriminate some which are very different in their nature or seat; . . . It is more particularly in diseases of the heart that we regret the insufficiency of this method and wish for something more precise.

The application of the hand affords some indications as to the extent, strength, and rhythm of the heart's motions; but these in general are by no means distinct, while in cases of considerable fatness or anasarca they become very obscure, or are altogether imperceptible. Within these few years some few physicians have, in those cases, attempted to gain further information by the application of the ear to the cardiac region. In this way the pulsations of the heart, perceived at once by the ear and touch, become, no doubt, more distinct. But even this method comes far short of what might be expected from it. . . . [I]ndependently of its deficiencies, there are other objections to its use: it is always inconvenient, both to the physician and patient; in the case of females it is not only indelicate, but often impracticable; and in that class of persons found in hospitals it is disgusting.

In 1816 I was consulted by a young woman labouring under general symptoms of a diseased heart, and in whose case percussion and the application of the hand were of little avail on account of the great degree of fatness. The other method just mentioned being rendered inadmissible by the age and sex of the patient, I happened to recollect a simple and well-known fact in acoustics, and fancied it might be turned to some use on the present occasion. The fact I allude to is the great distinctness with which we hear the scratch of a pin at one end of a piece of wood on applying our ear to the other. Immediately, on this suggestion, I rolled a quire of paper into a kind of cylinder and applied one end of it to the region of the heart and the other to my ear, and was not a little surprised and pleased to find that I could thereby perceive the action of the heart in a manner much more clear and distinct than I had ever been able to do by the immediate application of the ear. From this moment I imagined that the circumstance might furnish means for enabling us to ascertain the character, not only of the action of the heart, but of every species of sound produced by the motion of all the thoracic viscera and consequently for the exploration of the respiration, the voice, *the rhonchus,* and perhaps even the fluctuation of fluid extravasated in the pleura or the pericardium. With this conviction I forthwith commenced at the Hospital Necker a series of observations from which I have been able to deduce a set of new signs of diseases of the chest, for the most part certain, simple, and prominent, and calculated, perhaps, to render the diagnoses of the diseases of the lungs, heart, and pleura, as decided and circumstantial as the indications furnished to the surgeon by the introduction of the finger or sound, in the complaints wherein these are used.

The first instrument which I used was a cylinder of paper, formed of three quires, compactly rolled together, and kept in shape by paste. The longitudinal aperture which is always left in the centre of paper thus rolled led accidentally in my hands to an important discovery. This aperture is essential to the exploration of the voice. A cylinder without any aperture is best for the exploration of the heart: the same kind of instrument will, indeed, suffice for the respiration and rhonchus; but both these are most distinctly perceived by means of a cylinder which is perforated throughout and excavated into somewhat of a funnel shape, at one of its extremities, to the depth of an inch and a half.

Bodies of a moderate density, such as paper, the lighter kinds of wood, or Indian cane, are those which I always found preferable to others. This result is perhaps in opposition to an axiom in physics; it has, nevertheless, appeared to me one which is invariable. In consequence of these various experiments I now employ a cylinder of wood, an inch and a half in diameter and a foot long, perforated longitudinally by a bore three lines wide, and hollowed out into a funnel shape to the depth of an inch and a half at one of the extremities. It is divided into two portions, partly for the convenience of carriage and partly to permit its being used of half the usual length. The instrument in this form—that is, with the funnel-shaped extremity—is used in exploring the respiration and rhonchus: when applied to the exploration of the heart and the voice it is converted into a simple tube with thick sides by inserting into its excavated extremity a stopper or plug traversed by a small aperture, and accurately adjusted to the excavation. This instrument I have denominated *the stethoscope.* The dimensions mentioned are not a matter of indifference. A greater diameter renders its exact application to certain parts of the chest impracticable; greater length renders its retention in exact apposition more difficult, and when shorter, it is not so easy to apply it to the axilla, while it exposes the physician too closely to the patient's breath, and, besides, frequently obliges him to assume an inconvenient posture, a thing above all others to be avoided if we wish to observe accurately. The only case in which a shorter instrument is useful is where the patient is seated in bed or on a chair, the head or back of which is close to him: then it may be more convenient to employ the half-length instrument.

The use of this new method must not make us forget that of Auenbrugger; on the contrary, the latter acquires quite a fresh degree of value through the simultaneous employment of the former, and becomes applicable in many cases wherein its solitary application is either useless or hurtful. It is by this combination of the two methods that we obtain certain indications of emphysema of the lungs, pneumo-thorax, and of the existence of liquid extravasations in the cavity of the pleura.

In conclusion, I would beg to observe that it is only in an hospital that we can acquire, completely and certainly, the practice of this new art of observation; inasmuch as it is necessary to have occasionally verified, by examination after death, the diagnostics established by means of the cylinder in order that we may acquire confidence in the instrument and in our own observation, and that we may be convinced, by ocular demonstration, of the correctness of the indications obtained. It will be sufficient, however, to study any one disease in two or three subjects to enable us to recognise it with certainty; and the diseases of the lungs and heart are so common that a very brief attendance on an hospital will put it in the power of any one to obtain all the knowledge necessary for his guidance in this important class of affections.

CLAUDE BERNARD (1813–1878)

An Introduction to the Study
of Experimental Medicine

Born in Burgundy, Claude Bernard was apprenticed as a young man to an apothecary in Lyons, where he formed the aspiration to become a playwright. Failing to make headway as a writer, however, Bernard entered the Collège de France to learn medicine. He received his degree in 1843, and shortly after, became Magendie's assistant at the Hôtel Dieu. At the time, the study of physiology in France was completely dominated by Magendie, who had rejected the Vitalism of Bichat to embrace a purely positivistic view of natural phenomena. Like Magendie, Bernard disputed the existence of any "vital forces" in the human body and asserted that the organic world operated according to the same principles and laws that governed the inorganic. These principles guided Bernard's studies of physiological processes in his experimental work with living animals. Bernard's research on gastric juices, saliva, glycogen, and various poisons greatly enhanced medical understanding of metabolic processes, diseases such as diabetes, and the action of pharmaceutical agents, dramatically demonstrating the diverse and complex ways in which physiology is influenced by chemicals. As more and more organic substances began to be synthesized in laboratories, and as processes that once took place only inside the body were duplicated under artificial conditions outside of it, a new era of physiology entered upon the scene. Bernard's *Introduction à l'Étude de la Médecine Expérimentale* (1865) was, however, not only the starting point of a new scientific method but the impetus behind a new literary one; as Émile Zola commenced his project to document the operation of universal laws within human behavior and society, he credited Bernard with the principles that informed his enterprise and the new genre it engendered—*le roman expérimental*.

Only within very narrow boundaries can man observe the phenomena which surround him; most of them naturally escape his senses, and mere observation is not enough. To extend his knowledge, he has had to increase the power of his organs by means of special appliances; at the same time he has equipped himself with various instruments enabling him to penetrate inside of bodies, to dissociate them and to study their hidden parts. A necessary order may thus be established among the different processes of investigation or research, whether simple or complex: the first apply to those objects easiest to examine, for which our senses suffice; the second bring within our observation, by various means, objects and phenomena which would

From *An Introduction to the Study of Experimental Medicine*, trans. Henry Copley Green, intro. Lawrence J. Henderson (1927; reprint, New York: Dover Publications, 1957).

otherwise remain unknown to us forever, because in their natural state they are beyond our range. Investigation, now simple, again equipped and perfected, is therefore destined to make us discover and note the more or less hidden phenomena which surround us.

But man does not limit himself to seeing; he thinks and insists on learning the meaning of the phenomena whose existence has been revealed to him by observation. So he reasons, compares facts, puts questions to them, and by the answers which he extracts, tests one by another. This sort of control, by means of reasoning and facts, is what constitutes experiment, properly speaking; and it is the only process that we have for teaching ourselves about the nature of things outside us.

In the philosophic sense, observation shows, and experiment teaches.

VARIOUS DEFINITIONS OF OBSERVATION AND EXPERIMENT

We should set up a sort of contrast, in this way, between observers and experimenters: the first being passive in the appearance of phenomena; the second, on the other hand, taking a direct and active part in producing them. Cuvier expressed the same thought in saying: "The observer listens to nature; the experimenter questions and forces her to unveil herself."

This definition of experiment necessarily assumes that experimenters must be able to touch the body on which they wish to act, whether by destroying it or by altering it, so as to learn the part which it plays in the phenomena of nature. . . . It is on this very possibility of acting, or not acting, on a body that the distinction will exclusively rest between sciences called sciences of observation and sciences called experimental.

EXPERIMENTERS MUST DOUBT, AVOID FIXED IDEAS, AND ALWAYS KEEP THEIR FREEDOM OF MIND

The first condition to be fulfilled by men of science, applying themselves to the investigation of natural phenomena, is to maintain absolute freedom of mind, based on philosophic doubt. Yet we must not be in the least sceptical; we must believe in science, i.e., in determinism; we must believe in a complete and necessary relation between things, among the phenomena proper to living beings as well as in all others; but at the same time we must be thoroughly convinced that we know this relation only in a more or less approximate way, and that the theories we hold are far from embodying changeless truths. When we propound a general theory in our sciences, we are sure only that, literally speaking, all such theories are false. They are only partial and provisional truths which are necessary to us, as steps on which we rest, so as to go on with investigation; they embody only the present state of our knowledge, and consequently they must change with the growth of science, and all the more often when sciences are less advanced in their evolution.

THE INDEPENDENT CHARACTER OF
THE EXPERIMENTAL METHOD

The revolution which the experimental method has effected in the sciences is this: it has put a scientific criterion in the place of personal authority.

The experimental method is characterized by being dependent only on itself, because it includes within itself its criterion,—experience. It recognizes no authority other than that of facts and is free from personal authority.

The result of this is that when we have put forward an idea or a theory in science, our object must not be to preserve it by seeking everything that may support it and setting aside everything that may weaken it. On the contrary, we ought to examine with the greatest care the facts which apparently would overthrow it, because real progress always consists in exchanging an old theory which includes fewer facts for a new one which includes more. This proves that we have advanced, for in science the best precept is to alter and exchange our ideas as fast as science moves ahead. Our ideas are only intellectual instruments which we use to break into phenomena; we must change them when they have served their purpose, as we change a blunt lancet that we have used long enough.

The ideas and theories of our predecessors must be preserved only in so far as they represent the present state of science, but they are obviously destined to change, unless we admit that science is to make no further progress, and that is impossible.

In the experimental sciences, a mistaken respect for personal authority would be superstition and would form a real obstacle to the progress of science: at the same time, it would be contrary to the examples given us by the great men of all time. Great men, indeed, are precisely those who bring with them new ideas and destroy errors. They do not, therefore, respect the authority of their own predecessors, and they do not expect us to treat them otherwise.

In the experimental sciences, great men are never the promoters of absolute and immutable truths. Each great man belongs to his time and can come only at his proper moment, in the sense that there is a necessary and ordered sequence in the appearance of scientific discoveries. Great men may be compared to torches shining at long intervals, to guide the advance of science. They light up their time, either by discovering unexpected and fertile phenomena which open up new paths and reveal unknown horizons, or by generalizing acquired scientific facts and disclosing truths which their predecessors had not perceived. If each great man makes the science which he vitalizes take a long step forward, he never presumes to fix its final boundaries, and he is necessarily destined to be outdistanced and left behind by the progress of successive generations. Great men have been compared to giants upon whose shoulders pygmies have climbed, who nevertheless see further than they.

To sum up, the experimental method draws from within itself an impersonal authority which dominates science. It forces this authority even on great men, instead of seeking, like the scholastics, to prove from texts that they are infallible and that they have seen, said or thought everything discovered after them.

. . . [T]he names of promoters of science disappear little by little, and the further science advances, the more it takes an impersonal form and detaches itself from the past. To avoid a mistake which has sometimes been committed, I hasten to add that

I mean to speak here of the evolution of science only. In art and letters, personality dominates everything. There we are concerned with a spontaneous creation of the mind, that has nothing in common with the noting of natural phenomena, in which the mind must create nothing. The past keeps all its worth in the creations of art and letters; each individuality remains changeless in time and cannot be mistaken for another. A contemporary poet has characterized this sense of the personality of art and of the impersonality of science in these words,—"Art is myself; science is ourselves."

Physics and chemistry, as established sciences, offer us the independence and impersonality which the experimental method demands. But medicine is still in the shades of empiricism and suffers the consequences of its backward condition. We see it still more or less mingled with religion and with the supernatural. Superstitution and the marvellous play a great part in it. Sorcerers, somnambulists, healers by virtue of some gift from Heaven, are held as the equals of physicians. Medical personality is placed above science by physicians themselves; they seek their authority in tradition, in doctrines or in medical tact. This state of affairs is the clearest of proofs that the experimental method has by no means come into its own in medicine.

VIVISECTION

We have succeeded in discovering the laws of inorganic matter only by penetrating into inanimate bodies and machines; similarly we shall succeed in learning the laws and properties of living matter only by displacing living organs in order to get into their inner environment. After dissecting cadavers, then, we must necessarily dissect living beings, to uncover the inner or hidden parts of the organisms and see them work; to this sort of operation we give the name of vivisection, and without this mode of investigation, neither physiology nor scientific medicine is possible; to learn how man and animals live, we cannot avoid seeing great numbers of them die, because the mechanisms of life can be unveiled and proved only by knowledge of the mechanisms of death.

The prejudices clinging to respect for corpses long halted the progress of anatomy. In the same way, vivisection in all ages has met with prejudices and detractors. . . . [H]ave we a right to perform experiments and vivisections on man? Physicians make therapeutic experiments daily on their patients, and surgeons perform vivisections daily on their subjects. Experiments, then, may be performed on man, but within what limits? It is our duty and our right to perform an experiment on man whenever it can save his life, cure him or gain him some personal benefit. The principle of medical and surgical morality, therefore, consists in never performing on man an experiment which might be harmful to him to any extent, even though the result might be highly advantageous to science, i.e., to the health of others. But performing experiments and operations exclusively from the point of view of the patient's own advantage does not prevent their turning out profitably to science.

A cowardly assassin, a hero and a warrior each plunges a dagger into the breast of his fellow. What differentiates them, unless it be the ideas which guide their hands? A surgeon, a physiologist and Nero give themselves up alike to mutilation of living beings. What differentiates them also, if not ideas? I therefore shall not follow the example of LeGallois, in trying to justify physiologists in the eyes of strangers to science who reproach them with cruelty; the difference in ideas explains everything. A physiologist is not a man of fashion, he is a man of science, absorbed by the scientific idea which he pursues: he no longer hears the cry of animals, he no longer sees the blood that flows, he sees only his idea and perceives only organisms concealing problems which he intends to solve. Similarly, no surgeon is stopped by the most moving cries and sobs, because he sees only his idea and the purpose of his operation. Similarly again, no anatomist feels himself in a horrible slaughter house; under the influence of a scientific idea, he delightedly follows a nervous filament through stinking livid flesh, which to any other man would be an object of disgust and horror. After what has gone before we shall deem all discussion of vivisection futile or absurd. It is impossible for men, judging facts by such different ideas, ever to agree; and as it is impossible to satisfy everybody, a man of science should attend only to the opinion of men of science who understand him, and should derive rules of conduct only from his own conscience.

ROBERT KOCH (1843–1910)

"The Aetiology of Tuberculosis"

A German physician born in Hanover and educated at Göttingen, Robert Koch not only discovered the etiology of infectious diseases but established a model of bacteriological research that is still in place today. Koch insisted that before one could claim that a specific agent was the immediate cause of a disease, one had to demonstrate its presence in the infected host, isolate and cultivate that agent outside the host, and then infect a healthy organism with it. Following these principles, Koch's 1876 paper on anthrax demonstrated that the condition was caused by a specific bacillus. A meticulous description of the bacillus's life cycle and method of propagation, Koch's paper fully documented for the first time the "ethology" of a bacteriological culture. Only after Koch's signal findings regarding anthrax did it become possible to infer that all infectious diseases are caused by specific pathogenic organisms. A series of breakthroughs soon followed in the wake of Koch's discoveries: In 1879 alone, Neisser identified the gonococcus, Eberth and Gaffky the typhoid bacillus, Hansen the cause of leprosy, and Laveran that of malaria. In 1882, however, came the most momentous advance along this frontier: Koch's discovery and isolation of the tubercle bacillus, the microorganism that had during the nineteenth century ravaged close to one third of the world's adult population. In addition to making the bacilli visible for the first time by means of a new staining technique, Koch taught researchers how to identify, breed, and safely handle them. Eager to track other species of bacteria, Koch set out to study them in their natural habitats, traveling widely throughout the topics. In Egypt, he hunted the cholera vibrio, and in Java the malaria-causing parasite, plasmodium; in South Africa, he followed the trail of rinderpest and in Bombay that of bubonic plague. Medical research into the causation and transmission of such diseases went hand in hand with the era of European colonization, opening up regions of the globe whose endemic microorganisms had previously made settlement by Europeans close to impossible. In 1891, Koch became chief of Berlin's Institute for Infectious Disorders, where he continued his bacteriological and epidemiological studies until he retired in 1904, having literally converted the world into his laboratory.

If the number of victims which a disease claims is the measure of its significance, then all diseases, particularly the most dreaded infectious diseases, such as bubonic plague, Asiatic cholera, etc., must rank far behind tuberculosis. Statistics teach that one-seventh of all human beings die of tuberculosis, and that, if one considers only

Trans. Berna Pinner and Max Pinner. From *The American Review of Tuberculosis* 25 (3) (March 1932):285–323.

the productive middle-age groups, tuberculosis carries away one-third and often more of these. Public hygiene has therefore reason enough to devote its attention to so destructive a disease. . . .

There have been repeated attempts to fathom the nature of tuberculosis, but thus far without success. The so frequently successful staining methods for the demonstration of pathogenic microörganisms have failed in regard to this disease, and, to date, the experiments designed to isolate and cultivate a tubercle virus cannot be considered successful. . . .

The aim of the study had to be directed first toward the demonstration of some kind of parasitic forms, which are foreign to the body and which might possibly be interpreted as the cause of the disease. This demonstration became successful, indeed, by means of a certain staining process, which disclosed characteristic and heretofore unknown bacteria in all tuberculous organs. It would take us too far afield to tell of the road by which I arrived at this new process, and I shall therefore immediately give its description.

The objects for study are prepared in the usual fashion for the examination for pathogenic bacteria. They are either spread on the cover-slip, dried and heated, or they are cut in sections after being hardened in alcohol. The cover-slips or sections are put in a staining solution of the following formula: 200 cc. of distilled water are mixed with 1 cc. of a concentrated alcoholic methylene-blue solution, and with repeated shaking 0.2 cc. of a 10 per cent potassium-hydrate solution is added.

Under the microscope all constituents of animal tissue, particularly the nuclei and their disintegration products, appear brown, with the tubercle bacilli, however, beautifully blue. With the exception of leprosy bacilli, all other bacteria which I have thus far examined in this respect assume a brown color with this staining method. The color contrast between the brown-stained tissue and the blue tubercle bacilli is so striking, that the latter, which are frequently present only in very small numbers, are nevertheless seen and identified with the greatest certainty.

Incidentally, the bacteria can be stained not only with methylene-blue, but they take also other aniline dyes, with the exception of brown dyes, under the simultaneous action of an alkali; but their staining is not so beautiful by far as with methylene-blue.

In several respects the bacteria made visible by this process exhibit a characteristic behavior. They are rod-shaped, and they belong to the group of *bacilli*. They are very thin and one-fourth to one-half as long as the diameter of a red blood-corpuscle, although they may sometimes reach a greater length,—up to the full diameter of an erythrocyte. In shape and size they bear a striking similarity to leprosy bacilli. They are differentiated from the latter by being a bit more slender and by having tapered ends. Further, leprosy bacilli are stained by Weigert's nuclear stain, while the tubercle bacilli are not. Wherever the tuberculous process is in recent evolution and is rapidly progressing, the bacilli are present in large quantities; they usually form, then, densely bunched and frequently small braided groups, often intracellular; and they present at times the same picture as leprosy bacilli accumulated in cells.

If giant cells occur in the tuberculous tissue the bacilli are by predilection within these formations. In very slowly progressing tuberculous processes, the interior of giant cells is usually the only place in which bacilli are to be found. In this case the majority of giant cells enclose one or a few bacilli; and it produces a surprising impression to find repeatedly in large areas of the section groups of giant cells, most of which contain one or two tiny blue rods in the centre, and within the wide space enclosed by brown-stained nuclei. . . . [I]t may be assumed that the bacilli, acting as foreign bodies, are enclosed by giant cells; therefore it seems justifiable to assume that, even when the giant cell is found empty while all other features indicate processes as tuberculous, the giant cell was formerly the host of one or several bacilli, and that the latter have been responsible for their formation.

In regard to the occurrence of bacilli in the various tuberculous manifestations in human beings and animals it has been possible to examine the following material thus far:

1. *From Human Beings:*
   Eleven cases of miliary tuberculosis
   Twelve cases of caseous bronchitis and pneumonia (in 6 cases cavity-formation)
   One case of solitary tubercle in the brain, larger than a hazel-nut
   Two cases of intestinal tuberculosis
   Three cases of freshly excised scrofulous lymph nodes
   Four cases of fungoid arthritis
2. *From Animals:*
   Ten cases of Perlsucht with calcified nodules in the lungs, in several cases also in the peritoneum and once on the pericardium
   Three cases in which the lungs of cattle contained, not the well-known calcified nodules with knobby surface, as usually seen in Perlsucht, but smooth-walled, spherical nodes, filled with a thick, cheesy material

In addition to these cases of spontaneous tuberculosis, I could avail myself of a not inconsiderable number of animals which had been infected by inoculation with the most varied tuberculous materials: as, for instance, with gray and caseated tubercles from human lungs, with sputum from consumptives, with tuberculous masses from spontaneously diseased monkeys, rabbits, and guinea pigs, with masses of calcified or caseated lesions form *Perlsucht* in cattle, and finally with material from lesions obtained by animal-passage. The number of animals so infected amounted to 172 guinea pigs, 32 rabbits and 5 cats. In the majority of these cases the demonstration of bacilli had to be limited to the examination of tubercles in the lungs which were always present in large numbers. Here bacilli never failed to be found: frequently they were extraordinarily numerous, and sometimes spore-bearing, but in some preparations only a few yet unmistakable individual forms were observed.

Considering the regularity of the presence of tubercle bacilli it is striking that so far they have not been seen by anyone. But this is explained by the fact that the bacilli are extraordinarily small formations, and are usually so scanty in number, particularly when their occurrence is limited to the interior of giant cells, that for this reason alone they are not detectable by the most attentive observer without the use of quite specific staining-reactions. When present in larger numbers, they are mixed with a finely granular detritus, and obscured by it in such a manner that their visualization is made difficult in the highest degree.

Incidentally, there exist some reports about the finding of microörganisms in tuberculous tissue. For example, Schüller, in his paper on scrofulous and tuberculous arthropathies, mentions that he has constantly found micrococci. Just as the very small motile granules which were found in tubercles by Klebs, these micrococci are undoubtedly something entirely different from the tubercle bacilli seen by me, which are nonmotile and rod-shaped. Furthermore, in the first issue of his pathological reports Aufrecht states that, besides two different types of micrococcus, he has seen short, rod-like formations whose length was twice their breadth. He saw these rods in the centre of tubercles in three of a series of rabbits which he had infected with *Perlsucht* and tuberculous material. But tubercle bacilli are at least five times as long as they are thick, and often much longer yet in relation to their thickness; furthermore, in cases of uncomplicated tuberculosis they never occur mixed with micrococci or other bacteria in the tubercles. For this reason it is extremely unlikely that Aufrecht saw the real tubercle bacilli; had he done so, he would then have necessarily demonstrated their occurrence in human tubercles and in lungs with *Perlsucht*, and he could not have escaped noticing the conspicuous relationship between the bacilli and the giant cells.

On the basis of my numerous observations I consider it established that, in all tuberculous affections of man and animals, there occur constantly those bacilli which I have designated *tubercle bacilli* and which are distinguishable from all other microörganisms by characteristic properties. However, from the mere coincidental relation of tuberculous affections and bacilli it may not be concluded that these two phenomena have a causal relation, notwithstanding the not inconsiderable degree of likelihood for this assumption that is derivable from the fact that the bacilli occur by preference where tuberculous processes are incipient or progressing, and that they disappear where the disease comes to a standstill.

To prove that tuberculosis is a parasitic disease, that it is caused by the invasion of bacilli and that it is conditioned primarily by the growth and multiplication of the bacilli, it was necessary to isolate the bacilli from the body; to grow them in pure culture until they were freed from any disease-product of the animal organism which might adhere to them; and, by administering the isolated bacilli to animals, to reproduce the same morbid condition which, as known, is obtained by inoculation with spontaneously developed tuberculous material.

Disregarding the many preliminary experiments which served for the solution of this task, here again the finished method will be described. Its principle rests on the use of a solid transparent medium, which retains its solid consistence at incubator temperature. The advantages of this method of pure culture which I have introduced into bacteriology I have explained in detail in an earlier publication. That the really complicated task of growing tubercle bacilli in pure culture was achieved by this method is to me a new proof of its efficiency.

Serum from sheep- or cattle-blood, separated as pure as possible, is put into test-tubes closed with a cotton stopper and heated every day to 58°C. for six subsequent days. It is not always possible to sterilize the serum completely by this process, but in most cases it suffices. Then the serum is heated to 65°C. during several hours, or sufficiently long for it to be just coagulated and solidified. After this treatment it appears as an amber-yellow, completely transparent or only slightly opalescent, solid, jelly-like mass; and after several days at incubator temperature it must not show the slightest development of bacterial colonies. If the heating exceeds 75°C. or if it lasts too long, the serum becomes opaque. In order to obtain a large surface for the preparation of the cultures the serum is solidified in test-tubes slanted as much as possible. For those cultures intended for direct microscopical examination the serum is solidified in flat watch-crystals or in small hollow glass blocks.

Upon this solidified blood-serum, which forms a transparent medium that remains solid at incubator temperature, the tuberculous materials are applied in the following manner:

The simplest case in which the experiment is successful is presented, almost without exception, when an animal which has just died of tuberculosis, or a tuberculous animal which has just been killed for this purpose, is at one's disposal. First, the skin is deflected over the thorax and abdomen with instruments flamed just before use. With similarly prepared scissors and forceps, the ribs are cut in the middle, and the anterior chest-wall is removed without opening the abdominal cavity, so that the lungs are to a large extent laid free. Then the instruments are again exchanged for freshly disinfected ones and single tubercles or particles of them, of the size of a millet-seed, are quickly excised with scissors from the lung tissue, and immediately transferred to the surface of the solidified blood-serum with a platinum wire, which has been melted into a glass rod which must be flamed immediately before use. Of course, the cotton stopper may be removed for only a minimal time. In this manner a number of test-tubes, about six to ten, are implanted with tuberculous material, because, with even the most cautious manipulation, not all test-tubes remain free from accidental contamination.

Cultures that result from a growth of tubercle bacilli do not appear to the naked eye until the second week after the seeding, and ordinarily not until after the tenth day. They come into view as very small points and dry-looking scales.

With the aid of a 30- to 40-times magnification one can perceive the bacterial colonies as soon as toward the end of the first week. They appear as very neat spindle- and usually S-shaped or similarly curved formations, which consist of the well-known most tenuous bacilli when spread on a cover-slip, and stained and examined with high magnifications. Up to a certain degree their growth proceeds for a period of 3 to 4 weeks, as they enlarge to flat scale-like bits, usually not reaching the size of a poppy seed, and lie loosely on the medium, which they never invade or liquefy. Furthermore, the bacillary colony forms such a compact mass that its small scale can easily be removed with a platinum wire from the solidified blood-serum as a whole, and can be crushed only upon the application of a certain pressure.

In regard to these pure cultures I must mention that Klebs, Schüller, and Toussaint have also cultivated microörganisms from tuberculous masses. All three investigators found that, after their infection with tuberculous material, the nutritive-media fluids became cloudy as early as within two to three days, and contained numerous bacteria. In Klebs's experiments small motile rods developed rapidly, while Schüller and Toussaint obtained micrococci. I have convinced myself repeatedly that tubercle bacilli grow only very sparsely in liquids, that they never cloud the latter because they are totally nonmotile and that, if growth occurs, it becomes recognizable only after three or four weeks. The authors mentioned must therefore have dealt with organisms other than tubercle bacilli.

Up to this point it was established by my studies that the occurrence of characteristic bacilli is regularly coincidental with tuberculosis and that these bacilli can be obtained and isolated in pure cultures from tuberculous organs. It remained to answer the important question whether the isolated bacilli when again introduced into the animal body are capable of reproducing the morbid process of tuberculosis.

In order to exclude every error in the solution of this question, which contains the principal point in the whole study of the tubercle virus, many different series of experiments were done, which, on account of the significance of the point at issue, will be enumerated.

First, were done experiments involving the simple inoculation of bacilli in the previously described manner.

First Experiment: Of 6 recently bought guinea pigs which were kept in the same cage, four were inoculated on the abdomen with bacillary culture material derived from human lungs with miliary tubercles and grown in five transfers for fifty-four days. Two animals remained uninoculated. In the inoculated animals the inguinal lymph nodes swelled after fourteen days, the site of inoculation changed into an ulcer, and the animals became emaciated. After thirty-two days one of the inoculated animals died, and after thirty-five days the rest were killed. The inoculated guinea pigs, the one that had died spontaneously as well as the three killed ones, showed far-advanced tuberculosis of the spleen, liver and lungs; the inguinal nodes were much swollen and caseated; the bronchial lymph nodes were but little swollen. The two noninoculated animals displayed no trace of tuberculosis in lungs, liver or spleen.

Second Experiment: Of 8 guinea pigs, six were inoculated with bacillary culture material, derived from the tuberculous lung of an ape, and cultivated in eight transfers for ninety-five days. Two animals remained uninoculated as controls. The course was exactly the same as in the first experiment.

Third Experiment: Of 6 guinea pigs, five were inoculated with culture material, derived from a *Perlsucht* lung, and seventy-two days old and transferred six times.

Fourth Experiment: A number of animals (mice, rats, hedgehogs, hamsters, pigeons, frogs), whose susceptibility to tuberculosis is not known, were inoculated with cultures derived from the tuberculous lung of a monkey which had been cultivated for 113 days outside the animal body.

Fifth Experiment: Three rabbits were inoculated with a small crumb of a culture (derived from a caseous pneumonia in a human lung and cultivated for 89 days) in the anterior ocular chamber. An intense iritis developed after a few days, and the cornea soon became clouded and discolored to a yellowish-gray.

Sixth Experiment: Of three rabbits, one received an injection of pure blood-serum into the anterior chamber of the eye, and the two others an injection of the same blood-serum, in which, however, a small crumb of a culture (originating from a lung with *Perlsucht* and cultivated 91 days) had been suspended.

Seventh Experiment: Of 4 rabbits, the first received pure blood-serum in the anterior eye chamber; in the case of the second the needle, which contained blood-serum with a bacillary culture (from monkey tuberculosis, cultivated 132 days), was introduced into the anterior chamber of the eye, but the plunger was not moved, so that only a minimal amount of the fluid could get into the aqueous humor.

Eighth Experiment: Six rabbits were infected in the same manner as in the preceding experiment, using culture from a human lung with miliary tuberculosis, which had been cultivated 105 days.

I did not content myself with this, but began further experiments comprising injections of bacillary cultures into the abdominal cavity or directly into the blood-stream, and attempted, finally, to make tuberculous, with the artificially grown virus, such animals whose infection with tuberculosis was not easily accomplished.

The tubercles obtained by inoculation or injection of bacillary cultures were examined microscopically many times, and found entirely identical with the ordinary tubercles formed in the same animal species spontaneously or after infection with tuberculous masses. They had absolutely the same arrangement of cellular elements, and frequently contained giant cells which, just as in the case of the spontaneous tubercles, enclosed bacilli. Furthermore, from these tubercles, which were derived by means of the bacillary culture, the bacilli were again isolated in pure culture, and with these, as well as with the tubercles, inoculation experiments were done, which had entirely the same result as infection with human tubercles or with *Perlsucht.* Therefore, in this regard also, the tubercles obtained through infection with cultures behaved like those occurring naturally.

Looking back on these experiments, it is seen that a not inconsiderable number of experimental animals that received the bacillary cultures in very different ways—namely, through simple inoculation in the subcutaneous tissues, through injection into the abdominal cavity or the anterior chamber of the eye, or directly into the blood-stream—became tuberculous without exception. Not only were single nodules formed, but the extraordinary number of tubercles was in proportion to the large number of bacilli introduced. It was successful with other animals, through infection in the anterior ocular chamber with as small a number of bacilli as possible, to give rise to the very same tuberculous iritis as in the well known experiments of Cohnheim and Salomonsen, and Baumgarten, which were so decisive on the question of inoculation tuberculosis and which were performed with true tuberculous material only.

A confusion with spontaneous tuberculosis, or a chance undesigned infection with tuberculous virus is impossible in these experiments for the following reasons: In the first place, neither a spontaneous tuberculosis nor a chance infection could cause such massive eruptions of tubercles in so short a time. In the second place, the control animals, which were treated in exactly the same way as the infected animals, with only the single difference that they received no bacillary culture, remained healthy. In the third place, in the case of numerous guinea pigs and rabbits, infected and injected with other substances in the same way, for other purposes of research, there never occurred this typical picture of miliary tuberculosis, which can only exist when the body is suddenly overwhelmed with a large number of bacilli.

All these facts, taken together, justify the statement that the bacilli present in tuberculous substances are not only coincidental with the tuberculous process, but are the cause of the process, and that we have in the bacilli the real tuberculous virus.

This establishes the possibility of defining the boundaries of the diseases to be understood as tuberculosis, which could not be done with certainty until now. A definite criterion for tuberculosis was lacking. One author would reckon miliary tuberculosis, phthisis, scrofulosis, *Perlsucht,* etc., as tuberculosis; another would hold, perhaps with quite as much right, that all these morbid processes were different. In future it will not be difficult to decide what is tuberculous and what is not tuberculous. The decision will be established, not by the typical structure of the tubercle, nor its avascularity, nor the presence of giant cells, but by the demonstration of tubercle bacilli, whether in the tissues by staining-reactions or by culture on coagulated blood-serum. Taking this criterion as decisive, miliary tuberculosis, caseous pneumonia, caseous bronchitis, intestinal and lymph-node tuberculosis, *Perlsucht* in cattle, spontaneous and infectious tuberculosis in animals, must, according to my investigations, be declared identical. My investigations of scrofulosis and fungoid joint affections are not numerous enough to make a decision possible. In any event, a large number of scrofulous lymph nodes and joint affections belong to true tuberculosis. Perhaps they belong entirely to tuberculosis. The demonstration of tubercle bacilli in the caseated lymph node of a hog, or in the tubercles of a hen, permits the inference that tuberculosis has a wider dissemination among domestic animals than is commonly supposed. It is very desirable to learn exactly the distribution of tuberculosis in this respect.

Since the parasitic nature of tuberculosis is proved, it is still necessary for the completion of its aetiology to answer the questions of where the parasites come from and how they enter the body.

In regard to the first question it must be decided whether the infectious materials can propagate only under such conditions as prevail in the animal body or whether they may undergo a development independent of the animal organism, somewhere in free nature, such as, for example, is the case with anthrax bacilli.

In several experiments it was found that the tubercle bacilli grow only at temperatures between 30° and 41°C. Below 30° and above 42° not the slightest growth occurred within three weeks, while anthrax bacilli, for example, grow vigourously at 20° and between 42° and 43°C. The question mentioned can already be decided on the basis of this fact. In temperate climates there is no opportunity offered outside the animal body for an even temperature of above 30°C. of at least two weeks' duration. It may be concluded that, in their development, tubercle bacilli are dependent exclusively upon the animal organism; that they are true and not occasional parasites; and that they can be derived only from the animal organism.

Also the second question, as to how the parasites enter the body, can be answered. The great majority of all cases of tuberculosis begin in the respiratory tract, and the infectious material leaves its mark first in the lungs or in the bronchial lymph nodes. It is therefore very likely that tubercle bacilli are usually inspired with the air, attached to dust particles. There can hardly be any doubt about the manner by which they get into the air, considering in what excessive numbers tubercle bacilli present in cavity-contents are expectorated by consumptives and scattered everywhere.

In order to gain an opinion about the occurrence of tubercle bacilli in phthisical sputum I have examined repeatedly the sputum of a large series of consumptives and have found that in some of them no bacilli are present, and that, however, in approximately one-half of the cases, extraordinarily numerous bacilli are present, some of them sporogenic. Incidentally, it may be remarked that, in a number of specimens of sputum of persons not diseased with phthisis, tubercle bacilli were never found. Animals inoculated with fresh bacilliferous sputum become tuberculous as certainly as following inoculations with miliary tubercles.

Also, such infectious sputa did not lose their virulence after drying. Four guinea pigs were inoculated with two-weeks-old dried sputum, and 4 guinea pigs with sputum kept in the same way for 8 weeks; they all became tuberculous in the same manner as following infection with fresh material. It can therefore be assumed that phthisical sputum dried on the floor, clothes, etc., retains for a considerable time its virulence, and that, if it enters the lung in a pulverized state, it can produce tuberculosis there. Presumably the durability of its virulence is dependent upon the spore-formation of the tubercle bacilli, and it must be considered in this regard that the spore-formation, as we have seen in several examples, occurs already in the animal organism, and not, as in anthrax bacilli, outside of it.

It would lead too far into the realm of hypothesis to attempt to discuss here the conditions of acquired and inherited disposition, which undoubtedly play a significant rôle in the aetiology of tuberculosis. In this connection thorough studies are still required before a judgment is warranted. I wish to draw attention only to one point, which may serve as explanation for many puzzling phenomena: that is, the exceedingly slow growth of the tubercle bacilli. This is most probably the reason why the bacilli cannot infect the body through every little wound in such a way as do the unusually fast-growing anthrax bacilli. If one wishes to render an animal tuberculous with certainty, the infectious material must be brought into the subcutaneous tissue, into the peritoneal cavity, into the ocular chamber; in brief, into a place where the bacilli have the opportunity to propagate in a protected position and where they can focalize. Infections form superficial skin wounds not penetrating into the subcutaneous tissue, or from the cornea, are only exceptionally successful. The bacilli are eliminated again before they are able to implant themselves.

This explains why autopsies on tuberculous bodies do not cause infection, even when small cuts on the hand come in contact with tuberculous masses. Small superficial cuts are not suitable inoculation wounds for the invasion of bacilli. Similar conditions prevail probably for the implantation of bacilli which have reached the lungs. It is probable that certain peculiar factors favoring the implantation of bacilli, such as stasis of secretions, desquamation of epithelium, etc., must aid to make infection possible. It would be hardly understandable otherwise that tuberculosis is not much more frequent than it really is, since practically everybody, particularly in densely populated places, comes more or less in contact with tuberculosis.

If we ask further what significance belongs to the results gained in this study of tuberculosis it must be considered a gain for science that it has been possible for the first time to establish the complete proof of the parasitic nature of a human infectious disease, and this of the most important one. So far such proof was established only for anthrax, while in a number of other infectious diseases in human beings, for example, relapsing fever, wound infections, leprosy, gonorrhoea, it was only known that parasites occur simultaneously with the pathological process, but the causal connection between the two has not been established. It may be expected that the elucidation of the aetiology of tuberculosis will provide new viewpoints for the study of other infectious diseases, and that the research methods which have stood the test in the investigation of the aetiology of tuberculosis will be of advantage for the work in other infectious diseases. Quite particularly may this hold true for studies of those diseases, which, like syphilis and glanders, are most closely related to tuberculosis, and form with it the group of infectious tumors.

How far pathology and surgery can utilize the knowledge about the properties of the tuberculosis parasite it is not my duty to define. It remains to be seen whether, for example, the demonstration of tubercle bacilli in the sputum can be used for diagnostic purposes, or whether the certain diagnosis of many localized tuberculous affections will be of influence in their surgical treatment, and whether therapy may profit from further experiences about the living conditions of the tubercle bacilli. My studies have been done in the interest of public health, and I hope that this will derive the largest profit from them.

Tuberculosis has so far been habitually considered to be a manifestation of social misery, and it has been hoped that an improvement in the latter would reduce the disease. Measures specifically directed against tuberculosis are not known to preventive medicine. But in future the fight against this terrible plague of mankind will deal no longer with an undetermined something, but with a tangible parasite, whose living conditions are for the most part known and can be investigated further. The fact that this parasite finds the conditions for its existence only in the animal body and not, as with anthrax bacilli, also outside of it under usual, natural conditions, warrants a particularly favorable outlook for success in the fight against tuberculosis. First of all, the sources from which the infectious material flows must be closed as far as this is humanly possible. One of these sources, and certainly the most essential one, is the sputum of consumptives, whose disposal and change into a harmless condition has thus far not been accomplished. It cannot be connected with great difficulties to render such phthisical sputum harmless by suitable procedures of disinfection, and to eliminate thereby the largest part of the infective tuberculous material. Besides this, the disinfection of clothes, beds, etc., which have been used by tuberculous patients, must certainly be considered.

Another source of infection with tuberculosis is undoubtedly tuberculosis of domestic animals,—in the first rank, *Perlsucht*. Herewith, too, is indicated the position which public health has to assume in future on the question of the danger of meat and milk from animals with *Perlsucht*. *Perlsucht* is identical with tuberculosis in man, and is therefore a disease transmissible to man. It must therefore be treated exactly the same way as other diseases transmissible from animals to man. Be the danger of meat and milk from animals with *Perlsucht* ever so great or ever so little, it is present, and it must therefore be avoided. It is sufficiently known that anthrax-infected meat has been eaten by many persons, and often for a long time, and without any ill effects, and still no one will conclude therefrom that the trade in such meat should be permitted.

In regard to milk from cows with *Perlsucht* it is noteworthy that the extension of the tuberculous process to the mammary gland has been observed not rarely by veterinarians, and it is therefore quite possible that in such cases the tuberculous virus may be mixed directly with the milk.

Still further viewpoints might be mentioned in regard to measures which could serve to limit the disease on the basis of our present knowledge of the aetiology of tuberculosis but the discussion here would lead too far. When the conviction that tuberculosis is an exquisite infectious disease has become firmly established among physicians, the question of an adequate campaign against tuberculosis will certainly come under discussion and it will develop by itself.

Hearings before the Senate Subcommittee on Health: *Quality of Health Care— Human Experimentation, 1973*

In 1973, fueled by the growing controversy concerning both medicine's new technologies and the mounting scandals in its research community, Congress created a national commission charged with formulating policies that would govern experimentation with human subjects. The committee was, in large part, established through the efforts of Senator Walter Mondale, who in 1968 had introduced a bill recommending that Congress investigate the ethical, legal, and social implications of biomedical advances. In the intervening years, Mondale had gathered the support of several key senators, whose increasing disillusionment with medicine's inability to regulate itself culminated in the spring of 1973 with a series of hearings on the "Quality of Health Care—Human Experimentation." Immediately dispelling the notion that research and health care existed in two separate realms, Senator Edward Kennedy's opening remarks asserted that "Human experimentation is part of the routine practice of medicine." In the following weeks, the truth of his statement was borne out by disturbing testimony. Among the many research protocols presented before the Senate, three were particularly shocking: the Tuskegee Syphilis Study; a clinical trial using the drug Depo-Provera; and another involving the drug DES (diethylstilbestrol). The first project, conducted by the United States Public Health Service from the 1930s to the 1970s, examined a group of Alabama black men suffering from secondary syphilis. No subject was treated during the study, even after 1945, when penicillin became widely available. In the second study, Depo-Provera was administered to welfare mothers as a contraceptive without FDA approval and with no information provided to the subjects about its dangerous side effects; and in the third, more than a dozen university health clinics prescribed DES to female students as a morning-after pill without informing them that it carried the risk of cancer for them and their future children. As one witness testifying before the Senate observed, the subjects who had been used for experimentation shared "a common sense of captivity," whether they were blacks, poor people, women, or prisoners.

From *Quality of Health Care—Human Experimentation, 1973*, Hearings before the Senate Subcommittee on Health, 93d Cong., 1st sess., pt. 1, February 21 and 22, 1973; pt. 4, April 30, June 28, 29, and July 10, 1973 (Washington, D.C.: GPO, 1973).

WEDNESDAY, FEBRUARY 21, 1973

Senator KENNEDY. Today, as we begin this important set of oversight hearings on biomedical research and human experimentation, scientists may stand on the threshold of being able to re-create man. They will soon have the power to modify and control his behavior—indeed they can already do so in certain controlled, clinical settings.

In the last decade, we have witnessed an unparalleled expansion of our technological capabilities. The technology of biomedical research is the technology of man. Today, we have more biomedical research scientists at work on more kinds of projects than at any time in our history. Their success in these endeavors has taken us beyond the frontiers of man's understanding. And the gap between the development of the technology of man, and our capacity to understand the nature and implications of that technology, widens every day.

In the last decade, we have seen a surgeon hold a human heart in his hands and transplant it into another person's body; we have seen scores of surgeons renew life for thousands of people by the transplantation of kidneys; we have seen scientists unravelling the mysteries of the genetic code, learning how to alter the very structure of the building blocks of life; we have seen scientists begin to unlock the mysteries of the brain and begin to understand the physical basis of feelings—of sorrow and joy, of pain and pleasure, of anger and understanding; we have seen a breakthrough in the treatment of Hodgkins disease, a dreaded cancer of the lymph nodes; we have seen a vaccine developed to eliminate measles. We have all been touched by, and have all profited by, the fruits of biomedical research.

In the next decades scientists will place even more powerful tools in our hands. We will, as a society, have to be ready to answer many questions:

Under what conditions, if any, would genetic manipulation of our population be allowed?

Under what conditions, if any, would neurosurgical or pharmacologic modifications of behavior be allowed?

What constitutes death?

Who will have access to lifesaving equipment if it is in short supply—like kidney dialysis machines, or artificial hearts?

When may a society expose some of its members to harm in order to seek benefits for the rest of its people?

This set of hearings will explore many of these questions. We will hear from those who believe these new and powerful tools will help us realize our full potential as a nation and as a people; we will hear from others who feel that our basic and most cherished freedoms are threatened by the technology of man. . . .

The first panel this morning consists of Anna Burgess, Monterey, Tenn.; Marcia Greenberger, Center for Law and Social Policy, Washington, D.C.; and Nathan Kase, Yale University School of Medicine.

Miss Burgess is a participant in one of the programs we are exploring this morning. She will be able to offer some significant testimony.

Marsha Greenberger is from the Center for Law and Social Policy in Washington, and recently traveled to Tennessee to investigate the way Depo-Provera is being used.

Dr. Kase is chairman of the obstetrics and gynecology department at the Yale Medical School. He too, went to Tennessee to study the patterns of practice with Depo-Provera.

Ms. BURGESS. My name is Anna Burgess. I was born September 11, 1951. I live in a three room house. We have no running water, no electricity. In July of 1971, I was called to the welfare office. The welfare lady asked me if I had signed up for family planning. I was not on it then, and she said I ought to be taking something or other. She said they'd rather feed one youngun as two. She made arrangements for me to go to the health department. She said the shot would be the best because I wouldn't have to worry about forgetting it. She said it would last 6–8 months. I didn't go the first two times she arranged it because I was scared a little. In August or September one, I went to family planning at the health department. I signed up with them, that's all I ever signed. I sat and waited a while, and they called me into a back room. They weighed me, took my blood pressure and asked about my blood. They didn't take any blood because my baby wasn't three months old yet. I went out front and waited a few minutes and they called me back into another room. A nurse who I don't know told me to take my clothes off and put a paper gown on. They asked if I'd had a Pap smear. I said no. The doctor took one. He also checked my chest with a stethoscope. Then he told me to turn on my left side and gave me the shot. My hip hurt for two weeks. The next month I started spotting for about 3 days. They had told me I would have no period for 6–8 months. I started getting nervous, not acting like myself. I went to a private doctor. He didn't know nothing about the shot. He called the health department and then he gave me a shot to start my period, but he said he didn't know if it'd work. About a week later my period started. It lasted three to four weeks. I passed about a pound of flesh. The welfare called me in for another interview and asked how the shot was working. I told them everything that had happened. They suggested I go back to the health department and get the coil or pills. I went to the health department after I got two letters. My blood was low, so they gave tonic. This happened twice. I didn't take all the tonic. After that, I got tired of messing with them and went to a private doctor.

Senator KENNEDY. You took the drug. Did the doctors tell you at any time that it was an experimental drug?

Ms. BURGESS. No, they did not.

Senator KENNEDY. Did the doctors tell you at any time of the potential side effects of the drug?

Ms. BURGESS. No, they did not. They did not tell me nothing, except the impression it was safe.

Senator KENNEDY. They told you it was perfectly safe?

Ms. BURGESS. Right.

Senator KENNEDY. Do you feel the social workers were pressuring you to take the drug?

Ms. BURGESS. If it had not been for them, I would not have took it. If it had not been for the welfare people, I would not have taken the stuff in the first place.

Senator KENNEDY. Why do you feel they wanted you to take the drug?

Ms. BURGESS. To keep from having another child.

Senator KENNEDY. The welfare people wanted what?

Ms. BURGESS. They wanted me to take the birth control shot so there would not be no more children.

Senator KENNEDY. They were urging you to take it so you would not have any more children?

Ms. BURGESS. Right.

Senator KENNEDY. And you felt that you should take it because of their suggestion.

Ms. BURGESS. Well, it seemed the way I took it was, I thought they would take the check or something.

Senator KENNEDY. I am sorry, I did not hear you?

Ms. BURGESS. From the impression I got, if I did not take birth control, they would take the check.

Senator KENNEDY. If you did not take the Depo-Provera they were perhaps going to threaten your assistance program?

Ms. BURGESS. In a way, because they said they would rather pay one child as two.

Senator KENNEDY. Maybe you could tell us again what you feared. If you did not take the drug, what did you think might happen to you?

Ms. BURGESS. I thought they would take my check at that time. At that time I could not work and take care of the baby—

Senator KENNEDY. Take your check away?

Ms. BURGESS. That is what I thought they would do if I did not take the birth control that they suggested.

Senator KENNEDY. They urged you to take it, and they did not indicate to you that it was an experimental drug, that it has any dangerous side effects?

Ms. BURGESS. They did not.

Senator KENNEDY. Would you tell us about the impact the drug had on you?

Ms. BURGESS. I could not stand my own self and could not stand to hear the baby cry. If anybody comes in, and company comes in, I would have to walk off and leave them to keep from talking to them.

About a month later I started spotting. Then I went to a private doctor and ask him to give me a shot to start my period, and he said he did not know whether it would work or not, he would call the health department and find out about the shot, because he said he did not know about that.

After that, my period started and I bled for about three or four weeks and passed a half a pound of flesh and still bled for quite a while.

I finally went to my own doctor.

Senator KENNEDY. Did I understand you correctly that when you did go to your doctor you mentioned this to him, but he had never heard of the drug?

Ms. BURGESS. That is right. He had never heard of it.

Senator KENNEDY. Now, if you can just tell me again the effect of the drug on your personality. You felt it made you more nervous?

Ms. BURGESS. I was so nervous I couldn't stand nothing.

Senator KENNEDY. After you took the drug?

Ms. BURGESS. After I took it. I stand around and hear my baby crying—I couldn't stand to hear the baby cry or nothing else.

Senator KENNEDY. And before taking drug—

Ms. BURGESS. I didn't have no trouble at all.

Senator KENNEDY. And after you had the drug?

Ms. BURGESS. I was real nervous and couldn't stand myself and nobody else hardly.

Senator KENNEDY. Are you glad you took the drug?

Ms. BURGESS. No.

THURSDAY, FEBRUARY 22, 1973

Senator KENNEDY. Today we will learn of patterns of practice that have developed in this country with regard to DES. Yesterday the Commissioner of the Food and Drug Administration, Dr. Edwards, said that the widespread use of DES in university centers would be of great concern, that concern is justified, and we will demonstrate that today.

Our first witnesses this morning are Dr. Sidney Wolfe and Ms. Anita Johnson.

Ms. JOHNSON. I am Anita Johnson, an attorney with the Health Research Group in Washington, D.C., and this is Dr. Sidney Wolfe, a physician with the same group.

I wish to insert into the record at the outset a report on the "Morning after Pill" which we released December 8, 1972.

Diethylstilbestrol (DES) has long been known to be carcinogenic in animals and since 1969 has been known to cause cancer in humans administered DES in utero. Last summer FDA banned use of DES in animal feed because there were small residues of the substance in meat intended for human consumption. Although FDA long ago approved DES as a drug for certain circumscribed purposes it has never approved DES for use as a postcoital contraceptive. DES has never been shown to be safe and effective for this purpose.

Under these circumstances, doctors should not administer DES to women, if at all, only under the most stringent and careful conditions. All women should be informed that DES may cause cancer in their offspring if the Morning After Pill is not effective, and that animal tests have shown it causes cancer in animals administered the drug. No doctors should administer the pill unless they have filed an investigational new drug application with the FDA, are engaged in a research study involving meticulous short- and long-term followup of each patient, are under continuous institutional peer review of the experiment, keep complete records, and administer the drug only to patients who are fully informed of the risks of the experiment. Use of the Morning After Pill cannot even arguably be justified unless in the context of a well-designed and well-protected research study.

Yet the DES Morning After Pill is widely used. In cases we know about, it is used with unacceptable carelessness, in some cases without even the most elemental requirements of a genuine experiment.

Advocates for Medical Information, an Ann Arbor student group, reported to us last November that the health service at the University of Michigan was dispensing DES like water. At that time, women were not warned of possible side effects other than nausea, or of its unapproved status. Only nine out of the 69 cases studied by Advocates for Medicine Information were followed up, and these were voluntary followups by the patient. Although a family history of breast or genital cancer vastly increases the risk of DES, only three of the women were asked about this. Only 10 stated that their doctors inquired about exposure to other estrogens such as birth control pills or DES in utero. Doctors as a rule did not inquire about the possibility of pregnancy from the prior month—in which case DES would not abort and could damage the fetus—and did not assess the likelihood of pregnancy at the time of prescription.

At the University of Vermont, followup is lackadaisical. "If the woman becomes pregnant," said one doctor, "we assume she will return to the infirmary and tell us." When asked what warnings the women get at the health center, the doctor replied, "We don't dwell on the risks because one-shot use of DES presents no risk to the woman." Even if the woman becomes pregnant after DES use, she is not told of the evidence of risk to the fetus. Doctors there do not check the medical or family history of the woman for evidence of increased risk, "because the pill doesn't generate problems."

At the University of Oregon, the health service director stated that women are informed about the risk of cancer to female offspring, and are questioned about their family history before the pill is dispensed. There is no formal followup. "If she's had unprotected intercourse and asks for the pills, she gets it unless she has the counter indications," the director said.

At Oregon State, the health center gynecologist does not believe that DES is a proven human carcinogen. "I tell the women that Ralph Nader believes DES is dangerous, but that I don't." Women are not asked for family histories of cancer, and they are dispensed the pill for any unprotected intercourse. Asked whether the women are informed that it is an unapproved use, the doctor stated: "We tell the girls that FDA is studying DES."

At Indiana University the health service has prepared a written informed consent form which states that because of a strong possibility of cancer in offspring, "it is probably unwise to continue pregnancy" if DES is not effective. The form states that DES has not been approved for this use, that the long-term and some of the short-term effects of the pill are not known, and that the use of well studied methods of birth control is preferable. This consent form has only been available since December 14, 1972. Physicians there use the form only at their option. One doctor said that women are checked to be sure they are not already pregnant, and are discouraged from taking DES if their chances of pregnancy are not great. The Indiana Public Interest Research Group reports that at least one woman was given DES in 1972 with none of the above cautions except that she was informed that it was experimental.

At Princeton University women are apparently warned that the offspring may get cancer, but they are not warned of a risk to themselves, are not told that the pills are experimental, and are not asked for family histories.

Scripps College in California has dispensed the Morning After Pill with no warnings but that of nausea, with no medical or family histories or other inquiries made.

At Tufts and Boston Universities, the pill has been dispensed with no cancer warnings given. At UCLA, health service doctors told the *L.A. Times* that histories were taken and followup made, but a student there reported she had been given no cancer warnings.

At Syracuse, DES is dispensed. There are no regulations on dispensing DES, and no records are kept. At the request of the Syracuse Public Interest Research Group, the director agreed to issue a fact sheet to women who requested the pill. At Toronto, women are counseled to have an abortion if they become pregnant, and told that DES should not be used for routine contraception. At Cal State, a reporter was told that "universal procedures" were followed.

Other centers distributing the Morning After Pill are Minnesota, Harvard and Iowa State, and the Feminist Women's Health Center in L.A. Here in Washington, our Office manager was able to get a prescription for the Morning After Pill over the phone with no questions asked and no warnings given.

MONDAY, APRIL 30, 1973

Senator KENNEDY. Next we hear from a panel of witnesses. Mr. Fred Gray, who testified before the subcommittee on the Tuskegee study during the course of our hearings last March, is the attorney representing some of the victims of the experiment. He is also a member of the Alabama legislature, representing Barbour-Macon County.

Mr. GRAY. Mr. Chairman, on behalf of more than 40 of the surviving participants of the Tuskegee Syphilis Study, and on behalf of over 20 families of some of the deceased participants of the Tuskegee Study, I would like to express their appreciation for the invitation to return to this subcommittee and present the current status of their plight as a result of their participation in the Tuskegee Study.

I have with me Mr. Shaw, who was inadvertently taken to Birmingham, Ala. in the 1940's to be treated for syphilis, only to discover upon his arrival in Birmingham, that he was one of the participants in the Tuskegee study. He was denied treatment, sent away from the hospital, and placed on a bus home. We also have Mr. Carter Howard, another one of the participants. Both of these gentlemen have come to us for us to represent them since they received the letter from the Center for Disease Control on April 13, 1973.

Mr. SHAW. Mr. Chairman, would you like to know how I became involved in the study?

Senator KENNEDY. Yes, in your own words.

Mr. SHAW. For those who are living and remember, and for those who just read about it, in 1932 we began to emerge from what was known as the Hoover panic. We did not have adequate money, in other words, to care for our families. This offer was made in 1932 as free medication known as a blood test. I entered it in 1932 and was affiliated with it ever since.

Every 4 years they would take our blood. They would transport us to the Tuskegee VA hospital and give us a thorough examination.

In the late 1940's—I do not remember the exact date—they sent me to Birmingham. We left about 2 o'clock and we got to Birmingham before dark. They gave us our supper and put us to bed. The next morning they gave us breakfast. I saw a nurse roaming through the crowd. She said she had been worried all night. She said that she had been looking for a man that was not supposed to be here and his name is Herman Shaw. Naturally I stood up. She said come here.

She said what are you doing up here? I said I do not know, they sent me here. They got me a bus and sent me back home. When I notified the nurse of what happened in Macon County, I did not get any response.

Senator KENNEDY. Did you feel during this period that you were being cured, that they were looking after your medical needs?

Mr. SHAW. I have never had any treatment whatever.

Senator KENNEDY. What did they tell you when they looked at your blood? Did they tell you it looked good or looked bad?

Mr. SHAW. I just got a slap on the back and they said you are good for 100 years. That is all I ever had.

Senator KENNEDY. How many years have they been slapping you on your back?

Mr. SHAW. Forty years.

Senator KENNEDY. You were in this study for 40 years?

Mr. SHAW. Yes, sir.

Senator KENNEDY. Did they give you any kind of compensation while they were doing this study?

Mr. SHAW. No sir, with the exception of a 25-year certificate.

Senator KENNEDY. Twenty-five year what?

Mr. SHAW. Twenty-five year health certificate. They gave us a dollar a year, $25.

Senator KENNEDY. A dollar a year?

Mr. SHAW. Yes sir. Up to that time, from 1932, up until the time the 25-year limit ran out.

Senator KENNEDY. So the only compensation you have received has been the $25?

Mr. SHAW. That is right.

Senator KENNEDY. And the certificate of merit?

Mr. SHAW. Yes, sir.

Senator KENNEDY. What was the certificate of merit for?

Mr. SHAW. I do not know, sir. It was for regular attendance, that is all I can figure.

Senator KENNEDY. Do you think it is because you kept going back to the nurse or the doctor and letting them take your blood as they told you to do?

Mr. SHAW. Yes, sir.

Senator KENNEDY. When you were told to go back, did you think this was a check up and that since they didn't prescribe medication, that therefore you were healthy? What did you assume?

Mr. SHAW. Every year they would give us a white tablet for pain and a little vial— I guess it was some type of tonic. Every year for 40 years up to now, we had two different doctors. We would never get the same doctor back each time.

Senator KENNEDY. Different doctors?

Mr. SHAW. Different doctor every year.

Senator KENNEDY. When was the last time you were at a clinic?

Mr. SHAW. Last year.

Senator KENNEDY. What did they tell you last year?

Mr. SHAW. Slap on the back and said I was good for 100 years. I guess it was routine.

Senator KENNEDY. They gave you tablets in case you had any pain?

Mr. SHAW. Yes.

Senator KENNEDY. Did you ever have to take those tablets?

Mr. SHAW. Sometimes. Sometimes they would stay in the bottle until they were brown as that wall.

Senator KENNEDY. What did you think when you read about the news of the story, when the story broke about this experiment that you were a part of? What was your reaction to it?

Mr. SHAW. Being personally acquainted with Attorney Gray, I went to his office for advice and carried him the information I had received.

Senator KENNEDY. Were you surprised to read that this experiment was taking place and that you had been a part of it?

Mr. SHAW. Yes, sir; I certainly was surprised.

Senator KENNEDY. Mr. Howard, we want to welcome you here. Maybe you could tell us a little bit about your experience.

Mr. HOWARD. About who has been at my place?

Senator KENNEDY. Tell us a little bit about how you got involved.

Mr. HOWARD. I hardly know how I got involved in it. I was involved in it in 1932. They were having school in the church, and I think the teacher put out a notice for everybody in the community to meet out there on a certain date. Dr. Smith and I were the first two, I remember. At the end of a 2 hour meeting, they started taking blood, checking temperatures, heartbeat, blood system, and all of that. I got the same thing for about 40 years, I guess. I did get $25, and I do not know if it was for appreciation or they just decided they would give me something because I was so good about meeting them every time.

Senator KENNEDY. You met with them every time you were supposed to?

Mr. HOWARD. Yes, sir.

Senator KENNEDY. They gave you $25 too?

Mr. HOWARD. They gave me $25 and a 25-year certificate for being with them that long. I think I got that in 1958.

Senator KENNEDY. When was the last time you saw the doctor?

Mr. HOWARD. I saw him last year in June.

Senator KENNEDY. June of this past year?

Mr. HOWARD. Yes, sir, last year in June.

Senator KENNEDY. What did the doctor tell you?

Mr. HOWARD. He just gave me some pills and some medicine out of a bottle and said he would see me soon. That was last year in June, and I have not seen him since.

Senator KENNEDY. What did you think was happening when you saw these doctors over the period of these years? Did you think they were giving you a clean bill of health?

Mr. HOWARD. I hardly know. I had bad blood and they said they were working on it.

Senator KENNEDY. What do you think you need? What do you want them to do for you?

Mr. HOWARD. I need some money, that is what I need.

Senator KENNEDY. You think you ought to be compensated like others in the country are compensated when they are made a part of tests like that? You are asking that you be treated the same as other people are treated in this respect, is that right?

Mr. HOWARD. Yes.

Senator KENNEDY. I want to thank both of you gentlemen, Mr. Howard and Mr. Shaw, for coming up here. As we indicated, we are going to pursue this issue and work with you to make sure that justice is done in this case.

Our last witness this morning is Dr. Vernal Cave. Dr. Cave is director of the Bureau of Venereal Disease Control of the New York City Department of Health.

Dr. CAVE. Thank you, Mr. Chairman. I am the chairman of the board of trustees of the National Medical Association and chairman of its special committee investigating the Tuskegee study. This committee will make its report to the annual convention of the association in New York City in August.

I am not authorized to speak for any individual or any group, so it should be clear from the outset that the remarks and observations that follow are my responsibility alone.

What, if anything, did the study add to the body of medical knowledge? While some information was added to medical knowledge, as indeed information from experimental animals might add to medical knowledge, it was chiefly confirmatory information—information that could be and was acquired by far more humane means.

First and foremost, I would say that the information provided by this study confirmed what had been known for ages and had been previously reconfirmed by the Oslo study—that syphilis has a deleterious effect on the health and welfare of its victims.

Senator KENNEDY. In effect they knew this in 1932?

Dr. CAVE. Yes, sir. The study illustrated what was already known—that some persons whose syphilis is untreated will end up as disabled or insane or crippled human beings and that some will die. It was apparent from this study that the illnesses of individuals with untreated syphilis included significantly higher incidences of sometimes fatal diseases not thought to be related directly to syphilis. Thus, the presence of untreated syphilitic infection apparently predisposed its victims to other illnesses. The study also confirmed that some victims of untreated syphilis live on without developing any of the late manifestations of this disease. However, since we don't possess the Divine wisdom that would let us know which syphilitics are chosen to escape its late manifestations, the fact that some cases escape late disease cannot be used to justify withholding the administration of a known cure, any more than, for example, the knowledge that the body's defenses may overcome a pneumonia infection would justify withholding a known cure from a person suffering from pneumonia.

I have used the term "untreated syphilis." But at this point I must state that fortunately the information shows that most of the participants in this study received antibiotic treatment at some point in their lives either for syphilis by some doctor who was not aware of the study or for some other illness. This was a source of dismay to some of the administrators of this study. Incidentally, the fact that a majority of the patients were given antibiotic treatment, albeit inadequate therapy, at some point in their lives compromised the objective of this study to follow the course of truly untreated syphilis. One must bear this fact in mind in evaluating. There are other considerations from a strictly scientific point of view that brand this study as not very productive of scientific information that I will mention shortly.

The first report on the study to appear in the medical literature in 1936, 4 years after the study commenced, made it quite clear that the results of no treatment would be disastrous to a significant portion of the group. Cardiovascular, central nervous system and bone and joint system abnormalities were found to be about four times greater in the syphilitic group under age 40, when compared to the control group. The study revealed that only in one-fourth of the untreated syphilitics were no additional abnormalities found. At this point a comparison was made between 86 inadequately treated blacks and 26 of the untreated patients. It was clear then that even inadequate therapy was preferable to no treatment at all since only 1.2 percent of the inadequately treated individuals had evidence of cardiovascular involvement compared to 7.7 percent of those who received no treatment at all. In the interests of humaneness and compassion, surely the evidence obtained at the end of 4 years cried out that the study should be terminated.

Nevertheless, the study continued. A report published in 1946 dealing with 12 years of observations revealed that 25 percent of the syphilitic group and 14 percent of the controls of comparable ages had died. Thus, the writers concluded that an untreated black male syphilitic of age 25 would have a reduction in life expectancy of approximately 20 percent. Bear in mind that we were now in the period of penicillin therapy. Whether due to bureaucratic inertia, or zeal to publish more papers, or a blocking out of ethical principles, or—and we must consider this aspect—a sinister climate of racism, the study continued.

PART 8

The Institutionalization of Doctors and Patients

PHILIPPE PINEL (1745–1826)

The Clinical Training of Doctors

In the aftermath of the French Revolution, sweeping reforms in medical education and clinical teaching were undertaken, culminating in the legislation of 19 Ventose Year XI, the 1803 law that would oversee the practice of medicine in France for close to a century. As physician, teacher, and hospital administrator, Philippe Pinel played a vital role in the reorganization of his profession and its institutions. His essay "The Clinical Training of Doctors," submitted in a competition sponsored by the Society of Medicine in 1783, was a pivotal contribution to the reform and standardization of hospital teaching in France. Guided by both the British Empiricists and his French Idéologue colleagues, Pinel stressed the importance of experience, observation, and documentation. Rejecting the stagnant systems and outmoded theories of the past, he set forth an educational agenda that translated the intellectual aims of the Revolution into the organizing principles of modern medicine.

INTRODUCTION

Medicine must be taught in the hospitals—The healing art should be taught only in hospitals: this assertion needs no proof. Only in the hospital can one follow the evolution and progress of several illnesses at the same time and study variations of the same disease in a number of patients. This is the only way to understand the true history of diseases. In these shelters for suffering humanity, young students can analyze the influence of the seasons and of each year's medical constitution. And only in a hospital can the physician be certain that patients receive the specific diet and medication he prescribes, and that nascent symptoms are carefully observed.

General hospitals inadequate for medical teaching—Are the requisite facilities available in general hospitals? These are filled with cases that cannot be precisely diagnosed and that are often examined in a cursory and incomplete manner. Even an exact diagnosis may lead nowhere, because of the superficiality and negligence with which the nature of diseases is established, on the basis of trivial and often misleading signs. In less than an hour's visit, the physician examines hundreds of general hospital patients who present vague and confusing data: he seems to parody rather than to practice medicine. The prevalent negligence of the staff, mistakes in the diet, lack of cleanliness, unhealthy air, the proximity of certain contagious cases complicate illnesses in many ways and interfere with prognosis and therapy. Complex and often non-specific medication, the lack of supervision regarding the quantity and quality of food and drink are added sources of confusion. And in the end young students find that they have wasted several years in the presence of hospital physicians.

From *The Clinical Training of Doctors: An Essay of 1793*, ed. and trans. Dora B. Weiner (Baltimore: Johns Hopkins University Press, 1980).

Young doctors then restrict themselves to a few formulas and spend the rest of their lives in the narrow circle of blind routine worse, perhaps, than utter ignorance.

Need for an appropriate teaching hospital—This is why all modern medical schools have emphasized observation as a characteristic aspect of medicine when it is viewed as a major branch of the natural sciences. Leyden, Edinburgh, Vienna, Pavia, etc., have stressed the need of selecting a small number of patients for didactic purposes and grouping them on teaching wards. This offers the advantage of focusing the students' attention on a small number of well-defined cases that they must watch with greatest care, without neglecting any aspect of cleanliness or health.

Project for a teaching hospital: Proposal by the Society of Medicine—At a time when education is being restored in France and public instruction organized, the Society of Medicine turns its attention to a matter of supreme importance, the creation of teaching hospitals. Only clinical teaching can spread knowledge of the healing art in a uniform manner and restore the rigorous, oft-neglected principles of observation. All other public teaching of medicine by the lecture method is pointless and unproductive. Not content to indicate a simple question regarding the best possible organization of clinical schools, this learned company has proposed several points each of which might be discussed at length. But since the primary objective is to make the most accurate and precise observations at the sickbed and to help young students perceive the true character of illnesses so as to determine therapy, I shall limit myself to this simple proposition which solves the greatest number of questions posed by the Society: I shall examine

1) matters outside the clinical wards that might influence illnesses and modify them;

2) matters germane to the clinical wards and their internal administration;

3) the best method to train the students' judgment rather than their memory, and to focus their attention on perceivable evidence.

I

Topography of the hospital site—Hippocrates always keenly felt the need for an exact topographic description of the place where a physician intends to practice medicine. In his treatise on *Airs, Waters, Places,* the Father of Medicine insists that the physician ascertain whether the inhabitants obtain their water from a stagnant pool, a running stream or a source, whether the land is hilly and the climate very hot, or at a great elevation and naturally cold. Hippocrates advocates a careful look at the food, the occupation, and the usual way of life of the patient. Thus enlightened, the physician will be well prepared to understand the true nature of endemic and prevalent seasonal diseases.

Main aspects of this topography—Progress in the natural sciences of course provides modern physicians with resources for topographic research that the Father of Medicine lacked. They can gather exact information on the elevation of a terrain above sea level, its latitude and longitude, the air currents and their direction, the rivers, the nature of the soil, the hot or cold mineral waters, the mines, quarries, swamps, lakes, woods and mountains, their location, elevation, and their productivity in the three realms of nature. Topographic research should be undertaken by the physician at the beginning of his duties on a teaching ward. This knowledge will later decisively influence his treatment of illnesses because he will better understand their nature.

Nosologic meteorology—Meteorologic observations were imperfect in Hippocrates' time. Nevertheless, this great physician never fails to use them in beginning his descriptions of epidemics. It is in fact undeniable that sudden changes in atmospheric pressure, temperature, and humidity sometimes produce very noticeable effects and these are easier to study on several patients suffering from different diseases.

Meteorologic instruments for teaching wards—In order to render meteorologic observations as complete as possible, I propose that the physician take care to provide teaching wards with 1) a barometer; 2) a double thermometer, one outside, one inside; 3) a comparative hygrometer, for example that of M. Saussure; 4) an outdoor raingauge, to know the number of aqueous meteors during a given time; 5) an electrometer, since it is undeniable that atmospheric electricity acts on the animal economy; 6) an anemometer to record the direction of the winds; 7) a magnetic needle, to observe its variations. Notes on celestial observations, meteors, and the phases of the moon should complement the daily recordings from these instruments.

Influence of the air on physical health—The third book of Hippocrates' *Aphorisms* is almost entirely devoted to the different illnesses caused by seasonal variations. The illnesses do not always correspond to the same seasons: therefore Hippocrates resorts to occult and quasi-supernatural causes, *"quid divinum,"* in his book *On Prognosis*. He concedes that these might alter the air and cause illnesses of a particular kind at a specific time. Baillou, Septalius, Vallesius, Ramazzini and other famous physicians have also seen in specific alterations of the air the origin of acute illnesses prevalent in certain seasons. But no author has treated this subject with as much sagacity and depth as Sydenham who deserves the title of "English Hippocrates." Indeed it is well-known that, in his observations *On Epidemic Diseases,* he admits "annual constitutions" independent of temperature, humidity, or dryness, but related to unknown and inexplicable qualities of the air, undoubtedly caused by specific miasmata. Each "constitution" is identified with a particular fever that Sydenham called *stationary*. He named *intercurrent* other fevers prevalent at the same time and seemingly caused by abrupt changes in temperature or other tangible atmospheric conditions. It is clear that this part of medicine requires keen observation in a teaching hospital, great sagacity in distinguishing slight details, a ban on one's own imagination, and total reliance on sensory evidence.

Principles of contagion: are they found in the air?—In order to elucidate and confirm Sydenham's distinction between stationary and intercurrent fevers, one should compare the condition of patients, such as those assembled in a teaching hospital, with patients on the outside, subject to the same diseases. But, whatever the authority of a great name, it is difficult to believe that the principle of stationary fever resides in miasmata scattered in the air. On the contrary, all the facts concerning the propagation of plague, of smallpox, etc. indicate that their causative principles, far from being disseminated in the air, on the contrary adhere to furniture and clothing and are easily propagated by all kinds of threads, of cotton or wool. This is how, in

Cairo, Tunis, and other Levantine ports, French traders escape the ravages of plague by placing simple barricades around their quarters and receiving nothing from the outside that has not previously been dipped in water.

Location and plan of the teaching hospital—The site of the building figures among the external factors that can influence the condition of patients in teaching hospitals. The best exposure, says M. Tissot, is South, since one enjoys seeing the sun during the harshest season and is not exposed to extreme heat in the summer. But the location of teaching wards is so often subordinated to questions of economy or convenience that one will doubtless but rarely be free to choose the best possible exposure.

Subdivision of teaching wards to distribute patients—One must never lose sight of an important aim in teaching hospitals, which is that patients should be cared for as if they were at home. This supplies to regular, clean, and prompt service, and to the isolation of patients so that nothing complicates nor deflects the course of the illness by causing new symptoms to appear. It is therefore important that not only the whole section of the teaching hospital reserved for women be separate from that for men, but also that everything related to kitchen, laundry, and pharmacy be entirely independent so that it can be subjected to strict supervision.

Physicians must supervise diet closely—We know that dietetics was the first, the chief, and often the only part of medicine used by Hippocrates for the cure of illnesses. Experimentation with diets is not dangerous for patients and can be extraordinarily useful—but only if the physician has acquired an extensive knowledge of botany. He must have analyzed the classes of plants that can provide him with starches, gums, emulsions, oils, acids, aromatics, wines of different qualities, etc. He can then apply these appropriately to cure illnesses. It is thus the kitchen rather than the pharmacy that the doctor must often visit.

Materia medica of extreme simplicity, appropriate for a teaching hospital—The physician's medication should be equally simple and scientific. It should comprise only uncomplicated substances such as alkalis of soda and potash, ammonia, mineral acids, a few neutral salts, oxides of antimony, iron, mercury, etc., prepared with the greatest precision. As for the *materia medica* derived from the plant kingdom, it should be cleansed of the voluminous and utterly confusing hotchpotch that lacks the exact characteristics specified by botanists. It would be helpful to have a small garden near the teaching hospital. . . . The professor would thus find close at hand all the plants he wishes to use and the students could learn to identify them, and recognize them later on.

Precepts concerning movement and rest—To aid recovery, it is helpful to observe some precepts concerning movement and rest. Daily practice teaches that one must often fight courageously against the patient's inactivity and his tendency to stay in his bed.

Each room must therefore be provided with a comfortable chair appropriate for the patient, even when he is still extremely weak. One must also use good judgment in seizing the precise stage of the illness when the patient should get up and stay up for a more or less long time. There should even be a common hall reachable from all the rooms, a gathering place for patients as soon as their strength enables them to walk. The pleasure of company or conversation might speed convalescence, and so might innocuous diversions. As soon as the progress of recovery permits, patients should go out into a garden where plants are grown and take short walks or even do a little easy gardening or other movements designed to promote the play of muscles and favor the return of their strength. It is thus essential that a teaching hospital provide a place for physical exercise, with a pool table, swings, *bocce,* or bowling games. There should be space to permit short walks, running, jumping, and other movements that help electrify the limbs as soon as the patient's strength allows it.

Remarks on psychologic remedies—During the years when I visited hospitals for my education, I often learned what should have been done by seeing what was not done. I often found that patients responded well to comforting words that reassured them about their illness. Frequently left to themselves, abandoned to dire thoughts about their fate, often isolated from their relatives and all they loved, disgusted by the crudity and harshness of the servants, often plunged into the blackest depression by the ever-present thought of a real or imagined danger, they expressed the liveliest gratitude toward those who empathized with their sufferings and tried to inspire them with confidence in their recovery. It is an excellent remedy to go to their bedside and ask how they are, express an interest in their ailments, encourage them to persevere and to believe in a prompt return to health. I should also like to discourage the custom that forces seriously ill patients to receive extreme unction and surround themselves with the most lugubrious images. I have occasionally made it a point to compare the mood of a patient before and after these religious ceremonies and have often found the most striking differences. I do not mean to deprive pious souls of the comforts of religion that they crave; on the contrary, joyful psychologic experiences should be considered as a powerful remedy. But one should not worsen the dark depression of a fearful patient who sees in the arrival of the priest a presage of his own imminent funeral.

Only well-defined diseases admissible to teaching ward—Still another factor one must heed in a teaching hospital is to admit only cases with well-defined symptoms. These diseases will be used to teach students who must confront clear and logical ideas. Therefore it is essential that the total disease picture be as coherent and typical as possible. The students must be shown case histories where a sequence of clearly defined symptoms leads to a favorable or fatal outcome, so that one can classify the illness by simple comparisons and relate it to cases in the literature or in medical practice.

Questions to ask upon admitting a patient—But it will nevertheless be necessary, at the admission of each patient to the teaching ward, to elicit in an orderly manner information regarding all previous and present aspects of the patient's condition by a series of discriminating and methodical questions. The *Collegium Casuale* of Edinburgh proceeds in the following way: one records 1) information regarding details about the patient's age, sex, temperament, and profession; 2) a description of the symptoms at the moment treatment will begin, including i) manifest signs; ii) the external and internal symptoms enumerated by the patient; iii) the state of his principal functions such as pulse, temperature, respiration, and excretions; 3) recollections regarding the onset of illness and its course, including i) circumstances surrounding its beginning; ii) early symptoms; iii) their duration; 4) an evaluation of long-range causes that might have influenced the illness. That is to say one asks about i) the conjectures of the patient regarding such causes; ii) factors to which the patient may have been exposed before onset of the illness; iii) his previous state of health; iv) sickness among his parents or the persons with whom he habitually lives; 5) an account of the medication already administered, recording i) remedies used; ii) their effects; iii) the regimen and condition of the patient since the onset of illness; iv) the results to date.

II

Arrangements conducive to precise observations—It is obvious that medical observations can be precise and conclusive only if the evidence is reduced to the smallest possible number of facts and to the plainest data. This procedure is followed in all other branches of the natural sciences. To facilitate observation, nothing should interfere with the course of the illness nor the progress of nature. The arrangement of the clinical wards, the distribution of patients in their beds, diligent attention to cleanliness and salubrity, the administration of simple remedies whether plant or mineral, a meticulous choice of food and drink, an untiring supervision of students and their attempts to comfort the patients, all the details of the domestic service, all these must be supervised by the physician with the strictest circumspection and greatest enlightenment without hindering the healing process.

Structure of a teaching hospital: General views—The large number of plans published in recent years regarding the construction and internal disposition of hospitals obviate the need to enter into details on that subject. M. Tissot in particular has published useful views regarding the construction of a teaching hospital in his essay *On Medical Studies.* As a model one might perhaps take one of the pavilions proposed as part of a large hospital by the commissioners of the Academy of Sciences charged in 1788 with examining the projects for such an establishment. It would suffice to add all the requirements for the public teaching of medicine to the general dispositions for service and treatment of patients. An assembly hall would be needed for the professor's regular lectures and for the discussion of specific aspects of therapy after medical rounds. In addition, space would be required for chemical analyses, anatomical dissections, and research in experimental physics applied to medicine.

Urgent need for teaching hospitals in France—We hope that the French nation, having just reconquered its most inalienable rights, will create a clinical school promptly. Such an establishment is an urgent and indispensable priority since one of the worst ills that can afflict humanity is ignorance and lack of principles on the part of physicians. We must therefore profit from the experience of other nations and also put the progress made in the other sciences to use in our new establishment. Good judgment and precision will render medical observations useful and conclusive.

Number of patients on teaching wards—On a teaching ward, painstaking care must be expended on each disease: therefore their number must not exceed the time-limit of medical rounds nor the physician's attention span. The teaching ward at Vienna holds only twelve patients; that at Edinburgh, thirty-two. This last number seems large to me, if one aims at rigorous observation. It is very demanding to see fifteen or twenty patients consecutively. And we wish to banish the disgraceful ease with which the most mediocre doctor seems to run for the door when he makes rounds.

Grouping of patients on teaching wards—This holds equally true for the two sexes. One should first establish two general divisions, one for men, the other for women. The first would be subdivided into 1) boys up to puberty; 2) adults to about fifty years of age; 3) men from the climacteric to senescence. The women's section would be subdivided in a similar way and would comprise 1) childhood up to menstruation; 2) the whole period of fertility, that is, from onset to the end of menstruation; 3) from menopause to what is called *femina effeta.* Each of these subdivisions might hold three or four patients, a total of eighteen to twenty-four, a maximum, if one wishes to avoid hasty judgment caused by an excess of work.

Choice of a good professor essential but difficult—The most perfect organization of public teaching will be useless for medicine if the man in charge is merely a pedantic mediocrity with brilliant talents of elocution. I therefore propose the abolition of those arbitrary nominations obtained by intrigue, and also an end to all those competitions where facile talk and expert delivery often favor mediocrity to the detriment of true genius. I propose a different method uniquely designed to discover talent: as soon as the teaching hospital is organized, according to my own or some other appropriate method, let a competition be announced. Let each candidate provisionally fill the role of professor for a month or two and then publish his case histories. The lessons being public and the observations printed, it will be easy enough to identify the man superior to his competitors and worthy of the appointment— especially in a city as enlightened as the capital.

III

The best method to teach medicine and pitfalls to avoid—The true method to teach medicine is the one appropriate to all the natural sciences: focus the students' attention on concrete situations, impart high standards of accuracy for their perceptions and observations, warn them against hasty judgments and fanciful reasoning; choose readings that confirm their taste for rigor, and impose an orderly progression on their studies—in a word, train their judgment rather than their memory and inspire them with that noble enthusiasm for the healing art that masters all difficulties.

The clinical professor should not consider teaching of secondary importance, as so many doctors do in order to become fashionable and wealthy. He should devote himself to teaching as one of the most sacred and noble tasks to be fulfilled in society. The professor should have unlimited power of inspection over all patient needs and provide continuous and tireless supervision together with the hospital administrators, who alone manage the budget.

His detachment from any other commitment and the need constantly to follow the cold process of observation will help him avoid many errors that have plagued all teaching staffs in the past and have prevented the spread of sound ideas. Among these errors is the subservience to the opinions of famous men who are passionately dogmatic, filled with the ambition to lead a sect, and skilled at courting the admiration of the younger generation, so susceptible to blind devotion.

First year of academic studies—The first year of academic studies should be used chiefly for anatomy in the amphitheatres and for the study of some elementary works on physiology and hygiene. We know that anatomy is only learned well through the study and dissection of cadavers and by comparisons with zoology.

Physiology must not be divorced from hygiene: as one studies a specific function, one should think of the many ways in which the "things non-natural" might affect it. For instance, if one wishes to know the number of pulsations per minute in the radial artery of various individuals, one should study the variations that can be produced by hard liquor, violent exercise, sleep, or strong passion. Or, if one studies the phenomenon of digestion, one should examine the special characteristics of foodstuffs locally available and their propitious or damaging influence on various individuals. Observation would thus constantly complement reading.

Main studies in the second year—I think that second-year students should not be admitted to clinical lessons right away. They have not yet mastered the general principles of practical medicine nor acquired the habit of grasping pathologic symptoms. They have not yet reached the level that diagnosis and prognosis require. I would therefore propose that these students spend a great deal of time during their second year attending medical rounds on the general hospital wards. In order to train them to see for themselves, one might encourage them to follow three or four patients closely. They could write a history of these illnesses while profiting from the remarks of the physician on rounds or from those of some more advanced student.

Third year studies: structure of sickbed lessons—Students who have mastered the first two years of medical school will have the maturity needed for clinical lessons. They are worthy of learning from the clinical professor according to their ability and knowledge. He will be able to identify the particularly talented students who can assist him in the strict supervision and care of patients.

Means of training the students' judgement rather than their memory—The physician's visit to the clinical ward thus essentially consists of listening to the student in charge report on the illness of each patient. In the third year of medical school especially, the progress of the students' knowledge and the acquired habit of observation relieves the professor from going into a host of details. He can be content to remedy omissions, rectify errors, and offer new thoughts on difficult cases. Thus patient care can be prompt, attentive, and enlightened, and at the same time the students can gain experience, a solid foundation for further progress.

The several patients whom they successively supervise in the same room would thus allow students to investigate and master several diseases in the course of one year.

The present sketch of a teaching hospital seems to me based on principles prized by medical observers throughout history. Their implementation will hasten progress in medicine along the lines followed by all the other natural sciences. Medicine has lost this advantage in France because it has lacked a solid basis for teaching. Also, permission to practice has been granted with shameful ease, after a few pedantic efforts of memorization. It is a crime against humanity that the most difficult practical science, constantly toying with human lives, should have become a totally ve-nal profession, so numerous among us that the title of doctor is almost ridiculous. Only in a teaching hospital, under the eyes of a dedicated and enlightened profes-sor, can eager young students pursue the exact observation of pathologic phenom-ena and investigate the complex factors that exert a more or less marked influence on the animal economy. What exquisite judgment, cultivated talents, and deep knowl-edge of ancient and modern medicine such a professor must possess to be equal to his task! I dare say that, only once in a hundred years, will such a supremely diffi-cult position be filled in a worthy manner.

DOROTHEA L. DIX (1802–1887)

On Behalf of the Insane Poor

The granddaughter of a Boston physician, Dorothea L. Dix embarked on her life's work in 1841, determined to bring the plight of the insane into the glare of public attention. After spending two years documenting their conditions in Massachusetts prisons, almshouses, and places of correction, she undertook a national investigation in 1842, traveling more than ten thousand miles. During the next three years, in addition to visiting hospitals, she visited eighteen state penitentiaries, three hundred county jails, and more than five hundred almshouses. During her nearly fifty years of service on behalf of the insane, Dix did much to rouse the conscience of the nation with regard to their sufferings and treatment. Through her singlehanded efforts, public perception of the insane changed as they were gradually distinguished from criminals and derelicts and placed in state institutions mandated to care for them. Arguing that mental illness was the result neither of Divine will nor inborn defect but rather of society's failings, Dix doggedly and repeatedly posed the same question before numerous state legislatures: "Should not society, then, make compensation which alone can be made for these disastrous fruits of its social organization?"

MEMORIAL: TO THE LEGISLATURE
OF MASSACHUSETTS

GENTLEMEN.

I respectfully ask to present this Memorial, believing that the *cause,* which actuates to and sanctions so unusual a movement, presents no equivocal claim to public consideration and sympathy. Surrendering to calm and deep convictions of duty my habitual views of what is womanly and becoming, I proceed briefly to explain what has conducted me before you unsolicited and unsustained, trusting, while I do so, that the memorialist will be speedily forgotten in the memorial.

About two years since leisure afforded opportunity, and duty prompted me to visit several prisons and alms-houses in the vicinity of this metropolis. I found, near Boston, in the Jails and Asylums for the poor, a numerous class brought into unsuitable connexion with criminals and the general mass of Paupers. I refer to Idiots and Insane persons, dwelling in circumstances not only adverse to their own physical and moral improvement, but productive of extreme disadvantages to all other persons brought into association with them. I applied myself diligently to trace the causes of these evils, and sought to supply remedies. As one obstacle was surmounted, fresh difficulties appeared. Every new investigation has given depth to the conviction that

From *Memorial to the Legislature of Massachusetts, 1843* (Boston, 1904), reprinted in *On Behalf of the Insane Poor: Selected Reports* (New York: Arno Press and the New York Times, 1971).

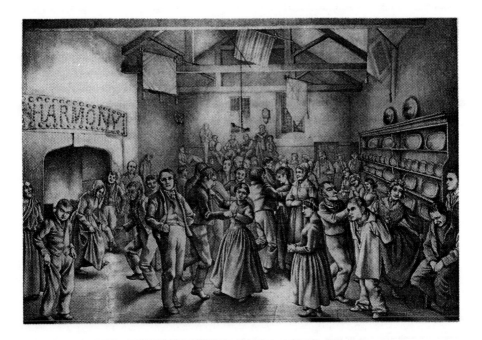

22. *Katherine Drake,* Lunatic's Ball, Somerset County Asylum, *lithograph after a drawing, 1848. Wellcome Institute Library, London. This lunatic's ball captures all of our ambivalence toward the insane. At first glance, the illustration presents a scene of benevolent images. Drake uses the dance as a symbol of the new asylum, where harmony reigned not through punishment and physical restraint but through social activities and diversions that keepers hoped would serve to mark the asylum as a microcosm of civilized life. However, as we look closer at the faces, demeanor, and gestures of the figures, the print takes on the aura of a parody: it is* as if *the insane are like the rest of us.*

it is only by decided, prompt, and vigorous legislation the evils to which I refer, and which I shall proceed more fully to illustrate, can be remedied. I shall be obliged to speak with great plainness, and to reveal many things revolting to the taste, and from which my woman's nature shrinks with peculiar sensitiveness. But truth is the highest consideration. *I tell what I have seen*—painful and shocking as the details often are—that from them you may feel more deeply the imperative obligation which lies upon you to prevent the possibility of a repetition or continuance of such outrages upon humanity. If I inflict pain upon you, and move you to horror, it is to acquaint you with sufferings which you have the power to alleviate, and make you hasten to the relief of the victims of legalized barbarity.

I come to present the strong claims of suffering humanity. I come to place before the Legislature of Massachusetts the condition of the miserable, the desolate, the outcast. I come as the advocate of helpless, forgotten, insane and idiotic men and women; of beings, sunk to a condition from which the most unconcerned would start with real horror; of beings wretched in our Prisons, and more wretched in our Alms-Houses. And I cannot suppose it needful to employ earnest persuasion, or stubborn argument, in order to arrest and fix attention upon a subject, only the more strongly pressing in its claims, because it is revolting and disgusting in its details.

I must confine myself to few examples, but am ready to furnish other and more complete details, if required. If my pictures are displeasing, coarse, and severe, my subjects, it must be recollected, offer no tranquil, refined, or composing features. The condition of human beings, reduced to the extremest states of degradation and misery, cannot be exhibited in softened language, or adorn a polished page.

I proceed, Gentlemen, briefly to call your attention to the *present* state of Insane Persons confined within this Commonwealth, in *cages, closets, cellars, stalls, pens! Chained, naked, beaten with rods,* and *lashed* into obedience!

As I state cold, severe *facts,* I feel obliged to refer to persons, and definitely to indicate localities. But it is upon my subject, not upon localities or individuals, I desire to fix attention; and I would speak as kindly as possible of all Wardens, Keepers, and other responsible officers, believing that *most* of these have erred not through hardness of heart and wilful cruelty, so much as want of skill and knowledge, and want of consideration. Familiarity with suffering, it is said, blunts the sensibilities, and where neglect once finds a footing other injuries are multiplied. This is not all, for it may justly and strongly be added that, from the deficiency of adequate means to meet the wants of these cases, it has been an absolute impossibility to do justice in this matter. Prisons are not constructed in view of being converted into County Hospitals, and Alms-Houses are not founded as receptacles for the Insane. And yet, in the face of justice and common sense, Wardens are by law compelled to receive, and the Masters of Alms-Houses not to refuse, Insane and Idiotic subjects in all stages of mental disease and privation.

It is the Commonwealth, not its integral parts, that is accountable for most of the abuses which have lately, and do still exist. I repeat it, it is defective legislation which perpetuates and multiplies these abuses.

In illustration of my subject, I offer the following extracts from my Note-Book and Journal:—

The use of cages all but universal; hardly a town but can refer to some not distant period of using them; chains are less common; negligences frequent; wilful abuse less frequent than sufferings proceeding from ignorance, or want of consideration. I encountered during the last three months many poor creatures wandering reckless and unprotected through the country. Innumerable accounts have been sent me of persons who had roved away unwatched and unsearched after; and I have heard that responsible persons, controlling the almshouses, have not thought themselves culpable in sending away from their shelter, to cast upon the chances of remote relief, insane men and women. These, left on the highways, unfriended and incompetent to control or direct their own movements, sometimes have found refuge in the hospital, and others have not been traced. But I cannot particularize; in traversing the state I have found hundreds of insane persons in every variety of circumstance and condition; many whose situation could not and need not be improved; a less number, but that very large, whose lives are the saddest pictures of human suffering and degradation. I give a few illustrations; but description fades before reality.

Danvers. November; visited the almshouse; a large building, much out of repair; understand a new one is in contemplation. Here are from fifty-six to sixty inmates; one idiotic; three insane; one of the latter in close confinement at all times.

Long before reaching the house, wild shouts, snatches of rude songs, imprecations, and obscene language, fell upon the ear, proceeding from the occupant of a low building, rather remote from the principal building to which my course was directed. Found the mistress, and was conducted to the place, which was called *'the home'* of the *forlorn* maniac, a young woman, exhibiting a condition of neglect and misery blotting out the faintest idea of comfort, and outraging every sentiment of decency. She had been, I learnt, "a respectable person; industrious and worthy; disappointments and trials shook her mind, and finally laid prostrate reason and self-control; she became a maniac for life! She had been at Worcester Hospital for a considerable time, and had been returned as incurable." The mistress told me she understood that, while there, she was "comfortable and decent." Alas! what a change was here exhibited! She had passed from one degree of violence and degradation to another, in swift progress; there she stood, clinging to, or beating upon, the bars of her caged apartment, the contracted size of which afforded space only for increasing accumulations of filth, a *foul* spectacle; there she stood with naked arms and dishevelled hair; the unwashed frame invested with fragments of unclean garments, the air so extremely offensive, though ventilation was afforded on all sides save one, that it was not possible to remain beyond a few moments without retreating for recovery to the outward air. Irritation of body, produced by utter filth and exposure, incited her to the horrid process of tearing off her skin by inches; her face, neck, and person, were thus disfigured to hideousness; she held up a fragment just rent off; to my exclamation of horror, the mistress replied, "Oh, we can't help it; half the skin is off sometimes; we can do nothing with her; and it makes no difference what she eats, for she consumes her own filth as readily as the food which is brought her."

It is now January; a fortnight since, two visitors reported that most wretched outcast as "wallowing in dirty straw, in a place yet more dirty, and without clothing, without fire. Worse cared for than the brutes, and wholly lost to consciousness of decency!" Is the whole story told? What was seen, is; what is reported is not. These gross exposures are not for the pained sight of one alone; all, all, coarse, brutal men, wondering, neglected children, old and young, each and all, witness this lowest, foulest state of miserable humanity. And who protects her, that worse than Paria outcast, from other wrongs and blacker outrages? I do not *know* that such *have been.* I do know that they are to be dreaded, and that they are not guarded against.

Some may say these things cannot be remedied; these furious maniacs are not to be raised from these base conditions. I *know* they are; could give *many* examples; let *one* suffice. A young woman, a pauper, in a distant town, *Sandisfield,* was for years a raging maniac. A cage, chains, and *the whip,* were the agents for controlling her, united with harsh tones and profane language. Annually, with others (the town's poor) she was put up at auction, and bid off at the lowest price which was declared for her. One year, not long past, an old man came forward in the number of applicants for the poor wretch; he was taunted and ridiculed; "what would he and his old wife do with such a mere beast?" "My wife says yes," replied he, "and I shall take her." She was given to his charge; he conveyed her home; she was washed, neatly dressed, and placed in a decent bed-room, furnished for comfort and opening into the kitchen. How altered her condition! As yet *the chains* were not off. The first week she was somewhat restless, at times violent, but the quiet kind ways of the old people wrought a change; she received her food decently; forsook acts of violence, and no longer uttered blasphemous or indecent language; after a week, the chain was lengthened, and she was received as a companion into the kitchen. Soon she engaged in trivial employments. "After a fortnight," said the old man, "I knocked off the chains and made her a free woman." She is at times excited, but not violently; they are careful of her diet; they keep her very clean; she calls them "father" and "mother." Go there now and you will find her "clothed," and though not perfectly in her "right mind," so far restored as to be a safe and comfortable inmate.

Newburyport. Visited the almshouse in June last; eighty inmates; seven insane, one idiotic. Commodious and neat house; several of the partially insane apparently very comfortable; two very improperly situated, namely, an insane man, not considered incurable, in an out-building, whose room opened upon what was called 'the dead room,' affording in lieu of companionship with the living, a contemplation of corpses! The other subject was a woman in a *cellar*. I desired to see her; much reluctance was shown. I pressed the request; the Master of the House stated that she was *in the cellar*; that she was *dangerous to be approached*; that 'she had lately attacked his wife;' and *was often naked*. I persisted; 'if you will not go with me, give me the keys and I will go alone.' Thus importuned, the outer doors were opened. I descended the stairs from within; a strange, unnatural noise seemed to proceed from beneath our feet; at the moment I did not much regard it. My conductor proceeded to remove a padlock while my eye explored the wide space in quest of the poor woman. All for a moment was still. But judge my horror and amazement, when a door to a closet *beneath* the *staircase* was opened, revealing in the imperfect light a female apparently wasted to a skeleton, partially wrapped in blankets, furnished for the narrow bed on which she was sitting; her countenance furrowed, not by age, but suffering, was the image of distress; in that contracted space, unlighted, unventilated, she poured forth the wailings of despair; mournfully she extended her arms and appealed to me, "why am I consigned to hell? dark—dark—I used to pray, I used to read the Bible—I have done no crime in my heart; I had friends, why have all forsaken me!—my God! my God! why hast *thou* forsaken me!" Those groans, those wailings come up daily, mingling, with how many others, a perpetual and sad memorial. When the good Lord shall require an account of our stewardship, what shall all and each answer!

Perhaps it will be inquired how long, how many days or hours was she imprisoned in these confined limits? *For years!* In another part of the cellar were other small closets, only better, because higher through the entire length, into one of which she by turns was transferred, so as to afford opportunity for fresh whitewashing, &c.

Violence and severity do but exasperate the Insane: the only availing influence is kindness and firmness. It is amazing what these will produce. How many examples might illustrate this position: I refer to one recently exhibited in Barre. The town Paupers are disposed of annually to some family who, for a stipulated sum agree to take charge of them. One of them, a young woman, was shown to me well clothed, neat, quiet, and employed at needle-work. It is possible that this is the same being who, but last year, was a raving madwoman, exhibiting every degree of violence in action and speech; a very tigress wrought to fury; caged, chained, beaten, loaded with injuries, and exhibiting the passions which an iron rule might be expected to stimulate and sustain. It is the same person; another family hold her in charge who better understand human nature and human influences; she is no longer chained, caged, and beaten; but if excited, a pair of mittens drawn over the hands secures from mischief. Where will she be next year, after the annual sale?

Sudbury. First week in September last I directed my way to the poor-farm there. Approaching, as I supposed, that place, all uncertainty vanished, as to which, of several dwellings in view, the course should be directed. The terrible screams and imprecations, impure language and amazing blasphemies, of a maniac, now, as often heretofore, indicated the place sought after. I know not how to proceed! The English language affords no combinations fit for describing the condition of the happy wretch there confined. In a stall, built under a woodshed on the road, was a naked man, defiled with filth, furiously tossing through the bars and about the cage, portions of straw (the only furnishing of his prison) already trampled to chaff. The mass of filth within, diffused wide abroad the most noisome stench. I have never witnessed paroxysms of madness so appalling; it seemed as if the ancient doctrine of the possession of demons was here illustrated. I hastened to the house overwhelmed with horror. The mistress informed me that ten days since he had been brought from Worcester Hospital, where the town did not choose any longer to meet the expenses of maintaining him; that he had been "dreadful noisy and dangerous to go near," ever since; it was hard work to give him food at any rate, for what was not immediately dashed at those who carried it, was cast down upon the festering mass within. "He's a dreadful care; worse than all the people and work on the farm beside."

Westford. Not many miles distant from Wayland is a sad spectacle; was told by the family who kept the poorhouse, that they had twenty-six paupers; one idiot; one simple; and one insane, an incurable case from Worcester hospital. I requested to see her, but was answered that she "wasn't fit to be seen; she was naked, and made so much trouble they did not know how to get along." I hesitated but a moment; I must see her, I said. I cannot adopt descriptions of the condition of the insane secondarily; what I assert for fact, I must see for myself. On this I was conducted above stairs into an apartment of decent size, pleasant aspect from abroad, and tolerably comfortable in its general appearance; but the inmates!—grant I may never look upon another such scene! A young woman, whose person was partially covered with portions of a blanket, sat upon the floor; her hair dishevelled; her naked arms crossed languidly over the breast; a distracted, unsteady eye, and low, murmuring voice, betraying both mental and physical disquiet. *About the waist was a chain,* the extremity of which was fastened into the wall of the house. As I left the room the poor creature said, "I want my gown!" The response from the attendant might have roused to indignation one not dispossesed of reason, and owning self-control.

I may here remark that severe measures, in enforcing rule, have in many places been openly revealed. I have not seen chastisement administered by stripes, and in but few instances have I seen the *rods* and *whips,* but I have seen blows inflicted, both passionately and repeatedly.

I have been asked if I have investigated the causes of insanity? I have not; but I have been told that this most calamitous overthrow of reason, often is the result of a life of sin; it is sometimes, but rarely added, they must take the consequences; they deserve no better care! Shall man be more just than God; he who causes his sun, and refreshing rains, and life-giving influence, to fall alike on the good and the evil? Is not the total wreck of reason, a state of distraction, and the loss of all that makes life cherished a retribution, sufficiently heavy, without adding to consequences so appalling, every indignity that can bring still lower the wretched sufferer? Have pity upon those who, while they were supposed to lie hid in secret sins, "have been scattered under *a dark veil of forgetfulness*; over whom is spread a heavy night, and who unto themselves are more grievous than the darkness."

Of the dangers and mischiefs sometimes following the location of insane persons in our almshouses, I will record but one more example. In Worcester, has for several years resided a young woman, a lunatic pauper of decent life and respectable family. I have seen her as she usually appeared, listless and silent, almost or quite sunk into a state of dementia, sitting one amidst the family, 'but not of them.' A few weeks since, revisiting that almshouse, judge my horror and amazement to see her negligently bearing in her arms a young infant, of which I was told she was the unconscious parent!

Men of Massachusetts, I beg, I implore, I demand, pity and protection, for these of my suffering, outraged sex!—Fathers, Husbands, Brothers, I would supplicate you for this boon—but what do I say? I dishonor you, divest you at once of christianity and humanity—does this appeal imply distrust. If it comes burthened with a doubt of your righteousness in this Legislation, then blot it out; while I declare confidence in your honor, not less than your humanity. Here you will put away the cold, calculating spirit of selfishness and self-seeking; lay off the armor of local strife and political opposition; here and now, for once, forgetful of the earthly and perishable, come up to these halls and consecrate them with one heart and one mind to works of righteousness and just judgment. Become the benefactors of your race, the just guardians of the solemn rights you hold in trust. Raise up the fallen; succor the desolate; restore the outcast; defend the helpless; and for your eternal and great reward, receive the benediction. . . . "Well done, good and faithful servants, become rulers over many things!"

The conviction is continually deepened that Hospitals are the only places where insane persons can be at once humanely and properly controlled. Poorhouses, converted into madhouses, cease to effect the purposes for which they were established, and instead of being asylums for the aged, the homeless, and the friendless, and places of refuge for orphaned or neglected childhood, are transformed into perpetual bedlams.

This crying evil and abuse of institutions, is not confined to our almshouses. The warden of a populous prison near this metropolis, populous, not with criminals only, but with the insane in almost every stage of insanity, and the idiotic in descending states from silly and simple, to helpless and speechless, has declared that, since their admission under the Rev. Stat. of 1835, page 382, "the prison has often more resembled the infernal regions than any place on earth!" and, what with the excitement inevitably produced by the crowded state of the prisons, and multiplying causes, not subject to much modification, there has been neither peace nor order one hour of the twenty-four; if ten were quiet, the residue were probably raving. Almost without interval might, and *must,* these be heard, blaspheming and furious, and to the last degree impure and indecent; uttering language, from which the base and the profligate have turned shuddering aside, and the abandoned have shrunk abashed. I myself, with many beside, can bear sad witness to these things.

In relation to the confinement of the insane in prisons the Sheriff of Hampshire county wires as follows:—

"I concur fully in the sentiments entertained by you in relation to this unwise, not to say inhuman, provision of our law (see Rev. Stat. 382) authorizing the commitment of lunatics to our Jails and Houses of Correction.

"Indeed this feature of our law seems to me a relic of that ancient barbarism which regarded misfortune as a crime, and those bereft of reason as also bereft of all sensibility; as having forfeited not only all title to compassion but to *humanity, . . .* "

Gentleman, I commit to you this sacred cause.

Respectfully submitted,
D. L. Dix.

85 Mt. Vernon St. Boston.
January, 1843.

FLORENCE NIGHTINGALE (1820–1910)

Notes on Hospitals

Florence Nightingale was born in Florence, Italy, into one of Britain's wealthiest and most eminent families. By the age of sixteen, she felt herself to be called by God to nurse the sick. After an agonizing, nearly twenty-year-long struggle against her family's resistance, Nightingale finally took up her vocation in 1854 when she departed for the Crimea with thirty-eight other nurses in her charge. The sheer physical horror of what she encountered at its hospital barracks left her with a moral outrage that would continue to fuel her mission of reform until her death. Four miles of cots—packed so closely she could scarcely walk between them—held nearly three thousand naked and half-starved soldiers, lying in rot, maggots, and decaying human waste. Into this "sink of human misery" Nightingale introduced order, cleanliness, and compassion as she set about feeding, clothing, washing, and nursing the British common soldier, often at her own expense. In 1856, Nightingale returned to England haunted by the ghosts of the Crimean dead and vowing to expunge "the grand administrative evil" responsible for the horrors she had witnessed. During the next several years, Nightingale exposed to public view the incompetence of the British War Office and set in motion far-reaching military and civilian reforms in medical care and education: She founded modern nursing, masterminded Britain's renovation of its military barracks and hospitals, and produced *Notes on Hospitals,* the book that revolutionized the idea of the hospital and assured, as Lytton Strachey later observed, that no great hospital would henceforth fail to "bear upon it the impress of her mind."

Feeling very desirous of contributing whatever aid I can to improvement in Hospital construction and administration—especially at this time, when several new hospitals are being built—it has occurred to me to transmit a few notes on defects which have come under my own observation in an extended experience of these institutions.

No one, I think, who brings ordinary powers of observation to bear on the sick and maimed can fail to observe a remarkable difference in the aspect of cases, in their duration and in their termination in different hospitals. To the superficial observer there are two things only apparent—the disease and the remedial treatment, medical or surgical. It requires a considerable amount of experience, in hospitals of various constructions and varied administrations, to go beyond this, and to be able to perceive that conditions arising out of these have a very powerful effect indeed upon the ultimate issue of cases which pass through the wards.

It is sometimes asserted that there is no such striking difference in the mortality

From *Notes on Hospitals* (London, 1859).

of different hospitals as one would be led to infer from their gre
ence in sanitary condition. There is, undoubtedly, some difficulty
rect statistical comparison to exhibit this. For, in the first place, (
receive very different proportions of the same class of diseases. The
pital may differ considerably from the ages in another. And the stat
admission may differ very much in each hospital. These elements, ⸏ ⸏uuot, affect
considerably the results of treatment, altogether apart from the sanitary state of
hospitals.

In the next place accurate hospital statistics are much more rare than is generally
imagined, and at the best they only give the mortality which has taken place *in* the
hospitals, and take no cognizance of those cases which are discharged in a hopeless
condition, to a much greater extent from some hospitals than from others.

Again, the sanitary state of any hospital ought not to be inferred solely from the
greater or less mortality. In one set of metropolitan hospitals, for example, I find
the mortality about two and a-half per cent upon the cases treated, while in other
metropolitan hospitals the deaths reach from about twelve to sixteen per cent. To
judge by the mortality in these cases would be most fallacious. Because in the first
class of hospitals every ailment, however slight, constitutes a title to hospital admission, while, in the latter class of hospitals, special diseases only, at all times accompanied by a high rate of mortality, are admitted. Hence the duration of the cases
admitted, and the general course and aspect of disease afford important criteria
whereby to judge of the healthiness or unhealthiness of any hospital in addition to
that afforded by the mortality statistics. Besides, careful observers are now generally convinced that the origin and spread of fever in a hospital, or the appearance
and spread of hospital gangrene, erysipelas and pyaemia generally, are much better
tests of the defective sanitary state of a hospital than its mortality returns. But I would
go further, and state that to the experienced eye of a careful observing nurse, the
daily, I had almost said hourly, changes which take place in patients, and which
changes rarely come under the cognizance of the periodical medical visitor, afford a
still more important class of data, from which to judge of the general adaptation of
a hospital for the reception and treatment of sick. One insensibly allies together restlessness, languor, feverishness, and general *malaise,* with closeness of wards, defective ventilation, defective structure, bad architectural and administrative
arrangements, until it is impossible to resist the conviction that the sick are suffering from something quite other than the disease inscribed on their bed-ticket—and
the inquiry insensibly arises in the mind, what can be the cause? To this query many
years' experience of hospitals in various countries and climates enables me to answer explicitly as the result of my own observation, that, even admitting to the full
extent the great value of the hospital improvements of recent years, a vast deal of
the suffering, and some at least of the mortality in these establishments, is avoidable.

What, then, are those defects to which such results are to be attributed?

I should state at once that to original defects in the sites and plans of hospitals,
and to deficient ventilation and overcrowding accompanying such defects, is to be
attributed a large proportion of the evil I have mentioned.

The facts flow almost of necessity from ascertained sanitary experience. But it is not often, excepting perhaps in the case of intelligent house surgeons, that the whole process whereby the sick, who ought to have had rapid recoveries, are retained week after week, or perhaps month after month, in hospital, is continuously observed. I have known a case of slight fever received into hospital, the fever pass off in less than a week, and yet the patient, from the foul state of the wards, not restored to health at the end of eight weeks.

The defects to which such occurrences are mainly to be attributed are four:—

1. The agglomeration of a large number of sick under the same roof.
2. Deficiency of space.
3. Deficiency of ventilation.
4. Deficiency of light.

These are the four radical defects in hospital construction.

But on the very threshold of the subject we shall probably be told that not to these defects, but to 'contagion' and 'infection,' is much of the unhealthy condition of some hospitals attributable, at least so far as concerns the occurrence of zymotic diseases. On the very threshold, therefore, we are obliged to make a digression in order to discuss the meaning of these two familiar words, and to lay these spectres which have terrified almost all ages and nations.

This is the more necessary, because on the exact influence exercised by these two presumed causes of hospital sickness and mortality depends to a great degree the possibility of our introducing efficient hospital attendance and nursing. Unfortunately both nurses and medical men, as well as medical students, have died of zymotic diseases prevailing in hospitals. It is an all-important question to decide whether the propagation of such diseases is inevitable or preventible. If the former, then the whole question must be considered as to whether hospitals necessarily attended with results so fatal should exist at all. If the latter, then it is our duty to prevent their propagation.

The idea of 'contagion,' as explaining the spread of disease, appears to have been adopted at a time when, from the neglect of sanitary arrangements, epidemics attacked whole masses of people, and when men had ceased to consider that nature had any laws for her guidance. Beginning with the poets and historians, the word finally made its way into medical nomenclature, where it has remained ever since, affording to certain classes of minds, chiefly in the southern and less educated parts of Europe, a satisfactory explanation for pestilence and an adequate excuse for non-exertion to prevent its recurrence.

And now, what does 'contagion' mean? It implies the communication of disease from person to person by *contact*. It pre-supposes the existence of certain germs like the sporules of fungi, which can be bottled up and conveyed any distance attached to clothing, to merchandize, especially to woollen stuffs, for which it is supposed to have a particular affection, and to feathers, which of all articles it especially loves— so much so, that, according to quarantine laws, a live goose may be safely introduced from a plague country; but if it happen to be eaten on the voyage, its feathers cannot be admitted without danger to the entire community. There is no end to the absurdities connected with this doctrine. Suffice it to say, that in the ordinary sense of the word, there is no proof, such as would be admitted in any scientific inquiry, that there is any such thing as 'contagion.'

There are two or three diseases in which there is a specific virus, which can be seen, tasted, smelt, and analysed, and which in certain constitutions propagates the original disease by inoculation—such as small-pox, cow-pox, &c. But these are not 'contagions' in the sense supposed.

The word 'infection,' which is often confounded with 'contagion,' expresses a fact, and does not involve a hypothesis. But just as there is no such thing as 'contagion,' there is no such thing as *inevitable* 'infection.' Infection acts through the air. Poison the air breathed by individuals and there is infection. Shut up 150 healthy people in a Black-hole of Calcutta, and in twenty-four hours an infection is produced so intense that it will, in that time, have destroyed nearly the whole of the inmates. Sick people are more susceptible than healthy people; and if they be shut up without sufficient space and sufficient fresh air, there will be produced not only fever, but erysipelas, pyaemia, and the usual tribe of hospital-generated epidemic diseases.

In certain hospitals it has been the custom to set apart wards for what are called 'infectious' diseases, but in reality there ought to be no diseases so considered. With proper sanitary precautions, diseases reputed to be the most 'infectious' may be treated in wards among other sick without any danger. Without proper sanitary arrangements, a number of healthy people may be congregated together so as to become subject to the worst horrors of 'infection.'

No stronger condemnation of any hospital or ward could be pronounced than the simple fact that any zymotic disease has originated in it, or that such diseases have attacked other patients than those brought in with them. And there can be no stronger condemnation of any town than the outbreak of fatal epidemics in it. Infection, and incapable management, or bad construction, are in hospitals as well as in towns, convertible terms.

It was necessary to say thus much to show to what hospital diseases are *not* necessarily due. To the following defects in site, construction, and management, as we think, they are mainly to be attributed.

1. *The agglomeration of a large number of sick under one roof.*—It is a well-established fact that, other things being equal, the amount of sickness and mortality on different areas bears a ratio to the degree of density of the population.

Why should undue agglomeration of sick be any exception to this law? Is it not rather to be expected that, the constitutions of sick people being more susceptible than those of healthy people, they should suffer more from this cause?

But if anything were wanting in confirmation of this fact, it would be the enormous mortality in the hospitals which contained perhaps the largest number of sick ever at one time under the same roof, viz., those at Scutari. The largest of these too famous hospitals had at one time 2500 sick and wounded under its roof, and it has happened that of Scutari patients two out of every five have died.

All experience tells the same tale, both among sick and well. Men will have a high rate of mortality in large barracks, a low one in separate huts, even with a much less amount of cubic space.

2. *Deficiency of Space.*—Wherever cubic space is deficient, ventilation is bad. Cubic space and ventilation will therefore go hand in hand. The law holds good with regard to hospitals, barracks, and all inhabited places.

3. *Deficiency of Ventilation.*—The want of fresh air may be detected in the appearance of patients sooner than any other want. No care or luxury will compensate indeed for its absence. Unless the air *within* the ward can be kept as flesh as it is *without,* the patients had better be away. *No* artificial ventilation will do this. Although in badly-constructed hospitals, or in countries where fuel is dear, and the winter very cold, artificial ventilation may be necessary, it never can compensate for the want of the open window. . . . [The] ward should be at least sixteen feet high, and the distance between the opposite windows not more than thirty feet. Every adult exhales by the lungs and skin forty-eight ounces, or three pints of water in twenty-four hours. Sixteen men in a room would therefore exhale in eight hours sixteen pints of water, and 123 cubic feet of carbonic acid into the atmosphere of the room. With the watery vapour there is also exhaled a large quantity of organic matter, ready to enter into the putrefactive condition. This is especially the case during the hours of sleep, and as it is a vital law that all excretions are injurious to health if reintroduced into the system, it is easy to understand how the breathing of damp foul air of this kind, and the consequent re-introduction of excrementitious matter into the blood through the function of respiration will tend to produce diseases.

If this be so for the well, how much more will it be so for the sick?—for the sick, the exhalations from whom are always highly morbid and dangerous, as they are one of nature's methods of eliminating noxious matter from the body, in order that it may recover health.

4. *Deficiency of Light.*—What is the proportionate influence of the four defects enumerated in delaying recovery I am not competent to determine.

Second only to fresh air, however, I should be inclined to rank light in importance for the sick. Direct sunlight, not only daylight, is necessary for speedy recovery, except, perhaps, in certain ophthalmic and a small number of other cases. Instances could be given, almost endless, where, in dark wards or in wards with a northern aspect, even when thoroughly warmed, or in wards with borrowed light, even when thoroughly ventilated, the sick could not by any means be made speedily to recover.

Among kindred effects of light I may mention, from experience, as quite perceptible in promoting recovery, the being able to see out of a window, instead of looking against a dead wall; the bright colours of flowers; the being able to read in bed by the light of a window close to the bed-head. It is generally said that the effect is upon the mind. Perhaps so; but it is no less so upon the body on that account.

MASSACHUSETTS GENERAL HOSPITAL

By-Laws, Rules and Regulations, Acts and Resolves

The history of Massachusetts General Hospital begins with a rather modest document. On August 20, 1810, a letter was circulated by Drs. James Jackson and John C. Warren inviting subscriptions "for a hospital for the reception of lunatics and other sick persons." A year later, the hospital received its charter from the Massachusetts State Legislature, and in 1818, its cornerstone was laid. The first patient was received on September 1, 1821. Two years later, John McLean bequeathed more than one hundred thousand dollars to the hospital's asylum, which was renamed in his memory. At the time, few Americans had ever seen a hospital, much less been in one. Even as late as the mid–nineteenth century, the hospital still remained a place of last resort for the sick, and those who entered its doors were virtually without exception the poor, who often had to choose between it and the almshouse. The admission of patients—a matter largely under the control of trustees and administrators—was as much a social and moral decision as a medical one. It rested on a perceived distinction between the worthy and unworthy poor, between those deemed to be deserving of the hospital's charity and those who were not. Once inside the hospital, "free" patients were expected to submit to the authority of their benefactors and to follow a regimen designed not only to restore their physical health but to improve their moral character.

ADMISSION AND BOARD OF PATIENTS

ARTICLE 1. Applications for admission of patients, must be made at the Hospital in Blossom Street, between the hours of 9 and 10, A.M., on each day of the week, except Sundays. In urgent cases, however, application may be made at other times. The patient, if able, should in all cases appear at the Hospital in person. If not able to attend, the application may be made at the Hospital by a friend, and the patient will be visited by the Physician to out-door patients; and no one can be admitted without a permit, except in case of recent accident.

Applications from the country must be made in writing, addressed to the Resident Physician of the Hospital, by the attending physician of the patient, accompanied by a description of the case, and, when a free bed is desired, a statement of the pecuniary circumstances of the patient.

ART. 2. Incurable cases and those of long standing, which admit only of temporary alleviation, are not regarded, in general, as suitable subjects for admission; the

From *Massachusetts General Hospital: By-Laws, Rules and Regulations, Acts and Resolves* (Boston, 1861).

great object being to afford substantial medical and surgical relief to as large a number of patients as possible.

ART. 3. No patient shall be admitted having a contagious disease. Persons infected with Syphilis shall not be admitted, except by vote of the Board of Trustees, and when admitted, shall pay not less than double the usual rate of board.

ART. 5. The price of board shall in all instances be so low as to make the Hospital to as great extent a charitable institution as its funds will permit; and in each instance shall be graduated as nearly as possible, according to the circumstances of the patients, and to the accommodation they may receive. When a patient remains only one day, the charge shall be at least one dollar.

VISITORS AND PATIENTS

ARTICLE 1. No visitors (except as hereinbefore mentioned) shall be admitted to the Hospital without a special permit.

On each day of the week, Sundays excepted, from 11 to $12^1/_2$ o'clock, friends may be admitted to visit patients in the wards; it being understood that no patient in any ward shall receive more than one visitor at a time: and that no patient in any female ward, shall be visited by a male friend, other than her father, son, husband, or brother.

Patients in private rooms may be visited by their friends at any suitable hours in the daytime, by permission of the Resident Physician; and any patient in the wards may in like manner be visited by friends who reside more than six miles from the city, upon obtaining the like permission.

No one calling to visit any member of the Resident Physician's or Steward's family, or an attendant, shall be admitted to visit the wards without the special permission of the Resident Physician.

In all cases, however, the Resident Physician may exercise discretionary powers as to excluding or admitting visitors.

ART. 2. The patients are expected to be quiet and exemplary in their behavior, and to conform strictly to the rules and regulations of the Trustees and the orders and prescriptions of the various officers in the establishment; and no indecent or immoral conduct in any patient or other person connected with or resident in the Hospital, shall be tolerated by the Resident Physician, who shall forthwith report any such misconduct to the Visiting Committee.

ART. 3. Such free patients as are able, in the opinion of the Physicians and Surgeons, shall assist in nursing others, or in such services as the Resident Physician or Matron may require; and if any persons refuse to perform such acts, their names shall be forthwith reported to the Visiting Committee.

ART. 4. No person, except the Physicians or Surgeons of the Hospital, shall speak of the health of a patient in the presence of such a patient.

ART. 5. The smoking of Tobacco is prohibited in the Hospital.

FREE BEDS

ARTICLE 1. Any individual on the payment of one hundred dollars shall be entitled to a free bed at the Hospital for one year. And on payment of one thousand dollars, or of such sum as the applicant would be required to pay for an annuity of one hundred dollars on the principles of life insurance, he shall be entitled to a free bed for life.

ART. 2. The Trustees shall, at the beginning of each quarter, determine what number of free beds shall be allowed at the Hospital, including such as may have been subscribed for, or for which any permanent subscription or bequest may have been made: *the whole number never to be less than thirty-seven.*

GEORGE ORWELL (1903–1950)

"How the Poor Die"

Eric Blair, who used the pseudonym George Orwell, was an English essayist, journalist, and novelist. Orwell was born in Bengal, India, where his father was a minor official in the British Customs Service. After graduating from Eton, to which he had won a scholarship, Orwell left for Burma and joined the Indian Imperial Police in 1922, beginning a decisive phase in his life that left him bitterly disillusioned with colonial rule. In 1927, he retired from the force to return to Europe, where, living among the poor in squalid conditions, he took up writing, as well as the avocations of dishwasher, hop-picker, and tramp—experiences described in his first published book, *Down and Out in Paris and London* (1933). In addition to his two most famous novels, *Animal Farm* (1945) and *1984* (1949), Orwell wrote several prose masterpieces, including *The Road to Wigan Pier* (1937), a study of the unemployed among the working classes of northern England, and *Homage to Catalonia* (1938), an account of his experiences as a soldier during the Spanish Civil War in the militia unit of an independent Marxist workers' party. Severely wounded, and hunted by the Communist secret police, Orwell fled Spain with a dread and hatred of totalitarianism that stayed with him until his death in London from tuberculosis. Few forms of oppression—whether perpetrated in prison cells or on hospital wards—escaped Orwell's observation. He was, as V. S. Pritchett remarked, "the conscience of his generation," a designation whose truth is irrefutably borne out by his giving witness to how the poor die.

In the year 1929 I spent several weeks in the Hôpital X, in the fifteenth arrondissement of Paris. The clerks put me through the usual third degree at the reception desk, and indeed I was kept answering questions for some twenty minutes before they would let me in. If you have ever had to fill up forms in a Latin country you will know the kind of questions I mean. For some days past I had been unequal to translating Reaumur into Fahrenheit, but I know that my temperature was round about 103, and by the end of the interview I had some difficulty in standing on my feet. At my back a resigned little knot of patients, carrying bundles done up in colored handkerchiefs, waited their turn to be questioned.

After the questioning came the bath—a compulsory routine for all newcomers, apparently, just as in prison or the workhouse. My clothes were taken away from me, and after I had sat shivering for some minutes in five inches of warm water I was given a linen nightshirt and a short blue flannel dressing gown—no slippers,

---

they had none big enough for me, they said—and led out into the open air. This was a night in February and I was suffering from pneumonia. The ward we were going to was two hundred yards away and it seemed that to get to it you had to cross the hospital grounds. Someone stumbled in front of me with a lantern. The gravel path was frosty underfoot, and the wind whipped the nightshirt round my bare calves. When we got into the ward I was aware of a strange feeling of familiarity whose origin I did not succeed in pinning down till later in the night. It was a long, rather low, ill-lit room, full of murmuring voices and with three rows of beds surprisingly close together. There was a foul smell, fecal and yet sweetish. As I lay down I saw on a bed nearly opposite me a small, round-shouldered, sandy-haired man sitting half naked while a doctor and a student performed some strange operation on him. First the doctor produced from his black bag a dozen small glasses like wine glasses, then the student burned a match inside each glass to exhaust the air, then the glass was popped on to the man's back or chest and the vacuum drew up a huge yellow blister. Only after some moments did I realize what they were doing to him. It was something called cupping, a treatment which you can read about in old medical text-books but which till then I had vaguely thought of as one of those things they do to horses.

The cold air outside had probably lowered my temperature, and I watched this barbarous remedy with detachment and even a certain amount of amusement. The next moment, however, the doctor and the student came across to my bed, hoisted me upright, and without a word began applying the same set of glasses, which had not been sterilized in any way. A few feeble protests that I uttered got no more response than if I had been an animal. I was very much impressed by the impersonal way in which the two men started on me. I had never been in the public ward of a hospital before, and it was my first experience of doctors who handle you without speaking to you or, in a human sense, taking any notice of you. They only put on six glasses in my case, but after doing so they scarified the blisters and applied the glasses again. Each glass now drew out about a dessert-spoonful of dark-colored blood. As I lay down again, humiliated, disgusted, and frightened by the thing that had been done to me, I reflected that now at least they would leave me alone. But no, not a bit of it. There was another treatment coming, the mustard poultice, seemingly a matter of routine like the hot bath. Two slatternly nurses had already got the poultice ready, and they lashed it round my chest as tight as a straitjacket while some men who were wandering about the ward in shirt and trousers began to collect round my bed with half-sympathetic grins. I learned later that watching a patient have a mustard poultice was a favorite pastime in the ward. These things are normally applied for a quarter of an hour and certainly they are funny enough if you don't happen to be the person inside. For the first five minutes the pain is severe, but you believe you can bear it. During the second five minutes this belief evaporates, but the poultice is buckled at the back and you can't get it off. This is the period the onlookers enjoy most. During the last five minutes, I noted, a sort of numbness supervenes. After the poultice had been removed a waterproof pillow packed with ice was thrust beneath my head and I was left alone. I did not sleep, and to the best of my knowledge this was the only night of my life—I mean the only night spent in bed—in which I have not slept at all, not even a minute.

During my first hour in the Hôpital X I had had a whole series of different and contradictory treatments, but this was misleading, for in general you got very little treatment at all, either good or bad, unless you were ill in some interesting and instructive way. At five in the morning the nurses came round, woke the patients, and took their temperatures, but did not wash them. If you were well enough you washed yourself, otherwise you depended on the kindness of some walking patient. It was generally patients, too, who carried the bedbottles and the grim bedpan, nicknamed *la casserole.* At eight breakfast arrived, called army-fashion *la soupe.* It was soup, too, a thin vegetable soup with slimy hunks of bread floating about in it. Later in the day the tall, solemn, black-bearded doctor made his rounds, with an interne and a troop of students following at his heels, but there were about sixty of us in the ward and it was evident that he had other wards to attend to as well. There were many beds past which he walked day after day, sometimes followed by imploring cries. On the other hand if you had some disease with which the students wanted to familiarize themselves you got plenty of attention of a kind. I myself, with an exceptionally fine specimen of a bronchial rattle, sometimes had as many as a dozen students queuing up to listen to my chest. It was a very queer feeling—queer, I mean, because of their intense interest in learning their job, together with a seeming lack of any perception that the patients were human beings. It is strange to relate, but sometimes as some young student stepped forward to take his turn at manipulating you, he would be actually tremulous with excitement, like a boy who has at last got his hands on some expensive piece of machinery. And then ear after ear—ears of young men, of girls, of Negroes—pressed against your back, relays of fingers solemnly but clumsily tapping, and not from any one of them did you get a word of conversation or a look direct in your face. As a non-paying patient, in the uniform nightshirt, you were primarily *a specimen,* a thing I did not resent but could never quite get used to.

After some days I grew well enough to sit up and study the surrounding patients. The stuffy room, with its narrow beds so close together that you could easily touch your neighbor's hand, had every sort of disease in it except, I suppose, acutely infectious cases. My right-hand neighbor was a little red-haired cobbler with one leg shorter than the other, who used to announce the death of any other patient (this happened a number of times, and my neighbor was always the first to hear of it) by whistling to me, exclaiming "Numero 43!" (or whatever it was) and flinging his arms above his head. This man had not much wrong with him, but in most of the other beds within my angle of vision some squalid tragedy or some plain horror was being enacted. In the bed that was foot to foot with mine there lay, until he died (I didn't see him die—they moved him to another bed), a little weazened man who was suffering from I do not know what disease, but something that made his whole body so intensely sensitive that any movement from side to side, sometimes even the weight of the bedclothes, would make him shout out with pain. His worst suffering was when he urinated, which he did with the greatest difficulty. A nurse would bring him the bedbottle and then for a long time stand beside his bed, whistling, as grooms are said to do with horses, until at last with an agonized shriek of *"Je pisse!"* he would get started. In the bed next to him the sandy-haired man whom I had seen being cupped used to cough up blood-streaked mucus at all hours. My left-hand neighbor was a tall, flaccid-looking young man who used periodically to have a tube inserted into his back and astonishing quantities of frothy liquid drawn off from some part of his body. In the bed beyond that a veteran of the war of 1870 was dying, a handsome old man with a white imperial, round whose bed, at all hours when visiting was allowed, four elderly female relatives dressed all in black sat exactly like crows, obviously scheming for some pitiful legacy. In the bed opposite me in the further row was an old bald-headed man with drooping moustaches and greatly swollen face and body, who was suffering from some disease that made him urinate almost incessantly. A huge glass receptacle stood always beside his bed. One day his wife and daughter came to visit him. At sight of them the old man's bloated face lit up with a smile of surprising sweetness, and as his daughter, a pretty girl of about twenty, approached the bed I saw that his hand was slowly working its way from under the bedclothes. I seemed to see in advance the gesture that was coming—the girl kneeling beside the bed, the old man's hand laid on her head in his dying blessing. But no, he merely handed her the bedbottle, which she promptly took from him and emptied into the receptacle.

About a dozen beds away from me was Numero 57—I think that was his number—a cirrhosis of the liver case. Everyone in the ward knew him by sight because he was sometimes the subject of a medical lecture. On two afternoons a week the tall, grave doctor would lecture in the ward to a party of students, and on more than one occasion old Numero 57 was wheeled in on a sort of trolley into the middle of the ward, where the doctor would roll back his nightshirt, dilate with his fingers a huge flabby protuberance on the man's belly—the diseased liver, I suppose—and explain solemnly that this was a disease attributable to alcoholism, commoner in the wine-drinking countries. As usual he neither spoke to his patient nor gave him a smile, a nod or any kind of recognition. While he talked, very grave and upright, he would hold the wasted body beneath his two hands, sometimes giving it a gentle roll to and fro, in just the attitude of a woman handling a rolling-pin. Not that Numero 57 minded this kind of thing. Obviously he was an old hospital inmate, a regular exhibit at lectures, his liver long since marked down for a bottle in some pathological museum. Utterly uninterested in what was said about him, he would lie with his colorless eyes gazing at nothing, while the doctor showed him off like a piece of antique china. He was a man of about sixty, astonishingly shrunken. His face, pale as vellum, had shrunken away till it seemed no bigger than a doll's.

One morning my cobbler neighbor woke me up plucking at my pillow before the nurses arrived. "Numero 57!"—he flung his arms above his head. There was a light in the ward, enough to see by. I could see old Numero 57 lying crumpled up on his side, his face sticking out over the side of the bed, and toward me. He had died some time during the night, nobody knew when. When the nurses came they received the news of his death indifferently and went about their work. After a long time, an hour or more, two other nurses marched in abreast like soldiers, with a great clumping of sabots, and knotted the corpse up in the sheets, but it was not removed till some time later. Meanwhile, in the better light, I had had time for a good look at Numero 57. Indeed I lay on my side to look at him. Curiously enough he was the first dead

European I had seen. I had seen dead men before, but always Asiatics and usually people who had died violent deaths. Numero 57's eyes were still open, his mouth also open, his small face contorted into an expression of agony. What most impressed me, however, was the whiteness of his face. It had been pale before, but now it was little darker than the sheets. As I gazed at the tiny, screwed-up face it struck me that this disgusting piece of refuse, waiting to be carted away and dumped on a slab in the dissecting room, was an example of "natural" death, one of the things you pray for in the Litany. There you are, then, I thought, that's what is waiting for you, twenty, thirty, forty years hence: that is how the lucky ones die, the one who lives to be old. One wants to live, of course, indeed one only stays alive by virtue of the fear of death, but I think now, as I thought then, that it's better to die violently and not too old. People talk about the horrors of war, but what weapon has man invented that even approaches in cruelty some of the commoner diseases? "Natural" death, almost by definition, means something slow, smelly, and painful. Even at that, it makes a difference if you can achieve it in your own home and not in a public institution. This poor old wretch who had just flickered out like a candle end was not even important enough to have anyone watching by his deathbed. He was merely a number, then a "subject" for the students' scalpels. And the sordid publicity of dying in such a place! In the Hôpital X the beds were very close together and there were no screens. Fancy, for instance, dying like the little man whose bed was for a while foot to foot with mine, the one who cried out when the bedclothes touched him! I dare say *"Je pisse!"* were his last recorded words. Perhaps the dying don't bother about such things—that at least would be the standard answer: nevertheless dying people are often more or less normal in their minds till within a day or so of the end.

In the public wards of a hospital you see horrors that you don't seem to meet with among people who manage to die in their own homes, as though certain diseases only attacked people at the lower income levels. But it is a fact that you would not in any English hospitals see some of the things I saw in the Hôpital X. This business of people just dying like animals, for instance, with nobody standing by, nobody interested, the death not even noticed till the morning—this happened more than once. You certainly would not see that in England, and still less would you see a corpse left exposed to the view of the other patients. I remember that once in a cottage hospital in England a man died while we were at tea, and though there were only six of us in the ward the nurses managed things so adroitly that the man was dead and his body removed without our even hearing about it till tea was over. A thing we perhaps underrate in England is the advantage we enjoy in having large numbers of well-trained and rigidly disciplined nurses. No doubt English nurses are dumb enough, they may tell fortunes with tea leaves, wear Union Jack badges, and keep photographs of the Queen on their mantelpieces, but at least they don't let you lie unwashed and constipated on an unmade bed, out of sheer laziness. The nurses at the Hôpital X still had a tinge of Mrs. Gamp about them, and later, in the military hospitals of Republican Spain, I was to see nurses almost too ignorant to take a temperature. You wouldn't, either, see in England such dirt as existed in the Hôpital X. Later on, when I was well enough to wash myself in the bathroom, I found that there was kept there a huge packing case into which the scraps of food and dirty dressings from the ward were flung, and the wainscotings were infested by crickets.

When I had got back my clothes and grown strong on my legs I fled from the Hôpital X, before my time was up and without waiting for a medical discharge. It was not the only hospital I have fled from, but its gloom and bareness, its sickly smell and, above all, something in its mental atmosphere stand out in my memory as exceptional. I had been taken there because it was the hospital belonging to my arrondissement, and I did not learn till after I was in it that it bore a bad reputation. A year or two later the celebrated swindler, Madame Hanaud, who was ill while on remand, was taken to the Hôpital X, and after a few days of it she managed to elude her guards, took a taxi, and drove back to the prison, explaining that she was more comfortable there. I have no doubt that the Hôpital X was quite untypical of French hospitals even at that date. But the patients, nearly all of them working men, were surprisingly resigned. Some of them seemed to find the conditions almost comfortable, for at least two were destitute malingerers who found this a good way of getting through the winter. The nurses connived because the malingerers made themselves useful by doing odd jobs. But the attitude of the majority was: of course this is a lousy place, but what else do you expect? It did not seem strange to them that you should be woken at five and then wait three hours before starting the day on watery soup, or that people should die with no one at their bedside, or even that your chance of getting medical attention should depend on catching the doctor's eye as he went past. According to their traditions that was what hospitals were like. If you are seriously ill, and if you are too poor to be treated in your own home, then you must go into hospital, and once there you must put up with harshness and discomfort, just as you would in the army. But on top of this I was interested to find a lingering belief in the old stories that have now almost faded from memory in England—stories, for instance, about doctors cutting you open out of sheer curiosity or thinking it funny to start operating before you were properly "under." There were dark tales about a little operating room said to be situated just beyond the bathroom. Dreadful screams were said to issue from this room. I saw nothing to confirm these stories and no doubt they were all nonsense, though I did see two students kill a sixteen-year-old boy, or nearly kill him (he appeared to be dying when I left the hospital, but he may have recovered later) by a mischievous experiment which they probably could not have tried on a paying patient. Well within living memory it used to be believed in London that in some of the big hospitals patients were killed off to get dissection subjects. I didn't hear this tale repeated at the Hôpital X, but I should think some of the men there would have found it credible. For it was a hospital in which not the methods, perhaps, but something of the atmosphere of the nineteenth century had managed to survive, and therein lay its peculiar interest.

During the past fifty years or so there has been a great change in the relationship between doctor and patient. If you look at almost any literature before the later part of the nineteenth century, you find that a hospital is popularly regarded as much the same thing as a prison, and an old-fashioned, dungeon-like prison at that. A hospital is a place of filth, torture, and death, a sort of ante-chamber to the tomb. No one who was not more or less destitute would have thought of going into such a place for treatment. And especially in the early part of the last century, when medical science had grown bolder than before without being any more successful, the whole business of doctoring was looked on with horror and dread by ordinary people. Surgery, in particular, was believed to be no more than a peculiarly gruesome form of sadism, and dissection, possible only with the aid of body-snatchers, was even confused with necromancy. From the nineteenth century you could collect a large horror-literature connected with doctors and hospitals. Think of poor old George III, in his dotage, shrieking for mercy as he sees his surgeons approaching to "bleed him till he faints"! Think of the conversations of Bob Sawyer and Benjamin Allen, which no doubt are hardly parodies, or the field hospitals in *La Débâcle* and *War and Peace,* or that shocking description of an amputation in Melville's *Whitejacket!* Even the names given to doctors in nineteenth-century English fiction, Slasher, Carver, Sawyer, Fillgrave, and so on, and the generic nickname "sawbones," are about as grim as they are comic. The anti-surgery tradition is perhaps best expressed in Tennyson's poem, *The Children's Hospital,* which is essentially a pre-chloroform document though it seems to have been written as late as 1880. Moreover, the outlook which Tennyson records in this poem had a lot to be said for it. When you consider what an operation without anaesthetics must have been like, what it notoriously *was* like, it is difficult not to suspect the motives of people who would undertake such things. For these bloody horrors which the students so eagerly looked forward to ("A magnificent sight if Slasher does it!") were admittedly more or less useless: the patient who did not die of shock usually died of gangrene, a result which was taken for granted. Even now doctors can be found whose motives are questionable. Anyone who has had much illness, or who has listened to medical students talking, will know what I mean. But anaesthetics were a turning point, and disinfectants were another. Nowhere in the world, probably, would you now see the kind of scene described by Axel Munthe in *The Story of San Michele,* when the sinister surgeon in top-hat and frock-coat, his starched shirtfront spattered with blood and pus, carves up patient after patient with the same knife and flings the severed limbs into a pile beside the table. Moreover, national health insurance has partly done away with the idea that a working-class patient is a pauper who deserves little consideration. Well into this century it was usual for "free" patients at the big hospitals to have their teeth extracted with no anaesthetic. They didn't pay, so why should they have an anesthetic—that was the attitude. That too has changed.

And yet every institution will always bear upon it some lingering memory of its past. A barrack-room is still haunted by the ghost of Kipling, and it is difficult to enter a workhouse without being reminded of *Oliver Twist.* Hospitals began as a kind of casual ward for lepers and the like to die in, and they continued as places where medical students learned their art on the bodies of the poor. You can still catch a faint suggestion of their history in their characteristically gloomy architecture. I would be far from complaining about the treatment I have received in any English hospital, but I do know that it is a sound instinct that warns people to keep out of hospitals if possible, and especially out of the public wards. Whatever the legal position may be, it is unquestionable that you have far less control over your own treatment, far less certainty that frivolous experiments will not be tried on you, when it is a case of "accept the discipline or get out." And it is a great thing to die in your own bed, though it is better still to die in your boots. However great the kindness and the efficiency, in every hospital death there will be some cruel, squalid detail, something perhaps too small to be told but leaving terribly painful memories behind, arising out of the haste, the crowding, the impersonality of a place where every day people are dying among strangers.

The dread of hospitals probably still survives among the very poor, and in all of us it has only recently disappeared. It is a dark patch not far beneath the surface of our minds. I have said earlier that when I entered the ward at the Hôpital X I was conscious of a strange feeling of familiarity. What the scene reminded me of, of course, was the reeking, pain-filled hospitals of the nineteenth century, which I had never seen but of which I had a traditional knowledge. And something, perhaps the black-clad doctor with his frowsy black bag, or perhaps only the sickly smell, played the queer trick of unearthing from my memory that poem of Tennyson's, *The Children's Hospital,* which I had not thought of for twenty years. It happened that as a child I had had it read aloud to me by a sick-nurse whose own working life might have stretched back to the time when Tennyson wrote the poem. The horrors and sufferings of the old-style hospitals were a vivid memory to her. We had shuddered over the poem together, and then seemingly I had forgotten it. Even its name would probably have recalled nothing to me. But the first glimpse of the ill-lit murmurous room, with the beds so close together, suddenly roused the train of thought to which it belonged, and in the night that followed I found myself remembering the whole story and atmosphere of the poem, with many of its lines complete.

MICHEL FOUCAULT (1926–1984)

The Birth of the Clinic: An Archaeology of Medical Perception

French philosopher and historical scholar Michel Foucault examined a range of cultural discourses and institutions surrounding madness, medicine, incarceration, and sexuality. The son of a physician, Foucault was educated at the Sorbonne, and in 1970 he was appointed the chair of the History of Systems of Thought at the Collège de France, a position he held until his death. In his analyses of how particular types of knowledge and social institutions came to exist, Foucault always sought to identify the *arche,* the controlling principle that guided their formations, using a method he called "archaeology." *Madness and Civilization* (1961), for example, examined the Enlightenment's concept of reason and its central role in the definition and treatment of the mad, while *The Birth of the Clinic* (1963) traced the emergence of modern medical theory and practice as they took shape under the imperative of a new epistemological principle. The embodiment of this principle was what Foucault called the clinical "gaze," a form and method of knowing that divested the patient of subjectivity and reconfigured him as a semiological field of pathological signs. By the same token, the "gaze" transformed the poor into teaching and research material, objects whose bodies could be bartered for medical progress in exchange for free care.

Modern medicine has fixed its own date of birth as being in the last years of the eighteenth century. Reflecting on its situation, it identifies the origin of its positivity with a return—over and above all theory—to the modest but effecting level of the perceived. In fact, this supposed empiricism is not based on a rediscovery of the absolute values of the visible, nor on the predetermined rejection of systems and all their chimeras, but on a reorganization of that manifest and secret space that opened up when a millennial gaze paused over men's sufferings. Nonetheless the rejuvenation of medical perception, the way colours and things came to life under the illuminating gaze of the first clinicians is no mere myth. At the beginning of the nineteenth century, doctors described what for centuries had remained below the threshold of the visible and the expressible, but this did not mean that, after over-indulging in speculation, they had begun to perceive once again, or that they listened to reason rather than to imagination; it meant that the relation between the visible and invisible—which is necessary to all concrete knowledge—changed its structure, revealing through gaze and language what had previously been below and

From *The Birth of the Clinic: An Archaeology of Medical Perception,* trans. A. M. Sheridan Smith (New York: Pantheon, 1973). Copyright 1963 Presses Universitaires de France.

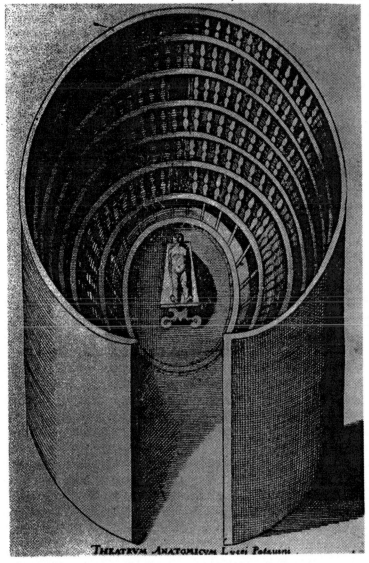

23. *Print of anatomical theater at Padua. From* M.D. *1:2, February 1957. Wellcome Institute Library, London. In 1537, the University of Padua created its first chair of anatomy for Andreas Vesalius, whose demonstrations and lectures soon became the city's most fashionable spectacles. In contrast to Gondouin's grandiose representation (fig. 6), this seventeenth-century print depicts the anatomical theater at Padua with a stark, almost brutal, simplicity. Although it harks back to medieval images of the encapsulated homunculus, the image is, at the same time, eerily modernistic, evoking Foucault's vision of the body subordinated to the "unimpeded empire of the gaze."*

beyond their domain. A new alliance was forged between words and things, enabling one *to see* and *to say*. Sometimes, indeed, the discourse was so completely 'naive' that it seems to belong to a more archaic level of rationality, as if it involved a return to the clear, innocent gaze of some earlier, golden age.

The eye becomes the depositary and source of clarity; it has the power to bring a truth to light that it receives only to the extent that it has brought it to light; as it opens, the eye first opens the truth: a flexion that marks the transition from the world of classical clarity—from the 'enlightenment'—to the nineteenth century. The gaze is no longer reductive, it is, rather, that which establishes the individual in his irreducible quality. And thus it becomes possible to organize a rational language around it. The *object* of discourse may equally well be a *subject*, without the figures of objectivity being in any way altered. It is this *formal* reorganization, *in depth,* rather than the abandonment of theories and old systems, that made *clinical experience* possible; it lifted the old Aristotelian prohibition: one could at last hold a scientifically structured discourse about an individual.

I should like to attempt here the analysis of a type of discourse—that of medical experience—at a period when, before the great discoveries of the nineteenth century, it had changed its materials more than its systematic form. The clinic is both a new 'carving up' of things and the principle of their verbalization in a form which we have been accustomed to recognizing as the language of a 'positive science.' Nonetheless, considered on an over-all basis, the clinic appears—in terms of the doctor's experience—as a new outline of the perceptible and statable. . . .

This new structure is indicated—but not, of course, exhausted—by the minute but decisive change, whereby the question: 'What is the matter with you?,' with which the eighteenth-century dialogue between doctor and patient began (a dialogue possessing its own grammar and style), was replaced by that other question: 'Where does it hurt?,' in which we recognize the operation of the clinic and the principle of its entire discourse.

This new definition of the clinic was bound up with a reorganization of the hospitals. A . . . hidden contract . . . was silently being formed about the same time between the hospital, where the poor were treated, and the clinic, in which doctors were trained. Once again, the thinking of those last days of the Revolution revived, sometimes word for word, what had been formulated in the period immediately preceding it. The most important moral problem raised by the idea of the clinic was the following: by what right can one transform into an object of clinical observation a patient whose poverty has compelled him to seek assistance at the hospital? He had asked for help of which he was the absolute subject, insofar as it had been conceived specifically for him; he was now required to be the object of a gaze, indeed, a relative object, since what was being deciphered in him was seen as contributing to a better knowledge of others. Furthermore, while observing, the clinic was also carrying out research; and this search for the new exposed it to a certain amount of risk: a doctor in private practice, Aikin remarked, must take care of his reputation; his way must be that of safety, if not of certainty; 'In the hospital he is not fettered in this way and his genius may express itself in a new way.' Does not the very essence of hospital aid become altered by the following principle: Hospital patients are, for several reasons, the most suitable subjects for an experimental course?

A certain balance must be kept, of course, between the interests of knowledge and those of the patient; there must be no infringement of the natural rights of the sick, or of the rights that society owes to the poor. The domain of the hospital was an ambiguous one: theoretically free, and, because of the non-contractual character of the relation between doctor and patient, open to the indifference of experiment, it bristled with obligations and moral limitations deriving from the unspoken—but present—contract binding man in general to poverty in its universal form. If, in the hospital, the doctor does not carry out theoretical experiments, free of all obligation to their human object, it is because, as soon as he sets foot in the hospital, he undergoes a decisive moral experience that circumscribes his otherwise unlimited practice by a closed system of duty.

But to look in order to know, to show in order to teach, is not this a tacit form of violence, all the more abusive for its silence, upon a sick body that demands to be comforted, not displayed? Can pain be a spectacle? Not only can it be, but it must be, by virtue of a subtle right that resides in the fact that no one is alone, the poor man less so than others, since he can obtain assistance only through the mediation of the rich. Since disease can be cured only if others intervene with their knowledge, their resources, their pity, since a patient can be cured only in society, it is just that the illnesses of some should be transformed into the experience of others; and that pain should be enabled to manifest itself: 'The sick man does not cease to be a citizen. . . . The history of the illnesses to which he is reduced is necessary to his fellow men because it teaches them by what ills they are threatened.' If he refused to offer himself as an object of instruction, the patient would be guilty of ingratitude, because 'he would have enjoyed the advantages resulting from sociability, without paying the tribute of gratitude.' And in accordance with a structure of reciprocity, there emerges for the rich man the utility of offering help to the hospitalized poor: by paying for them to be treated, he is, by the same token, making possible a greater knowledge of the illnesses with which he himself may be affected; what is benevolence towards the poor is transformed into knowledge that is applicable to the rich.

These, then, were the terms of the contract by which rich and poor participated in the organization of clinical experience. In a regime of economic freedom, the hospital had found a way of interesting the rich; the clinic constitutes the progressive reversal of the other contractual part; it is the *interest* paid by the poor on the capital that the rich have consented to invest in the hospital; an interest that must be understood in its heavy surcharge, since it is a compensation that is of the order of *objective interest* for science and of *vital interest* for the rich. The hospital became viable for private initiative from the moment that sickness, which had come to seek a cure, was turned into a spectacle. Helping ended up by paying, thanks to the virtues of the clinical gaze.

PART 9

The Construction of Pain, Suffering, and Death

FRANCES BURNEY
(MADAME D'ARBLAY) (1752–1840)

"A Mastectomy"

On September 30, 1811, Frances Burney, an English novelist married to General Alexander d'Arblay, underwent breast surgery to remove a tumor her physicians believed to be malignant. At the time, no anesthesia was available. Burney had been living in Paris since 1802, and on March 22, 1812—several months after her operation—she began composing an account of it for her family and friends in England. Attending Burney were two of the most eminent physicians in France: Antoine Dubois, obstetrician to the Empress, and Baron Dominique Jean Larrey, surgeon to Napoleon. To all appearances, the operation was a success, and in 1812, after the Battle of Waterloo, Burney returned to England, where she died at the age of eighty-eight. Like her novels *Evelina* (1778), *Cecilia* (1782), and *Camilla* (1796), Burney's epistolary narrative of her ordeal explores bodily and psychic violation within the context of a social decorum that demands women's self-abnegation in the face of public exposure and humiliation.

[*of* 30 September 1811]

To Esther (Burney) Burney

Separated as I have now so long—long been from my dearest Father—BROTHERS—SISTERS—NIECES, & NATIVE FRIENDS, I would spare, at least, their kind hearts any grief for me but what they must inevitably feel in reflecting upon the sorrow of such an absence to one so tenderly attached to all her first and for-ever so dear & regretted ties—nevertheless, if they should hear that I have been dangerously ill from any hand but my own, they might have doubts of my perfect recovery which my own alone can obviate. But to You, my beloved Esther, who, living more in the World, will surely hear it ere long, to you I will write the whole history.

About August, in the year 1810, I began to be annoyed by a small pain in my breast, which went on augmenting from week to week, yet, being rather heavy than acute, without causing me any uneasiness with respect to consequences: Alas, '*what was the ignorance?*' The most sympathising of Partners, however, was more disturbed: not a start, not a wry face, not a movement that indicated pain was unobserved, & so early conceived apprehensions to which I was a stranger. He pressed me to see some Surgeon; I revolted from the idea, & hoped, by care & warmth, to make all succour unnecessary. Thus passed some months, during which Madame de

---

Excerpts of a letter from Frances Burney (Madame D'Arblay) to Esther (Burney) Burney, September 30, 1811. The Henry W. and Albert A. Berg Collection, The New York Public Library, Astor, Lenox, and Tilden Foundations. From *The Journals and Letters of Frances Burney (Madame D'Arblay)*, ed. Joyce Hemlow, Vol. 6: *France 1803–1812* (Oxford: Clarendon Press, 1975).

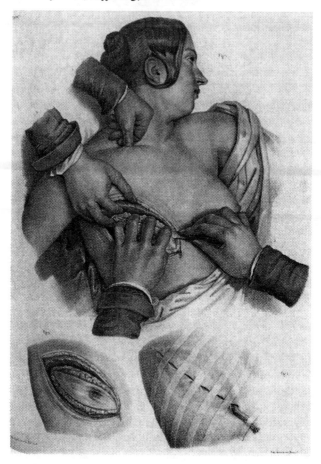

24. N. H. Jacob, Illustration of a mammectomy, from C. A. Delaunay, ed., Iconographie
d'Anatomie Chirurgicale et de Médecine Opératoire, par Le Docteur J. M. Bourgery
*(Paris: Librairie Anatomique, 1840). Special Collections, Health Sciences Library,
Columbia University. This plate from Bourgery's eight-volume series on anatomy and
surgery demonstrates the excision of a cancerous mass in the breast. While an assistant is stanching the blood flow with the thumb of his left hand, the surgeon separates
the tumor from its surrounding tissue with his lancet. The scene is at once disturbing
and aesthetically pleasing, portraying surgery as both a violation as well as a restoration of the integrity of the body. Underplaying the torture of surgery in a preanesthetic
era, the artist stresses the serenity of the woman's face and the flawless beauty of her
skin.*

Maisonneuve, my particularly intimate friend, joined with M. d'Arblay to press me to consent to an examination.

M. Dubois, the most celebrated surgeon of France, was then appointed accoucheur to the Empress, & already lodged in the Tuilleries, & in constant attendance: but nothing could slacken the ardour of M. d'A. to obtain the first advice. Fortunately for his kind wishes, M. Dubois had retained a partial regard for me from the time of his former attendance, &, when applied to through a third person, he took the first moment of liberty, granted by a *promenade* taken by the Empress, to come to me. It was now I began to perceive my real danger, M. Dubois gave me a prescription to be pursued for a month, during which time he could not undertake to see me again, & pronounced nothing—but uttered so many charges to me to be tranquil, & to suffer no uneasiness, that I could not but suspect there was room for terrible inquietude. My alarm was encreased by the non-appearance of M. d'A. after his departure. They had remained together some time in the Book room, & M. d'A. did not return—till, unable to bear the suspence, I begged him to come back. He, also, sought then to tranquilize me—but in words only; his looks were shocking! his features, his whole face displayed the bitterest woe. I had not, therefore, much difficulty in telling myself what he endeavoured not to tell me—that a small operation would be necessary to avert evil consequences!—Ah, my dearest Esther, for this I felt no courage—my dread & repugnance, from a thousand reasons *besides* the pain, almost shook all my faculties, &, for some time, I was rather confounded & stupified than affrighted.— Direful, however, was the effect of this interview; the pains became quicker & more violent, & the hardness of the spot affected encreased. I took, but vainly, my proscription, & every symtom grew more serious. At this time, M. de Narbonne spoke to M. d'A. of a Surgeon of great eminence, M. Larrey, who had cured a polonoise lady of his acquaintance of a similar malady. . . . M. Larrey came, though very unwillingly, & full of scruples concerning M. Dubois . . . & I was now put upon a new *regime*, & animated by the fairest hopes. In fine, I was much better, & every symtom of alarm abated. My good M. Larrey was enchanted, yet so anxious, that he forced me to see le Docteur Ribe, the first anatomist, he said, in France, from his own fear lest he was under any delusion, from the excess of his desire to save me. I was as rebellious to the first visit of this famous anatomist as Maria will tell you I had been to that of M. Dubois, so odious to me was this sort of process: however, I was obliged to submit: & M. Ribe confirmed our best hopes—Here, my dearest Esther, I must grow brief, for my theme becomes less pleasant—. . . . The good M. Larrey, when he came to me next . . . sadly announced his hope of dissolving the hardness [was] nearly extinguished. M. Ribe was now again called in—but he only corroborated the terrible judgement: yet they allowed to my pleadings some further essays, & the more easily as the weather was not propitious to any operation.

A Physician was now called in, Dr. Moreau, to hear if he could suggest any new means: but Dr. Larrey had left him no resources untried. A formal consultation now was held, of Larrey, Ribe, & Moreau—&, in fine, I was formally condemned to an operation by all Three. I was as much astonished as disappointed—for the poor breast was no where discoloured, & not much larger than its healthy neighbour. Yet I felt the evil to be deep, so deep, that I often thought if it could not be dissolved, it could only with life be extirpated. I called up, however, all the reason I possessed, or could assume, & told them—that if they saw no other alternative, I would not resist their opinion & experience:—the good Dr. Larrey, who, during his long attendance had conceived for me the warmest friendship, had now tears in his Eyes; from my dread he had expected resistance. He proposed again calling in M. Dubois. No, I told him, if I could not by himself be saved, I had no sort of hope elsewhere, &, if it must be, what I wanted in courage should be supplied by Confidence. The good man was now dissatisfied with himself, and declared I ought to have the First & most eminent advice his Country could afford. . . . Yet this modest man is premier chirugien de la Garde Imperiale, & had been lately created a Baron for his eminent services!— M. Dubois, he added, from his super-skill & experience, might yet, perhaps, suggest some cure. This conquered me quickly, ah—Send for him! Send for him! I cried—& Dr. Moreau received the commission to consult with him.—What an interval was this! Yet my poor M. d'A was more to be pitied than myself, thought he knew not the terrible idea I had internally annexed to the trial—but Oh what he suffered!—& with what exquisite tenderness he solaced all I had to bear! M. Dubois . . . appointed the earliest day in his power for a general & final consultation. I was informed of it only on the Same day, to avoid useless agitation. He met here Drs. Larrey, Ribe, & Moreau. The case, I saw, offered uncommon difficulties, or presented eminent danger, but, the examination over, they desired to consult together. I left them—what an half hour I passed alone!—M. d'A. was at his office. Dr. Larrey then came to summon me.

I came back, & took my seat, with what calmness I was able. All were silent, & Dr. Larrey, I saw, hid himself nearly behind my Sofa. My heart beat fast: I saw all hope was over. I called upon them to speak. M. Dubois then, after a long & unintelligible harangue, from his own disturbance, pronounced my doom.

All hope of escaping this evil being now at an end, I could only console or employ my Mind in considering how to render it less dreadful to M. d'A. M. Dubois had pronounced 'il faut s'attendre à souffrir, Je ne veux pas vous trompez—Vous Souffrirez—vous souffrirez *beaucoup*!—' M. Ribe had *charged* me to cry! to withhold or restrain myself might have seriously bad consequences, he said. M. Moreau, in ecchoing this injunction, enquired whether I had cried or screamed at the birth of Alexander—Alas, I told him, it had not been possible to do otherwise; Oh then, he answered, there is no fear!—What terrible inferences were here to be drawn! I desired, therefore, that M. d'A. might be kept in ignorance of the day till the operation should be over. To this they agreed. . . . I obtained with difficulty a promise of 4 hours warning, which were essential to me for sundry regulations.

From this time, I assumed the best spirits in my power, *to meet the coming blow*;— & support my too sympathising Partner. They would let me make no preparations, refusing to inform me what would be necessary. . . . M. d'A filled a Closet with Charpie, compresses, & bandages—All that to *me* was owned, as wanting, was an arm Chair & some Towels.—Many things, however, joined to the depth of my pains, assured me the business was not without danger. I therefore made my Will. . . .

In fine, One morning—the last of September, 1811, while I was still in Bed. . . . [A] letter was delivered to me . . . 'twas from M. Larrey, to acquaint me that at 10 o'clock he should be with me, properly accompanied, & to exhort me to rely as much upon his sensibility & his prudence, as upon his dexterity & his experience; he charged to secure the absence of M. d'A: & told me that the young Physician who would deliver me this *announce,* would prepare for the operation, in which he must lend his aid: & also that it had been the decision of the consultation to allow me but two hours notice.

I then, by the Maid, sent word to the young Dr. Aumont that I could not be ready till one o'clock: & I finished my breakfast, &—not with much appetite, you will believe! forced down a crust of bread, & hurried off, under various pretences, M. d'A. He was scarcely gone, when M. Du Bois arrived: I renewed my request for one o'clock: the rest came; all were fain to consent to the delay, for I had an apartment to prepare for my banished Mate. This arrangement, & those for myself, occupied me completely. Two engaged nurses were out of the way—I had a bed, Curtains, & heaven knows what to prepare—but business was good for my nerves. I was obliged to quit my room to have it put in order:—Dr. Aumont would not leave the house; he remained in the Sallon, folding linen!—He had demanded 4 or 5 old & fine left off under Garments. I strolled to the Sallon—I saw it fitted with preparations, & I recoiled—But I soon returned; to what effect disguise from myself what I must so soon know?—yet the sight of the immense quantity of bandages, compresses, spunges, Lint—Made me a little sick:—I walked backwards & forwards till I quieted all emotion, & became, by degrees, nearly stupid—torpid, without sentiment or consciousness:—& thus I remained till the Clock struck three.

I rang for my Maid & Nurses,—but before I could speak to them, my room, without previous message, was entered by 7 Men in black, Dr. Larrey, M. Dubois, Dr. Moreau, Dr. Aumont, Dr. Ribe, & a pupil of Dr. Larrey, & another of M. Dubois. I was now awakened from my stupor—& by a sort of indignation—Why so many? & without leave?—But I could not utter a syllable. M. Dubois acted as Commander in Chief. Dr. Larrey kept out of sight; M. Dubois ordered a Bed stead into the middle of the room. Astonished, I turned to Dr. Larrey, who had promised that an Arm Chair would suffice; but he hung his head, & would not look at me. Two *old mattrasses* M. Dubois then demanded, & an old Sheet. I now began to tremble violently, more with distaste & horrour of the preparations even than of the pain. These arranged to his liking, he desired me to mount the Bed stead. I stood suspended, for a moment, whether I should not abruptly escape. I called to my maid—she was crying, & the two Nurses stood, transfixed, at the door. Let those women all go! cried M. Dubois. This order recovered me my Voice—No, I cried, let them stay! *qu'elles restent!* M. Dubois now tried to issue his commands *en militaire,* but I resisted all that were resistable—I was compelled, however, to submit to taking off my long robe de Chambre, which I had meant to retain. My distress was, I suppose, apparent, though not my Wishes, for M. Dubois himself now softened, & spoke soothingly. Can *You,* I cried, feel for an operation that, to *You,* must seem so trivial?—Trivial? he repeated—taking up a bit of paper, which he tore, unconsciously, into a million of pieces, *oui—c'est peu de chose—mais—*' he stammered, & could not go on. No one else attempted to speak, but I was softened myself, when I saw even M. Dubois grow agitated, while Dr. Larrey kept always aloof, yet a glance shewed me he was pale as ashes.

I mounted . . . unbidden, the Bed stead—& M. Dubois placed me upon the Mattress, & spread a cambric handkerchief upon my face. It was transparent, however, & I saw, through it, that the Bed stead was instantly surrounded by the 7 men & my nurse. I refused to be held; but when, Bright through the cambric; I saw the glitter of polished Steel—I closed my Eyes. I would not trust to convulsive fear the sight of the terrible incision. A silence the most profound ensued, which lasted for some minutes, during which, I imagine, they took their orders by signs, & made their examination—Oh what a horrible suspension!—I did not breathe—& M. Dubois tried vainly to find any pulse. This pause, at length, was broken by Dr. Larrey, who, in a voice of solemn melancholy, said 'Qui me tiendra ce sein?—'

No one answered; at least not verbally; but this aroused me from my passively submissive state, for I feared they imagined the whole breast infected—feared it too justly,—for, again through the Cambric, I saw the hand of M. Dubois held up, while his fore finger first described a straight line from top to bottom of the breast, secondly a Cross, & thirdly a circle; intimating that the WHOLE was to be taken off. Excited by this idea, I started up, threw off my veil, &, in answer to the demand 'Qui me tiendra ce sein,? cried 'C'est moi, Monsieur!' & I held My hand under it, & explained the nature of my sufferings, which all sprang from one point, though they darted into every part. I was heard attentively, but in utter silence, & M. Dubois then re-placed me as before, &, as before, spread my veil over my face. How vain, alas, my representation! immediately again I saw the fatal finger describe the Cross—& the circle—Hopeless, then, desperate, & self-given up, I closed once more my Eyes, relinquishing all watching, all resistance, all interference, & sadly resolute to be wholly resigned.

. . . [T]his resolution once taken, was firmly adhered to, in defiance of a terror that surpasses all description, & the most torturing pain. Yet—when the dreadful steel was plunged into the breast—cutting through veins—arteries—flesh—nerves—I needed no injunctions not to restrain my cries. I began a scream that lasted unintermittingly during the whole time of the incision—& I almost marvel that it rings not in my Ears still! so excruciating was the agony. When the wound was made, & the instrument was withdrawn, the pain seemed undiminished, for the air that suddenly rushed into those delicate parts felt like a mass of minute but sharp & forked poniards, that were tearing the edges of the wound—but when again I felt the instrument—describing a curve—cutting against the grain, if I may so say, while the flesh resisted in a manner so forcible as to oppose & tire the hand of the operator, who was forced to change from the right to the left—then, indeed, I thought I must have expired. I attempted no more to open my Eyes,—they felt as if hermettically shut, & so firmly closed, that the Eyelids seemed indented into the Cheeks. The instrument this second time withdrawn, I concluded the operation over— Oh no! presently the terrible cutting was renewed—& worse than ever, to separate the bottom, the foundation of this dreadful gland from the parts to which it adhered— Again all description would be baffled—yet again all was not over,—Dr Larrey rested but his own hand, &—Oh Heaven!—I then felt the Knife <rack>ling against the breast bone—scraping it!—This performed, while I yet remained in utterly speechless torture, I heard the Voice of Mr. Larrey,—(all others guarded a dead silence) in a tone nearly tragic, desire every one present to pronounce if any thing more remained to be done; The general voice was Yes,—but the finger of Mr. Dubois—which I literally *felt* elevated over the wound, though I saw nothing, & though he touched nothing, so indescribably sensitive was the spot—pointed to some further requisition—& again began the scraping!—and, after this, Dr. Moreau thought he discerned a peccant attom—and still, & still, M. Dubois demanded attom after attom.

. . . [E]ven now, 9 months after it is over, I have a head ache from going on with the account! & this miserable account, which I began 3 Months ago, at least, I dare not revise, nor read, the recollection is still so painful. . . . [T]he operation, including the treatment & the dressing, lasted 20 minutes! a time, for sufferings so acute, that was hardly supportable—However, I bore it with all the courage I could exert, & never moved, nor stopt them, nor resisted, nor remonstrated, nor spoke—except once or twice, during the dressings, to say 'Ah Messieurs! que je vous plains!—' for indeed I was sensible to the feeling concern with which they all saw what I endured. . . . Twice, I believe, I fainted; at least, I have two total chasms in my memory of this transaction, that impede my tying together what passed. When all was done, & they lifted me up that I might be put to bed, my strength was so totally annihilated, that I was obliged to be carried, & could not even sustain my hands & arms, which hung as if I had been lifeless; while my face, as the Nurse has told me, was utterly colourless. This removal made me open my Eyes—& I then saw my good Dr. Larrey, pale nearly as myself, his face streaked with blood, & its expression depicting grief, apprehension, & almost horrour.

When I was in bed,—my poor M. d'Arblay—who ought to write you himself his own history of this Morning—was called to me—& afterwards our Alex.—

God bless my dearest Esther—I fear this is all written—confusedly, but I cannot read it—& I can write it no more, therefore I entreat you to let all my dear Brethren male & female take a perusal. . . .

WILLIAM COWPER (1731–1800)

"Memoir of the Early Life"

Trained as a British barrister, William Cowper became a poet of great distinction, combining religious sentiment with a celebration of nature's beauty. Cowper's mother died in childbirth when he was six, and four years later, he was sent to Westminster School, where he boarded until his graduation at the age of eighteen. In 1759, he was made Commissioner of Bankrupts but resigned the post several years later because of a moral and mental crisis that involved agonizing religious terrors. The publication in 1785 of Cowper's most well-known poem, "The Task," secured his fame as a poet and drew around him a devoted circle of admirers, friends, and relatives. Suffering intermittent bouts of mental collapse for the next two years, Cowper failed to recover from his last "attack" in 1787, after which he was frequently subject to delusions, voices, and bizarre imaginings. Cowper began to compose his narrative "memoir" in 1765, never intending it for general publication. Given his evangelical inclinations, he framed his ordeal as a spiritual autobiography, a tale of conversion in which the restoration of the mind was secondary to the redemption of the soul. Cowper's stated purpose in recording his experiences was to benefit his close friends and relatives, who, he hoped, would gain solace and draw useful lessons from seeing "the Sovereignty of God's free grace in the deliverance of a Sinfull Soul from the nethermost Hell."

At six years old I was taken from the nursery and from the immediate care of a most indulgent mother and sent to a considerable school in Bedfordshire. Here I had hardships of different kinds to conflict with, which I felt more sensibly in proportion to the tenderness with which I had been treated at home. But my chief affliction consisted in my being singled out from all the other boys by a lad about fifteen years of age as a proper project upon whom he might let loose the cruelty of his temper. I choose to forbear a particular recital of the many acts of barbarity with which he made it his business continually to persecute me; it will be sufficient to say that he had by his savage treatment of me impressed such a dread of his figure upon my mind that I well remember being afraid to lift up my eyes upon him higher than his knees, and that I knew him by his shoe-buckles better than any other part of his dress. May the Lord pardon him and may we meet in glory!

One day as I was sitting alone on a bench in the school, melancholy and almost ready to weep at the recollection of what I had already suffered and expecting at the same time my tormentor every moment, these words of the Psalmist came into my mind, "I will not be afraid of what man can do unto me." I applied this to my own

From "Memoir of William Cowper: An Autobiography," ed. Maurice J. Quinlan, *Proceedings of the American Philosophical Society* 97 (4) (September 1953):359–382.

case with a degree of trust and confidence in God that would have been no disgrace to a much more experienced Christian. Instantly I perceived in myself a briskness of spirits and a cheerfulness which I had never before experienced, and took several paces up and down the room with joyful alacrity—*his gift* in whom I trusted. Happy had it been for me if this early effort towards a dependence on the blessed God had been frequently repeated by me. But alas! it was the first and last instance of the kind between infancy and manhood. The cruelty of this boy, which he had long practised in so secret a manner that no creature suspected it, was at length discovered. He was expelled from the school and I was taken from it.

From hence at eight years old I was sent to Mr. D, an eminent surgeon and oculist, having very weak eyes and being in danger of losing one of them. I continued a year in this family, where religion was neither known nor practised, and from thence was dispatched to Westminster. Whatever seeds of religion I might carry thither before my seven years' apprenticeship to the classics was expired, they were all marred and corrupted; the duty of the school-boy swallowed up every other; and I acquired Latin and Greek at the expense of a knowledge much more important.

At the age of eighteen, being tolerably furnished with grammatical knowledge but as ignorant in all points of religion as the satchel at my back, I was taken from Westminster and, having spent about nine months at home, was sent to acquire the practice of the law with an attorney. There I might have lived and died without hearing or seeing anything that might remind me of a single Christian duty, had it not been that I was at liberty to spend my leisure time (which was well nigh all my time) at my uncle's in Southampton Row. By this means I had indeed an opportunity of seeing the inside of a church, whither I went with the family on Sundays, which probably I should otherwise never have seen.

At the expiration of this term I became in a manner complete master of myself and took possession of a complete set of chambers in the Temple at the age of twenty-one. This being a critical season of my life and one upon which much depended, it pleased my all-merciful Father in Jesus Christ to give a check to my rash and ruinous career of wickedness at the very onset. I was struck not long after my settlement in the Temple with such a dejection of spirits as none but they who have felt the same can have the least conception of. Day and night I was upon the rack, lying down in horror and rising up in despair. I presently lost all relish for those studies to which I had before been closely attached; the classics no longer had any charms for me; I had need of something more salutary than amusement, but I had no one to direct me where to find it.

A change of scene was recommended to me, and I embraced an opportunity of going with some friends to Southampton, where I spent several months. Soon after our arrival we walked to a place called Freemantle about a mile from the town; the morning was clear and calm; the sun shone bright upon the sea; and the country on the borders of it was the most beautiful I had ever seen. We sat down upon an eminence at the end of the arm of the sea which runs between Southampton and the New Forest. Here it was that on a sudden, as if another sun had been kindled that instant in the heavens on purpose to dispel sorrow and vexation of spirit, I felt the weight of all my misery taken off; my heart became light and joyful in a moment; I could have wept with transport had I been alone. I must needs believe that nothing less than the Almighty fiat could have filled me with such inexpressible delight, not by a gradual dawning of peace, but, as it were, with a flash of his life-giving countenance. I think I remember something like a glow of gratitude to the Father of mercies for this unexpected blessing and that I ascribed it to his gracious acceptance of my prayers. But Satan and my own wicked heart quickly persuaded me that I was indebted for my deliverance to nothing but a change of scene and the amusing varieties of the place. By this means he turned the blessing into a poison, teaching me to conclude that nothing but a continued circle of diversion and indulgence of appetite could secure me from a relapse.

By this time, my patrimony being well nigh spent and there being no appearance that I should ever repair the damage by a fortune of my own getting, I began to be a little apprehensive of approaching want. It was, I imagine, under some apprehensions of this kind that I one day said to a friend of mine, if the clerk to the journals of the House of Lords should die I had some hopes that my kinsman who had the place in his disposal would appoint me to succeed him. We both agreed that the business of that place, being transacted in private, would exactly suit me, and both expressed an earnest wish for his death that I might be provided for. Thus did I covet what God had commanded me not to covet and involved myself in still deeper guilt by doing it in the spirit of a murderer. It pleased the Lord to give me my heart's desire and with it an immediate punishment for my crime. The poor man died and by his death not only the clerkship of the journals became vacant but it became necessary to appoint officers to two other places. . . . I was bid to expect an examination at the bar of the House touching my sufficiency for the post I had taken. Being necessarily ignorant of the nature of that business, it became expedient that I should visit the office daily in order to qualify myself for the strictest scrutiny. All the horror of my fears and perplexities now returned. A thunderbolt would have been as welcome to me as this intelligence. The feelings of a man when he arrives at the place of execution are probably much like mine every time I set my foot in the office, which was every day for more than half a year together.

A thought would sometimes come across my mind that my sins had perhaps brought this distress upon me, that the hand of divine vengeance was in it, but in the pride of my heart I presently acquitted myself and thereby implicitly charged God with injustice, saying, "What sins have I committed to deserve this?"

I saw plainly that God alone could deliver me, but was firmly persuaded that he would not and therefore omitted to ask it.

I now began to look upon madness as the only chance remaining. I had a strong kind of foreboding that so it would one day fare with me, and I wished for it earnestly and looked forward to it with impatient expectation.

Now came the grand temptation, the point to which all the while Satan had been driving me, the dark and hellish purpose of self-murder. I grew more sullen and reserved, fled from all society, even from my most intimate friends, and shut myself up in my chambers.

Being reconciled to the apprehension of madness, I began to be reconciled to the apprehension of death. Though formerly in my happiest hours I had never been able to glance a single thought that way without shuddering at the idea of dissolution, I now wished for it and found myself but little shocked at the idea of procuring it myself. Perhaps, thought I, there is no God; or if there be, the scriptures may be false; if so then God has nowhere forbidden suicide. I considered life as my property and therefore at my own disposal. Men of great name, I observed, had destroyed themselves, and the world still retained the profoundest respect for their memories.

But above all I was persuaded to believe that if the act were ever so unlawful and even supposing Christianity to be true, my misery in hell itself would be more supportable. I well recollect, too, that when I was about eleven years of age my father desired me to read a vindication of self-murder and give him my sentiments upon the question. I did so and argued against it. My father heard my reasons and was silent, neither approving or disapproving, from whence I inferred that he sided with the author against me. . . . One evening in November, 1763, as soon as it was dark, affecting as cheerful and unconcerned an air as possible, I went into an apothecary's shop and asked for an half ounce phial of laudanum. The man seemed to observe me narrowly, but if he did I managed my voice and countenance so as to deceive him. I repaired to my room and having shut both the outer and inner door prepared myself for the last scene of the tragedy. I poured the laudanum into a small basin, set it on a chair by the bedside, half undressed myself, and laid down between the blankets, shuddering with horror at what I was about to perpetrate. I reproached myself bitterly with folly and rank cowardice for having suffered the fear of death to influence me as it had done and was filled with disdain at my own pitiful timidity: but still something seemed to overrule me and to say *"Think what you are doing! Consider and live."*

At length, however, with the most confirmed resolution, I reached forth my hand towards the basin, when the fingers of both hands were as closely contracted as if bound with a cord and became entirely useless. Still, indeed, I could have made shift with both hands, dead and lifeless as they were, to have raised the basin to my mouth, for my arms were not at all affected: but this new difficulty struck me with wonder; it had the air of a divine interposition.

I spent the rest of the day in a kind of stupid insensibility, undetermined as to the manner of dying but still bent on self-murder as the only possible deliverance.

I went to bed, as I thought, to take my last sleep in this world. I slept as usual and awoke about three o'clock. Immediately I arose and by the help of a rushlight found my penknife, took it into bed with me, and lay with it for some hours directly pointed against my heart. Twice or thrice I placed it upright under my left breast, leaning all my weight upon it, but the point was broken off and would not penetrate.

In this manner the time passed till the day began to break. I heard the clock strike seven, and instantly it occurred to me there was no time to be lost. . . . Not one hesitating thought now remained, but I fell greedily to the execution of my purpose. My garter was made of a broad scarlet binding with a sliding buckle being sewn together at the ends; by the help of the buckle I made a noose and fixed it about my neck, straining it so tight that I hardly left a passage for my breath or for the blood to circulate; the tongue of the buckle held it fast. At each corner of the bed was placed a wreath of carved work fastened by an iron pin which passed up through the midst of it. The other part of the garter which made a loop I slipped over one of these and hung by it some seconds, drawing up my feet under me that they might not touch the floor; but the iron bent, the carved work slipped off, and the garter with it. I then fastened it to the frame of the tester, winding it round and typing it in a strong knot. The frame broke short and let me down again.

The third effort was more likely to succeed. I set the door open, which reached within a foot of the ceiling; by the help of a chair I could command the top of it, and the loop, being large enough to admit a large angle of the door, was easily fixed so as not to slip off again. I pushed away the chair with my feet and hung at my whole length. While I hung there I distinctly heard a voice say three times, *" 'Tis over!"* Though I am sure of the fact and was so at the time, yet it did not at all alarm me or affect my resolution. I hung so long that I lost all sense, all consciousness of existence.

When I came to myself again I thought myself in hell; the sound of my own dreadful groans was all that I heard, and a feeling like that of flashes was just beginning to seize upon my whole body. In a few seconds I found myself fallen with my face to the floor. In about half a minute I recovered my feet and reeling and staggering I stumbled into bed again.

By the blessed providence of God the garter which had held me till the bitterness of temporal death was past broke just before eternal death had taken place upon me.

Soon after I got into bed I was surprised to hear a noise in the dining-room, where the laundress was lighting a fire; she had found the door unbolted, notwithstanding my design to fasten it, and must have passed the bed-chamber door while I was hanging on it and yet never perceived me.

To this moment I had felt no concern of a spiritual kind. Ignorant of original sin, insensible of the guilt of actual transgression, I understood neither the law nor the gospel—the condemning nature of the one nor the restoring mercies of the other. I was as much unacquainted with Christ in all his saving offices as if his blessed name had never reached me. Now, therefore, a new scene opened upon me. Conviction of sin took place, especially of that just committed; the meanness of it as well as its atrocity were exhibited to me in colours so inconceivably strong that I despised myself with a contempt not to be imagined or expressed for having attempted it. This sense of it secured me from the repetition of a crime which I could not now reflect on without abhorrence.

My sins were now set in an array against me, and I began to see and feel that I had lived without God in the world. As I walked to and fro in my chamber I said within myself, *"There never was so abandoned a wretch, so great a sinner."*

In every book I opened I found something that struck me to the heart. I remember taking up a volume of Beaumont and Fletcher which lay upon the table in my kinsman's lodgings and the first sentence which I saw was this, "The justice of the gods is in it." My heart instantly replied, "It is the truth," and I cannot but observe that as I found something in every author to condemn me so it was the first sentences in general I pitched upon. Everything preached to me, and everything preached the curse of the law.

I never went into the street but I thought the people stood and laughed at me and held me in contempt, and could hardly persuade myself but that the voice of my conscience was loud enough for every one to hear it. They who knew me seemed to avoid me, and if they spoke to me seemed to do it in scorn. I bought a ballad of one who was singing it in the street because I thought it was written on me.

I dined alone either at the tavern, where I went in the dark, or at the chop-house, where I always took care to hide myself in the darkest corner of the room. I slept generally an hour in the evening, but it was only to be terrified in dreams, and when I awoke it was some time before I could walk steadily through the passage into the dining-room. I reeled and staggered like a drunken man; the eyes of man I could not bear.

Another time I seemed to pronounce to myself, "Evil be thou my good." I verily thought that I had adopted that hellish sentiment—it seemed to come so directly from my heart. I rose from bed to look for my prayer-book and having found it endeavoured to pray, but immediately experienced the impossibility of drawing nigh to God unless he first draw nigh to us. I made many passionate attempts towards prayer but failed in all.

I felt a sense of burning in my heart like that of real fire and concluded it was an earnest of those eternal flames which would soon receive me. I laid myself down, howling with horror while my knees smote against each other.

In this condition my brother found me, and the first words I spoke to him were, "Oh! Brother, I am damned! think of eternity and then think what it is to be damned!" I had indeed a sense of eternity impressed upon my mind which seemed almost to amount to a full comprehension of it.

My brother, pierced to the heart with the sight of my misery, tried to comfort me, but all to no purpose. I refused comfort, and my mind appeared to me in such colours that to administer it to me was only to exasperate me and to mock my fears. I slept my three hours well and then awoke with ten times a stronger alienation from God than ever.

Satan plied me closely with horrible visions and more horrible voices.

At eleven o'clock my brother called upon me, and in about an hour after his arrival that distemper of mind which I had so ardently wished for actually seized me.

While I traversed the apartment in the most horrible dismay of soul, expecting every moment that the earth would open her mouth and swallow me, my conscience scaring me, the avenger of blood pursuing me, and the city of refuge out of reach and out of sight, a strange and horrible darkness fell upon me. If it were possible that a heavy blow could light on the brain without touching the skull, such was the sensation I felt. I clapped my hand to my forehead and cried aloud through the pain it gave me. At every stroke my thoughts and expressions became more wild and incoherent; all that remained clear was the sense of sin and the expectation of punishment. These kept undisturbed possession all through my illness without interruption or abatement.

My brother instantly observed the change and consulted with my friends on the best manner to dispose of me. It was agreed among them that I should be carried to St. Albans, where Dr. Cotton kept a house for the reception of such patients, and with whom I was known to have a slight acquaintance. Not only his skill as a physician recommended him to their choice but his well-known humanity and sweetness of temper. It will be proper to draw a veil over the secrets of my prison-house; let it suffice to say that the low state of body and mind to which I was reduced was perfectly well calculated to humble the natural vain-glory and pride of my heart.

These are the efficacious means which Infinite Wisdom thought meet to make use of for that purpose. A sense of self-loathing and abhorrence ran through all my insanity. Conviction of sin and expectation of instant judgment never left me from the 7th of December, 1763, until the middle of July following.

After five months of continual expectation that the divine vengeance would plunge me into the bottomless pit, I became so familiar with despair as to have contracted a sort of hardiness and indifference as to the event. I began to persuade myself that while the execution of the sentence was suspended it would be for my interest to indulge a less horrible train of ideas than I had been accustomed to muse upon. "Eat and drink for to-morrow thou shalt be in hell" was the maxim on which I proceeded. By this means I entered into conversation with the Doctor, laughed at his stories, and told him some of my own to match them—still, however, carrying a sentence of irrevocable doom in my heart.

In about three months more (July 25, 1764) my brother came from Cambridge to visit me. Dr. C. having told him that he thought me greatly amended, he was rather disappointed at finding me almost as silent and reserved as ever, for the first sight of him struck me with many painful sensations both of sorrow for my own remediless condition and envy of his happiness.

As soon as we were left alone he asked me how I found myself; I answered, "As much better as despair can make me." We went together into the garden. Here on expressing a settled assurance of sudden judgment, he protested to me that it was all a delusion and protested so strongly that I could not help giving some attention to him. I burst into tears and cried out, "If it be a delusion then am I the happiest of beings." Something like a ray of hope was shot into my heart, but still I was afraid to indulge it. We dined together, and I spent the afternoon in a more cheerful manner. Something seemed to whisper to me every moment, "Still there is mercy."

I went to bed and slept well. In the morning I dreamed that the sweetest boy I ever saw came dancing up to my beside; he seemed just out of leading-strings, yet I took particular notice of the firmness and steadiness of his tread. The sight affected me with pleasure and served at least to harmonize my spirits, so that I awoke for the first time with a sensation of delight on my mind. Still, however, I knew not where to look for the establishment of the comfort I felt; my joy was as much a mystery to myself as to those about me. The blessed God was preparing me for the clearer light of his countenance by this first dawning of that light upon me.

But the happy period which was to shake off my fetters and afford me a clear opening of the free mercy of God in Christ Jesus was now arrived. I flung myself into a chair near the window and, seeing a Bible there, ventured once more to apply to it for comfort and instruction. The first verse I saw was the 25th of the 3rd of Romans: "Whom God hath set forth to be a propitiation through faith in his blood to declare his righteousness for the remission of sins that are past through the forbearance of God."

Immediately I received strength to believe it, and the full beams of the Sun of Righteousness shone upon me. I saw the sufficiency of the atonement he had made, my pardon sealed in his blood, and all the fulness and completeness of his justification. In a moment I believed and received the gospel. My eyes filled with tears and my voice choked with transport, I could only look up to heaven in silent fear, overwhelmed with love and wonder. But the works of the Holy Ghost is best described in his own words. It is "joy unspeakable and full of glory." Thus was my heavenly Father in Christ Jesus pleased to give me the full assurance of faith and out of a strong, stony, unbelieving heart to raise up a child unto Abraham.

I now employed my brother to seek out an abode for me in the neighbourhood of Cambridge, being determined by the Lord's leave to see London, the scene of my former abominations, no more.

In the beginning of June, 1765, I received a letter from my brother to say he had taken lodgings for me at Huntingdon which he believed would suit me. Thought it was sixteen miles from Cambridge I was resolved to take them, for I had been two months in perfect health, and my circumstances required a less expensive way of life. It was with great reluctance, however, that I thought of leaving the place of my second nativity; I had so much leisure there to study the blessed word of God and had enjoyed so much happiness; but God ordered everything for me like an indulgent Father and had prepared a more comfortable place of residence than I could have chosen for myself.

I took possession of my new abode Nov. 11, 1765. I have found it a place of rest prepared for me by God's own hand, where he has blessed me with a thousand mercies and instances of his fatherly protection, and where he has given me abundant means of furtherance in the knowledge of our Lord Jesus, both by the study of his own word and communion with his dear disciples. May nothing but death interrupt our union!

"Answer to the Religious Objections Advanced against the Employment of Anaesthetic Agents in Midwifery and Surgery"

James Simpson received his medical degree from the University of Edinburgh and served as its professor of midwifery from 1840 until his death. Author of several works on gynecology and obstetrics, Simpson helped lay the foundations of these specialties by inventing the uterine sound—an examining instrument—and anticipating the development of ovariotomy. It is not, however, for these achievements that he is most re-membered. On November 4, 1847, Simpson, along with two colleagues, inhaled doses of chloroform, the anesthetic that would soon revolutionize not only childbirth but the whole of surgery. Simpson's experiment quickly sparked a prolonged and heated debate about the safety and moral advis-ability of administering chloroform to women in labor. Among the objec-tions physicians raised against anesthesia was its tendency to lift the patient's sexual inhibitions, creating situations in which the lying-in room was, in the words of one physician, "defiled by the most painful and obscene con-versation" and "sexual orgasm was substituted for . . . natural pains." Some physicians took another tack, arguing that these "natural" pains existed by virtue of God's will and that their amelioration was irrevocably prohibited by biblical injunction.

Along with many of my professional brethren in Scotland, and perhaps elsewhere, I have, during the last few months, often heard patients and others strongly object to the superinduction of anaesthesia in labour, by the inhalation of Ether or Chloro-form, on the assumed ground, that an immunity from pain during parturition was contrary to religion and the express commands of Scripture. Not a few medical men have, I know, joined in this same objection; and have refused to relieve their pa-tients from the agonies of childbirth, on the allegation that they believed that their employment of suitable anaesthetic means for such a purpose would be unscriptural and irreligious. And I am informed, that in another medical school, my conduct in introducing and advocating the superinduction of anaesthesia in labour has been pub-licly denounced *ex cathedra* as an attempt to contravene the arrangements and de-crees of Providence, hence reprehensible and heretical in its character, and anxiously

From *Anaesthesia, or the Employment of Chloroform and Ether in Surgery, Midwifery, Etc.* (Phila-delphia, 1849).

to be avoided and eschewed by all properly principled students and practitioners. I have been favoured with various earnest private communications to the same effect. Probably, therefore, I may be excused if I attempt, however imperfectly, to point out what I conscientiously conceive to be the errors and fallacies of those who thus believe that the practice in question ought in any degree to be opposed and rejected on religious grounds. I shall, therefore, in the first place, quote the words of it in full from the third chapter of Genesis. . . .

> GENESIS, chap. iii, v. 14.—"And the Lord God said unto the serpent,— Because thou hast done this, thou art cursed above all cattle, and above every beast of the field; upon thy belly shalt thou go, and dust shalt thou eat all the days of thy life.
>
> 15. "And I will put enmity between thee and the woman, and between thy seed and her seed; it shall bruise thy head and thou shalt bruise his heel.
>
> 16. "Unto the woman he said, I will greatly multiply thy sorrow (*'itztzabhon*) and thy conception, in sorrow (*'etzebh*) thou shalt bring forth children; and thy desire shall be to thy husband, and he shall rule over thee.
>
> 17. "And unto Adam he said,—Because thou hast hearkened unto the voice of thy wife, and hast eaten of the tree, of which I commanded thee, saying, Thou shalt not eat of it; cursed is the ground for thy sake: in sorrow (*'itztzabhon*) shalt thou eat of it all the days of thy life.
>
> 18. "Thorns also and thistles shall it bring forth to thee; and thou shalt eat the herb of the field.
>
> 19. "In the sweat of thy face shalt thou eat bread, till thou return unto the ground; for out of it wast thou taken: for dust thou art, and unto dust shall thou return."

I would begin by observing, that,—

The primeval curse is triple. It contains a judgment, First, upon the serpent (verses 14, 15); Secondly, upon the woman (v. 16); and, Thirdly, upon the ground for the sake of the man (v. 17–19). Those who, from the terms of the first curse, argue against the superinduction of anaesthesia in labour, aver that we are bound to take and act upon the words of the curse *literally* . . . "I will greatly multiply the sorrow *of* thy conception; in sorrow thou shall bring forth children."

Now if . . . the whole curse is, as it averred, to be understood and acted on literally, then man must be equally erring and sinning, when, as now, instead of his own sweat and personal exertions, he employs the horse and the ox—water and steam power—sowing, reaping, thrashing, and grinding machines, &c., to do this work for him, and elaborate the "bread" which he eats. The ever active intellect which God has bestowed upon man, has urged him on to the discovery of these and similar inventions. But if the first curse must be read and acted on literally, it has so far urged him on to these improper acts by which he thus saves himself from the effects of that curse. Nay, more; if some physicians hold that they feel conscientiously constrained not to relieve the agonies of a woman in childbirth, because it was ordained that she should bring forth in sorrow, then they ought to feel conscientiously constrained on the very same grounds not to use their professional skill and art to prevent man from dying; for at the same time it was decreed, by the same authority with the same force, that man should be subject to death,—"dust thou art, and unto dust shalt thou return."

But does the word sorrow ("in sorrow thou shalt bring forth children") really mean physical and bodily *pain,* as is taken for granted by those who maintain the improper and irreligious character of any means used to assuage and annul the sufferings of childbirth? Now, the word "sorrow" occurs there several times in two consecutive verses of the curse; (verses 16 and 17). The corresponding word, or rather words, in the original Hebrew . . . are *'etzebh,* and *'itztzabhon.* The meaning of the verb *'atzabh* (the root of these nouns) is 1. To *labour,* to *form,* to *fashion.* 2. To *toil with pain,* to *suffer,* to be *grieved;* used also of the mind." . . . In fact, the Hebrew word for *labour* (in the sense of work or toil) is exactly like the English word *labour,* used also to import the act of parturition. Certainly, the greatest characteristic of human parturition as compared with parturition in the lower animals, is the enormous amount of muscular action and effort (labour) provided for, and usually required for its consummation. The erect position (*vultus ad sidera erectus*) of the human body, renders a series of peculiar mechanical arrangements and obstructions necessary in the human pelvis, &c., for the prevention of abortion and premature labour, and for the well-being of the mother during pregnancy. But these same mechanical adaptations and arrangements . . . all render also, at last, the ultimate expulsion of the infant in labour, a far more difficult, and more prolonged process than in the quadruped, for instance, with its horizontal body. To overcome these greater mechanical obstacles, the human mother is provided with a uterus immensely more muscular and energetic than that of any of the lower animals. The uterus of woman is many times stronger and more powerful than the uterus, for example, of the cow. In other words, I repeat, the great characteristic of human parturition is the vastly greater amount of muscular effort, toil, or labour required for its accomplishment. The state of anaesthesia does not withdraw or abolish that muscular effort, toil, or labour; for if so, it would then stop, and arrest entirely the act of parturition itself. But it removes the physical pain and agony otherwise attendant on these muscular contractions and efforts.

From what I have stated under the two preceding heads, we are then, I believe, justly entitled to infer that the Hebrew term which, in our English translation of the primeval curse, is rendered "sorrow" (Genesis iii. 16), principally signifies the severe muscular *efforts* and *struggles* of which parturition—and more particularly human parturition—essentially consists; and does not specially signify the *feelings* or *sensations* of pain to which these muscular efforts or contractions give rise.

But even if . . . we were to admit that woman was, as the results of the primal curse, adjudged to the miseries of pure physical pain and agony in parturition, still, certainly under the Christian dispensation, the moral *necessity* of undergoing such anguish has ceased and terminated. Those who believe otherwise, must believe, in contradiction to the whole spirit and whole testimony of revealed truth, that the death and sacrifice of Christ was not, as it is everywhere declared to be, an all-sufficient sacrifice for all the sins and crimes of man. Christ, the "man of sorrows," who "hath given himself up for us an offering and a sacrifice to God," "surely hath borne our griefs and carried our sorrows"; for God "saw the travail of his soul, and was satis-fied." And He himself told and impressed on his disciples, that His mission was to introduce "mercy, and not sacrifice."

It may not be out of place to remind those who opposed the employment of anaesthetic means in labour on supposed religious grounds, that on the very same grounds many discoveries in sciences and art,—even in the medical art—have been opposed upon their first proposition; and yet, *now* that the first introduction is over, and the opinions and practices they inculcate are established, no one would be deemed exactly rational who would turn against the present or future *continuance* of their employment any such improper weapon. I might adduce many instances, but one may suffice for all. When small-pox inoculation was introduced . . . [it] was declared a "diabolical operation," and a discovery sent into the world by the Powers of Evil. And, again, when Dr. Jenner introduced vaccination, . . . theological reasons again were not wanting for calling in question the orthodoxy of this other new practice. "Small-pox (argued Dr. Rowley) is a visitation from God. . . . " And he subsequently proposed, "whether vaccination be agreeable to the will and ordinances of God, as a question worthy of the consideration of the contemplative and learned ministers of the gospel of Jesus Christ; and whether it be impious and profane, thus to wrest out of the hands of the Almighty the divine dispensation of Providence!"

I have heard objections urged against the state of anaesthesia as a counteraction to pain in surgery and midwifery, on other and different grounds from any I have yet noticed, viz., that in superinducting a temporary absence of *corporeal* sensibil-ity, we also superinduce, at the same time, a temporary absence of *mental* conscious-ness. And it is argued, that, as medical men, we are not entitled to put the activity and consciousness of the mind of any patient in abeyance, for the mere purpose of saving that patient from any bodily pain or agony. Some medical men even, have gravely pressed this argument. But if there were any propriety in it, why, then, these same medical men could never have been justified in doing what they have one and all of them done perhaps hundreds of times; viz., exhibit, by the mouth, opium and other narcotics and hyponotics to their patients, to mitigate pain and superinduce anaesthesia and sleep. There is no greater impropriety or sin in producing sleep and freedom from pain by exhibiting a medicine by the mouth than by exhibiting it by the lungs.

Besides those that urge, on a kind of religious ground, that an artificial or anaesthetic state of unconsciousness should not be induced merely to save frail hu-manity from the miseries and tortures of bodily pain, forget that we have the great-est of all examples set before us for following out this very principle of practice. I allude to that most singular description of the preliminaries and details of the first surgical operation ever performed on man, which is contained in Genesis ii. 21:—"And the Lord God caused a deep sleep to fall upon Adam; and he slept; and he took one of his ribs, and closed up the flesh instead thereof." In this remarkable verse the whole process of a surgical operation is briefly detailed. But the passage is prin-cipally striking, as affording evidence of our Creator himself using means to save poor human nature from the unnecessary endurance of physical pain. "It ought to be noted (observes Calvin in his commentary on this verse), that Adam was sunk into a profound sleep, in order that he might feel no pain."

ERNEST HEMINGWAY (1899-1961)

"Indian Camp"

Some of Ernest Hemingway's strongest memories of his childhood were of the hunting and fishing trips he took to Horton Bay, Michigan, with his father, a wealthy and prominent physician who committed suicide in 1928. Hemingway was later to shape these vivid recollections into the Nick Adams stories, introducing the character who would evolve into the spartan, suffering protagonists of his novels, beginning with Jake Barnes in *The Sun Also Rises* (1926) and Frederic Henry in *A Farewell to Arms* (1929). Based on his life abroad, the first novel portrayed the "lost generation" of Americans, uprooted and aimless in the wake of World War I, while the second, which drew on his experiences as an ambulance driver with the Italian army, recounted a love affair blighted by the horrors of war. *For Whom the Bell Tolls* (1940), set in the Spanish Civil War, is considered by many to be Hemingway's masterpiece, appearing at the end of the decade during which his influence on American writing came to dominate its style and psychological outlook. An abiding theme in Hemingway's life and work is human fortitude in the face of death, whether on the battlegrounds of war or in the bullring. It is a theme that surfaces with all its complex ironies in "Indian Camp," an early Nick Adams story published in the collection *In Our Time* (1925). Having just witnessed a gruesome death, the ten-year-old Nick, nestled in a rowboat with his father, is suddenly overcome by the conviction that he himself will never die. On July 2, 1961, Hemingway, in failing psychological and physical health, shot himself dead.

At the lake shore there was another rowboat drawn up. The two Indians stood waiting.

Nick and his father got in the stern of the boat and the Indians shoved it off and one of them got in to row. Uncle George sat in the stern of the camp rowboat. The young Indian shoved the camp boat off and got in to row Uncle George.

The two boats started off in the dark. Nick heard the oarlocks of the other boat quite a way ahead of them in the mist. The Indians rowed with quick choppy strokes. Nick lay back with his father's arm around him. It was cold on the water. The Indian who was rowing them was working very hard, but the other boat moved farther ahead in the mist all the time.

"Where are we going, Dad?" Nick asked.

"Over to the Indian camp. There is an Indian lady very sick."

"Oh," said Nick.

Across the bay they found the other boat beached. Uncle George was smoking a

From *In Our Time: Stories by Ernest Hemingway* (New York: Collier Books, 1986). Copyright 1925 by Charles Scribner's Sons; renewal copyright 1953 by Ernest Hemingway. Reprinted with permission of Charles Scribner's Sons, an imprint of Macmillan Publishing Company.

cigar in the dark. The young Indian pulled the boat way up the beach. Uncle George gave both the Indians cigars.

They walked up from the beach through a meadow that was soaking wet with dew, following the young Indian who carried a lantern. Then they went into the woods and followed a trail that led to the logging road that ran back into the hills. It was much lighter on the logging road as the timber was cut away on both sides. The young Indian stopped and blew out his lantern and they· all walked on along the road.

They came around a bend and a dog came out barking. Ahead were the lights of the shanties where the Indian bark-peelers lived. More dogs rushed out at them. The two Indians sent them back to the shanties. In the shanty nearest the road there was a light in the window. An old woman stood in the doorway holding a lamp.

Inside on a wooden bunk lay a young Indian woman. She had been trying to have her baby for two days. All the old women in the camp had been helping her. The men had moved off up the road to sit in the dark and smoke out of range of the noise she made. She screamed just as Nick and the two Indians followed his father and Uncle George into the shanty. She lay in the lower bunk, very big under a quilt. Her head was turned to one side. In the upper bunk was her husband. He had cut his foot very badly with an ax three days before. He was smoking a pipe. The room smelled very bad.

Nick's father ordered some water to be put on the stove, and while it was heating he spoke to Nick.

"This lady is going to have a baby, Nick," he said.

"I know," said Nick.

"You don't know," said his father. "Listen to me. What she is going through is called being in labor. The baby wants to be born and she wants it to be born. All her muscles are trying to get the baby born. That is what is happening when she screams."

"I see," Nick said.

Just then the woman cried out.

"Oh, Daddy, can't you give her something to make her stop screaming?" asked Nick.

"No. I haven't any anesthetic," his father said. "But her screams are not important. I don't hear them because they are not important."

The husband in the upper bunk rolled over against the wall.

The woman in the kitchen motioned to the doctor that the water was hot. Nick's father went into the kitchen and poured about half of the water out of the big kettle into a basin. Into the water left in the kettle he put several things he unwrapped from a handkerchief.

"Those must boil," he said, and began to scrub his hands in the basin of hot water with a cake of soap he had brought from the camp. Nick watched his father's hands scrubbing each other with the soap. While his father washed his hands very carefully and thoroughly, he talked.

"You see, Nick, babies are supposed to be born head first but sometimes they're not. When they're not they make a lot of trouble for everybody. Maybe I'll have to operate on this lady. We'll know in a little while."

When he was satisfied with his hands he went in and went to work.

"Pull back that quilt, will you, George?" he said. "I'd rather not touch it."

Later when he started to operate Uncle George and three Indian men held the woman still. She bit Uncle George on the arm and Uncle George said, "Damn squaw bitch!" and the young Indian who had rowed Uncle George over laughed at him. Nick held the basin for his father. It all took a long time.

His father picked the baby up and slapped it to make it breathe and handed it to the old woman.

"See, it's a boy, Nick," he said. "How do you like being an intern?"

Nick said, "All right." He was looking away so as not to see what his father was doing.

"There. That gets it," said his father and put something into the basin.

Nick didn't look at it.

"Now," his father said, "there's some stitches to put in. You can watch this or not, Nick, just as you like. I'm going to sew up the incision I made."

Nick did not watch. His curiosity had been gone for a long time.

His father finished and stood up. Uncle George and the three Indian men stood up. Nick put the basin out in the kitchen.

Uncle George looked at his arm. The young Indian smiled reminiscently.

"I'll put some peroxide on that, George," the doctor said.

He bent over the Indian woman. She was quiet now and her eyes were closed. She looked very pale. She did not know what had become of the baby or anything.

"I'll be back in the morning," the doctor said, standing up. "The nurse should be here from St. Ignace by noon and she'll bring everything we need."

He was feeling exalted and talkative as football players are in the dressing room after a game.

"That's one for the medical journal, George," he said. "Doing a Caesarian with a jackknife and sewing it up with nine-foot, tapered gut leaders."

Uncle George was standing against the wall, looking at his arm.

"Oh, you're a great man, all right," he said.

"Ought to have a look at the proud father. They're usually the worst sufferers in these little affairs," the doctor said. "I must say he took it all pretty quietly."

He pulled back the blanket from the Indian's head. His hand came away wet. He mounted on the edge of the lower bunk with the lamp in one hand and looked in. The Indian lay with his face toward the wall. His throat had been cut from ear to ear. The blood had flowed down into a pool where his body sagged the bunk. His head rested on his left arm. The open razor lay, edge up, in the blankets.

"Take Nick out of the shanty, George," the doctor said.

There was no need of that. Nick, standing in the door of the kitchen, had a good view of the upper bunk when his father, the lamp in one hand, tipped the Indian's head back.

It was just beginning to be daylight when they walked along the logging road back toward the lake.

"I'm terribly sorry I brought you along, Nickie," said his father, all his postoperative exhilaration gone. "It was an awful mess to put you through."

"Do ladies always have such a hard time having babies?" Nick asked.

"No, that was very, very exceptional."

"Why did he kill himself, Daddy?"

"I don't know, Nick. He couldn't stand things, I guess."

"Do many men kill themselves, Daddy?"

"Not very many, Nick."

"Do many women?"

"Hardly ever."

"Don't they ever?"

"Oh, yes. They do sometimes."

"Daddy?"

"Yes."

"Where did Uncle George go?"

"He'll turn up all right."

"Is dying hard, Daddy?"

"No, I think it's pretty easy, Nick. It all depends."

They were seated in the boat, Nick in the stern, his father rowing. The sun was coming up over the hills. A bass jumped, making a circle in the water. Nick trailed his hand in the water. It felt warm in the sharp chill of the morning.

In the early morning on the lake sitting in the stern of the boat with his father rowing, he felt quite sure that he would never die.

"The Interior Castle"

A novelist and short story writer whose work won the Pulitzer Prize in 1970, Jean Stafford was born in Covina, California, but spent most of her childhood in Colorado. After receiving a B.A. and M.A. from the University of Colorado, she traveled abroad to study philology at the University of Heidelberg in Germany, where she began to write in earnest. Upon her return to the United States, Stafford met the poet Robert Lowell, whom she married in 1940. Her first novel, *Boston Adventure* (1944), described the social and spiritual exile of Sonie, a young woman who aspires to redeem her humiliating past by making her mark in Boston society. *The Mountain Lion* (1947), planned as a sequel to Sonie's story, recounted the relationship between a brother and sister in which she sickens and declines while he thrives and grows into manhood. By the time the novel was published, Stafford and Lowell's marriage had fallen apart. In the winter of 1946, Stafford entered the Payne Whitney Clinic, where she was placed under the care of Drs. Gregory Zilboorg and Mary Jane Sherfey, who treated her for depression and alcoholism. At the time, "The Interior Castle" had just appeared in *Partisan Review.* Stafford had written an earlier version of the story in 1940, soon after Lowell had broken her nose in a drunken rage. The incident had sparked Stafford's memories of the excruciating surgery she had endured two years earlier when Lowell had smashed his car into a wall, leaving Stafford, who was sitting next to him, with a shattered face and skull. Acclaimed as one of Stafford's best short stories, "The Interior Castle" takes up a key theme in her work—the search for psychic inviolability—and conveys it through the uncanny "aesthetic distance she keeps between us and the untouchable otherness of her characters." The story's title is borrowed from a work by St. Theresa of Avila, who used the image to describe the innermost recesses of the soul.

I

Pansy Vanneman, injured in an automobile accident, often woke up before dawn when the night noises of the hospital still came, in hushed hurry, through her half-open door. By day, when the nurses talked audibly with the internes, laughed without inhibition, and took no pains to soften their footsteps on the resounding composition floors, the routine of the hospital seemed as bland and commonplace as that of a bank or a factory. But in the dark hours, the whispering and the quickly stilled clatter of glasses and basins, the moans of patients whose morphine was wearing off, the soft squeak of a stretcher as it rolled past in its way from the emergency ward— these suggested agony and death. Thus, on the first morning, Pansy had faltered to consciousness long before daylight and had found herself in a ward from every bed of which, it seemed to her, came the bewildered protest of someone about to die. A caged light burned on the floor beside the bed next to hers. Her neighbor was dying and a priest was administering Extreme Unction. He was stout and elderly and he suffered from asthma so that the struggle of his breathing, so close to her, was the basic pattern and all the other sounds were superimposed upon it. Two middle-aged men in overcoats knelt on the floor beside the high bed. In a foreign tongue, the half-gone woman babbled against the hissing and sighing of the Latin prayers. She played with her rosary as if it were a toy: she tried, and failed, to put it into her mouth.

Pansy felt horror, but she felt no pity. An hour or so later, when the white ceiling lights were turned on and everything—faces, counterpanes, and the hands that groped upon them—was transformed into a uniform gray sordor, the woman was wheeled away in her bed to die somewhere else, in privacy. Pansy did not quite take this in, although she stared for a long time at the new, empty bed that had replaced the other.

The next morning, when she again woke up before the light, this time in a private room, she recalled the woman with such sorrow that she might have been a friend. Simultaneously, she mourned the driver of the taxicab in which she had been injured, for he had died at about noon the day before. She had been told this as she lay on a stretcher in the corridor, waiting to be taken to the X-ray room; an interne, passing by, had paused and smiled down at her and had said, "Your cab-driver is dead. You were lucky."

Six weeks after the accident, she woke one morning just as daylight was showing on the windows as a murky smear. It was a minute or two before she realized why she was so reluctant to be awake, why her uneasiness amounted almost to alarm. Then she remembered that her nose was to be operated on today. She lay straight and motionless under the seersucker counterpane. Her blood-red eyes in her darned face stared through the window and saw a frozen river and leafless elm trees and a grizzled esplanade where dogs danced on the ends of leashes, their bundled-up owners stumbling after them, half blind with sleepiness and cold. Warm as the hospital room was, it did not prevent Pansy from knowing, as keenly as though she were one of the walkers, how very cold it was outside. Each twig of a nearby tree was stark. Cold red brick buildings nudged the low-lying sky which was pale and inert like a punctured sac.

In six weeks, the scene had varied little: there was promise in the skies neither of sun nor of snow; no red sunsets marked these days. The trees could neither die nor leaf out again. Pansy could not remember another season in her life so constant, when the very minutes themselves were suffused with the winter pallor as they dropped from the moon-faced clock in the corridor. Likewise, her room accomplished no alterations from day to day. On the glass-topped bureau stood two potted plants telegraphed by faraway well-wishers. They did not fade, and if a leaf turned brown and fell, it soon was replaced; so did the blossoms renew themselves. The roots, like the skies and like the bare trees, seemed zealously determined to maintain a status quo. The bedside table, covered every day with a clean white towel, though the one removed was always immaculate, was furnished sparsely with a water glass, a bent drinking tube, a sweating pitcher, and a stack of paper handkerchiefs. There were a few letters in the drawer, a hairbrush, a pencil, and some postal cards on which, from time to time, she wrote brief messages to relatives and friends: "Dr. Nash says that my reflexes are shipshape (*sic*) and Dr. Rivers says the frontal fracture has all but healed and that the occipital is coming along nicely. Dr. Nicholas, the nose doctor, promises to operate as soon as Dr. Rivers gives him the go-ahead sign (*sic*)."

The bed itself was never rumpled. Once fretful and now convalescent, Miss Vanneman might have been expected to toss or to turn the pillows or to unmoor the counterpane; but hour after hour and day after day she lay at full length and would not even suffer the nurses to raise the head-piece of the adjustable bed. So perfect and stubborn was her body's immobility that it was as if the room and the landscape, mortified by the ice, were extensions of herself. Her resolute quiescence and her disinclination to talk, the one seeming somehow to proceed from the other, resembled, so the nurses said, a final coma. And they observed, in pitying indignation, that she might as *well* be dead for all the interest she took in life. Amongst themselves they scolded her for what they thought a moral weakness: an automobile accident, no matter how serious, was not reason enough for anyone to give up the will to live or to be happy. She had not—to come down bluntly to the facts—had the decency to be grateful that it was the driver of the cab and not she who had died. (And how dreadfully the man had died!) She was twenty-five years old and she came from a distant city. These were really the only facts known about her. Evidently she had not been here long, for she had no visitors, a lack which was at first sadly moving to the nurses but which became to them a source of unreasonable annoyance: had anyone the right to live so one-dimensionally? It was impossible to laugh at her, for she said nothing absurd; her demands could not be complained of because they did not exist; she could not be hated for a sharp tongue nor for a supercilious one; she could not be admired for bravery or for wit or for interest in her fellow creatures. She was believed to be a frightful snob.

Pansy, for her part, took a secret and mischievous pleasure in the bewilderment of her attendants and the more they courted her with offers of magazines, crossword puzzles, and a radio that she could rent from the hospital, the farther she retired from them into herself and into the world which she had created in her long hours here and which no one could ever penetrate nor imagine. Sometimes she did not even answer the nurses' questions; as they rubbed her back with alcohol and steadily discoursed, she was as remote from them as if she were miles away. She did not think that she lived on a higher plane than that of the nurses and the doctors but that she lived on a different one and that at this particular time—this time of exploration and habituation—she had no extra strength to spend on making herself known to them. All she had been before and all the memories she might have brought out to disturb the monotony of, say, the morning bath, and all that the past meant to the future when she would leave the hospital, were of no present consequence to her. Not even in her thoughts did she employ more than a minimum of memory. And when she did remember, it was in flat pictures, rigorously independent of one another: she saw her thin, poetic mother who grew thinner and more poetic in her canvas deck-chair at Saranac reading *Lalla Rookh.* She saw herself in an inappropriate pink hat drinking iced tea in a garden so oppressive with the smell of phlox that the tea itself tasted of it. She recalled an afternoon in autumn in Vermont when she had heard three dogs' voices in the north woods and she could tell, by the characteristic minor key struck three times at intervals, like bells from several churches, that they had treed something: the eastern sky was pink and the trees on the horizon looked like some eccentric vascular system meticulously drawn on colored paper.

What Pansy thought of all the time was her own brain. Not only the brain as the seat of consciousness, but the physical organ itself which she envisaged, romantically, now as a jewel, now as a flower, now as a light in a glass, now as an envelope of rosy vellum containing other envelopes, one within the other, diminishing infinitely. It was always pink and always fragile, always deeply interior and invaluable. She believed that she had reached the innermost chamber of knowledge and that perhaps her knowledge was the same as the saint's achievement of pure love. It was only convention, she thought, that made one say "sacred heart" and not "sacred brain."

Often, but never articulately, the color pink troubled her and the picture of herself in the wrong hat hung steadfastly before her mind's eye. None of the other girls had worn hats and since autumn had come early that year, they were dressed in green and rusty brown and dark yellow. Poor Pansy wore a white eyelet frock with a lacing of black ribbon around the square neck. When she came through the arch, overhung with bittersweet, and saw that they had not yet heard her, she almost turned back, but Mr. Oliver was there and she was in love with him. She was in love with him though he was ten years older than she and had never shown any interest in her beyond asking her once, quite fatuously but in an intimate voice, if the yodeling of the little boy who peddled clams did not make her wish to visit Switzerland. Actually, there was more to this question than met the eye, for some days later Pansy learned that Mr. Oliver, who was immensely rich, kept an apartment in Geneva. In the garden that day, he spoke to her only once. He said, "My dear, you look exactly like something out of Katherine Mansfield," and immediately turned and within her hearing asked Beatrice Sherburne to dine with him that night at the Country Club. Afterward, Pansy went down to the sea and threw the beautiful hat onto the full tide and saw it vanish in the wake of a trawler. Thereafter, when she heard the clam boy coming down the road, she locked the door and when the knocking had stopped and her mother called down from her chaise longue, "Who was it, dearie?" she replied, "A salesman."

It was only the fact that the hat had been pink that worried her. The rest of the memory was trivial, for she knew that she could never again love anything as ecstatically as she loved the spirit of Pansy Vanneman, enclosed within her head.

But her study was not without distraction, and she fought two adversaries: pain and Dr. Nicholas. Against Dr. Nicholas, she defended herself valorously and in fear; but pain, the pain, that is, that was independent of his instruments, she sometimes forced upon herself adventurously like a child scaring himself in a graveyard.

Dr. Nicholas greatly admired her crushed and splintered nose which he daily probed and peered at, exclaiming that he had never seen anything like it. His shapely hands ached for their knives; he was impatient with the skull-fracture man's cautious delay.

He spoke of "our" nose and said "we" would be a new person when we could breathe again. His own nose was magnificent. Not even his own brilliant surgery could have improved upon it nor could a first-rate sculptor have duplicated its direct downward line which permitted only the least curvature inward toward the end; nor the delicately rounded lateral declivities; nor the thin-walled, perfectly matched nostrils.

Miss Vanneman did not doubt his humaneness nor his talent—he was a celebrated man—but she questioned whether he had imagination. Immediately beyond the prongs of his speculum lay her treasure whose price he, no more than the nurses, could estimate. She believed he could not destroy it, but she feared that he might maim it: might leave a scratch on one of the brilliant facets of the jewel, bruise a petal of the flower, smudge the glass where the light burned, blot the envelopes, and that then she would die or would go mad. While she did not question that in either eventuality her brain would after a time redeem its original impeccability, she did not quite yet wish to enter upon either kind of eternity, for she was not certain that she could carry with her her knowledge as well as its receptacle.

Blunderer that he was, Dr. Nicholas was an honorable enemy, not like the demon, pain, which skulked in a thousand guises within her head, and which often she recklessly willed to attack her and then drove back in terror. After the rout, sweat streamed from her face and soaked the neck of the coarse hospital shirt. To be sure, it came usually of its own accord, running like a wild fire through all the convolutions to fill with flame the small sockets and ravines and then, at last, to withdraw, leaving behind a throbbing and an echo. On these occasions, she was as helpless as a tree in a wind. But at the other times when, by closing her eyes and rolling up the eyeballs in such a way that she fancied she looked directly on the place where her brain was, the pain woke sluggishly and came toward her at a snail's pace. Then, bit by bit, it gained speed. Sometimes it faltered back, subsided altogether, and then it rushed like a tidal wave driven by a hurricane, lashing and roaring until she lifted her hands from the counterpane, crushed her broken teeth into her swollen lip, stared in panic at the soothing walls with her ruby eyes, stretched out her legs until she felt their bones must snap. Each cove, each narrow inlet, every living bay was flooded and the frail brain, a little hat-shaped boat, was washed from its mooring and set adrift. The skull was as vast as the world and the brain was as small as a seashell.

Then came calm weather and the safe journey home. She kept vigil for a while, though, and did not close her eyes, but gazing pacifically at the trees, conceived of the pain as the guardian of her treasure who would not let her see it; that was why she was handled so savagely whenever she turned her eyes inward. Once this watch was interrupted: by chance she looked into the corridor and saw a shaggy mop slink past the door, followed by a senile porter. A pair of ancient eyes, as rheumy as an old dog's, stared uncritically in at her and a toothless mouth formed a brutish word. She was so surprised that she immediately closed her eyes to shut out the shape of the word and the pain dug up the unmapped regions of her head with mattocks, ludicrously huge. It was the familiar pain, but this time, even as she endured it, she observed with detachment that its effect upon her was less than that of its contents, the by-products, for example, of temporal confusion and the bizarre misapplication of the style of one sensation to another. At the moment, for example, although her brain reiterated to her that *it* was being assailed, she was stroking her right wrist with her left hand as though to assusage the ache, long since dispelled, of the sprain in the joint. Some minutes after she had opened her eyes and left off soothing her wrist, she lay rigid experiencing the sequel to the pain, an ideal terror. For, as before on several occasions, she was overwhelmed with the knowledge that the pain had been consummated in the vessel of her mind and for the moment the vessel was unbeautiful: she thought, quailing, of those plastic folds as palpable as the fingers of locked hands containing in their very cells, their fissures, their repulsive hemispheres, the mind, the soul, the inscrutable intelligence.

The porter, then, like the pink hat and like her mother and the hounds' voices, loitered with her.

II

Dr. Nicholas came at nine o'clock to prepare her for the operation. With him came an entourage of white-frocked acolytes, and one of them wheeled in a wagon on which lay knives and scissors and pincers, cans of swabs and gauze. In the midst of these was a bowl of liquid whose rich purple color made it seem strange like the brew of an alchemist.

"All set?" the surgeon asked her, smiling. "A little nervous, what? I don't blame you. I've often said I'd rather break a leg than have a submucous resection." Pansy thought for a moment he was going to touch his nose. His approach to her was roundabout. He moved through the yellow light shed by the globe in the ceiling which gave his forehead a liquid gloss; he paused by the bureau and touched a blossom of the cyclamen; he looked out the window and said, to no one and to all, "I couldn't start my car this morning. Came in a cab." Then he came forward. As he came, he removed a speculum from the pocket of his short-sleeved coat and like a cat, inquiring of the nature of a surface with its paws, he put out his hand toward her and drew it back, gently murmuring, "You must not be afraid, my dear. There is no danger, you know. Do you think for a minute I would operate if there were?"

Dr. Nicholas, young, brilliant, and handsome, was an aristocrat, a husband, a father, a clubman, a Christian, a kind counselor, and a trustee of his preparatory school. Like many of the medical profession, even those whose specialty was centered on the organ of the basest sense, he interested himself in the psychology of his patients: in several instances, for example, he had found that severe attacks of sinusitis were coincident with emotional crises. Miss Vanneman more than ordinarily captured his fancy since her skull had been fractured and her behavior throughout had been so extraordinary that he felt he was observing at first hand some of the results of shock, that incommensurable element, which frequently were too subtle to see. There was, for example, the matter of her complete passivity during a lumbar puncture, reports of which were written down in her history and were enlarged upon for him by Dr. Rivers' interne who had been in charge. Except for a tremor in her throat and a deepening of pallor, there were no signs at all that she was aware of what was happening to her. She made no sound, did not close her eyes nor clench her fists. She had had several punctures; her only reaction had been to the very first one, the morning after she had been brought in. When the interne explained to her that he was going to drain off cerebrospinal fluid which was pressing against her brain, she exclaimed, "My God!" but it was not an exclamation of fear. The young man had been unable to name what it was he had heard in her voice; he could only say that it had not been fear as he had observed it in other patients.

Dr. Nicholas wondered about her. There was no way of guessing whether she had always had a nature of so tolerant and undemanding a complexion. It gave him a melancholy pleasure to think that before her accident she had been high-spirited and loquacious; he was moved to think that perhaps she had been a beauty and that when she had first seen her face in the looking glass she had lost all joy in herself. It was very difficult to tell what the face had been, for it was so bruised and swollen, so hacked-up and lopsided. The black stitches the length of the nose, across the saddle, across the cheekbone, showed that there would be unsightly scars. He had ventured once to give her the name of a plastic surgeon but she had only replied with a vague, refusing smile. He had hoisted a manly shoulder and said, "You're the doctor."

Much as he pondered, coming to no conclusions, about what went on inside that pitiable skull, he was, of course, far more interested in the nose, deranged so badly that it would require his topmost skill to restore its functions to it. He would be obliged not only to make a submucous resection, a simple run-of-the-mill operation, but to remove the vomer, always a delicate task but further complicated in this case by the proximity of the bone to the frontal fracture line which conceivably was not entirely closed. If it were not and he operated too soon and if a cold germ then found its way into the opening, his patient would be carried off by meningitis in the twinkling of an eye. He wondered if she knew in what potential danger she lay; he desired to assure her that he had brought his craft to its nearest perfection and that she had nothing to fear of him, but feeling that she was perhaps both ignorant and unimaginative and that such consolation would create a fear rather than dispel one, he held his tongue and came nearer to the bed.

Watching him, Pansy could already feel the prongs of his pliers opening her nostrils for the insertion of his fine probers. The pain he caused her with his instruments was of a different kind from that which she felt unaided: it was a naked, clean, and vivid pain that made her faint and ill and made her wish to die. Once she had fainted as he ruthlessly explored and after she was brought around, he continued until he had finished his investigation. The memory of this outrage had afterward several times made her cry.

This morning she looked at him and listened to him with hatred. Fixing her eyes upon the middle of his high, protuberant brow, she imagined the clutter behind it and she despised its obtuse imperfection. In his bland unawareness, this nobody, this nose-bigot, was about to play with fire and she wished him ill.

He said, "I can't blame you. No, I expect you're not looking forward to our little party. But you'll be glad to be able to breathe again."

He stationed his lieutenants. The interne stood opposite him on the left side of the bed. The surgical nurse wheeled the wagon within easy reach of his hands and stood beside it. Another nurse stood at the foot of the bed. A third drew the shades at the windows and attached a blinding light that shone down on the patient hotly, and then she left the room, softly closing the door. Pansy stared at the silver ribbon tied in a great bow round the green crepe paper of one of the flower pots. It made her realize for the first time that one of the days she had lain here had been Christmas, but she had no time to consider this strange and thrilling fact, for Dr. Nicholas was genially explaining his anesthetic. He would soak packs of gauze in the purple fluid, a cocaine solution, and he would place them then in her nostrils, leaving them there for an hour. He warned her that the packing would be disagreeable (he did not say "painful") but that it would be well worth a few minutes of discomfort not to be in the least sick after the operation. He asked her if she were ready and when she nodded her head, he adjusted the mirror on his forehead and began.

At the first touch of his speculum, Pansy's fingers mechanically bent to the palms of her hands and she stiffened. He said, "A pack, Miss Kennedy," and Pansy closed her eyes. There was a rush of plunging pain as he drove the sodden gobbet of gauze high up into her nose and something bitter burned in her throat so that she retched. The doctor paused a moment and the surgical nurse wiped Pansy's mouth. He returned to her with another pack, pushing it with his bodkin doggedly until it lodged against the first. Stop! Stop! cried all her nerves, wailing along the surface of her skin. The coats that covered them were torn off and they shuddered like naked people screaming, Stop! Stop! But Dr. Nicholas did not hear. Time and again he came back with a fresh pack and did not pause at all until one nostril was finished. She opened her eyes and saw him wipe the sweat off his forehead and saw the dark interne bending over her, fascinated. Miss Kennedy bathed her temples in ice water and Dr. Nicholas said, "There. It won't be much longer. I'll tell them to send you some coffee, though I'm afraid you won't be able to taste it. Ever drink coffee with chicory in it? I have no use for it."

She snatched at his irrelevancy and, though she had never tasted chicory, she said severely, "I love it."

Dr. Nicholas chuckled. "De gustibus. Ready? A pack, Miss Kennedy."

The second nostril was harder to pack since the other side was now distended and this passage was anyhow much narrower, as narrow, he had once remarked, as that in the nose of an infant. In such pain as passed all language and even the farthest fetched analogies, she turned her eyes inward thinking that under the obscuring cloak of the surgeon's pain, she could see her brain without the knowledge of its keeper. But Dr. Nicholas and his aides would give her no peace. They surrounded her with their murmuring and their foot-shuffling and the rustling of their starched uniforms, and her eyelids continually flew back in embarrassment and mistrust. She was claimed entirely by this present, meaningless pain and suddenly and sharply she forgot what she had meant to do. She was aware of nothing but her ascent to the summit of something; what it was she did not know, whether it was a tower or a peak or Jacob's ladder. Now she was an abstract word, now she was a theorem of geometry, now she was a kite flying, a top spinning, a prism flashing, a kaleidoscope turning.

But none of the others in the room could see inside when the surgeon was finished, the nurse at the foot of the bed said, "Now you must take a look in the mirror. It's simply too comical." And they all laughed intimately like old, fast friends. She smiled politely and looked at her reflection: over the gruesomely fattened snout, her scarlet eyes stared in fixed reproach upon her upturned lips, gray with bruises. But even in its smile of betrayal, the mouth itself was puzzled: it reminded her that something had been left behind, but she could not recall what it was. She was hollowed out and was as dry as a white bone.

III

They strapped her ankles to the operating table and put leather nooses round her wrists. Over her head was a mirror with a thousand facets in which she saw a thousand travesties of her face. At her right side was the table, shrouded in white, where lay the glittering blades of the many knives, thrusting out fitful rays of light. All the cloth was frosty; everything was white or silver and as cold as snow. Dr. Nicholas, a tall snowman with silver eyes and silver fingernails, came into the room soundlessly for he walked on layers and layers of snow that deadened his footsteps; behind him came the interne, a smaller snowman, less impressively proportioned. At the foot of the table, a snow figure put her frozen hands upon Pansy's helpless feet. The doctor plucked the packs from the cold, numb nose. His laugh was like a cry on a bitter, still night: "I will show you now," he called across the expanse of snow, "that you can feel nothing." The pincers bit at nothing, snapped at the air and cracked a nerveless icicle. Pansy called back and heard her own voice echo: "I feel nothing."

Here the walls were gray, not tan. Suddenly the face of the nurse at the foot of the table broke apart and Pansy first thought it was in grief. But it was a smile and she said, "Did you enjoy your coffee?" Down the gray corridors of the maze, the words rippled, ran like mice, birds, broken beads: Did you enjoy your coffee? your coffee? your coffee? Similarly once in another room that also had gray walls, the same voice had said, "Shall I give her some whisky?" She was overcome with gratitude that this young woman (how pretty she was with her white hair and her white face and her china-blue eyes!) had been with her that first night and was with her now.

In the great stillness of the winter, the operation began. The knives carved snow. Pansy was happy. She had been given a hypnotic just before they came to fetch her and she would have gone to sleep had she not enjoyed so much this trickery of Dr. Nicholas' whom now she tenderly loved.

There was a clock in the operating room and from time to time she looked at it. An hour passed. The snowman's face was melting; drops of water hung from his fine nose, but his silver eyes were as bright as ever. Her love was returned, she knew: he loved her nose exactly as she loved his knives. She looked at her face in the domed mirror and saw how the blood had streaked her lily-white cheeks and had stained her shroud. She returned to the private song: Did you enjoy your coffee? your coffee?

At the half-hour, a murmur, sanguine and slumbrous, came to her and only when she had repeated the words twice did they engrave their meaning upon her. Dr. Nicholas said, "Stand back now, nurse. I'm at this girl's brain and I don't want my elbow jogged." Instantly Pansy was alive. Her strapped ankles arched angrily; her wrists strained against their bracelets. She jerked her head and she felt the pain flare; she had made the knife slip.

"Be still!" cried the surgeon. "Be quiet, please!"

He had made her remember what it was she had lost when he had rammed his gauze into her nose: she bustled like a housewife to shut the door. She thought, I must hurry before the robbers come. It would be like the time Mother left the cellar door open and the robber came and took, of all things, the terrarium.

Dr. Nicholas was whispering to her. He said, in the voice of a lover, "If you can stand it five minutes more, I can perform the second operation now and you won't have to go through this again. What do you say?"

She did not reply. It took her several seconds to remember why it was her mother had set such store by the terrarium and then it came to her that the bishop's widow had brought her an herb from Palestine to put in it.

The interne said, "You don't want to have your nose packed again, do you?"

The surgical nurse said, "She's a good patient, isn't she, sir?"

"Never had a better," replied Dr. Nicholas. "But don't call me 'sir.' You must be a Canadian to call me 'sir.'"

The nurse at the foot of the bed said, "I'll order some more coffee for you."

"How about it, Miss Vanneman?" said the doctor. "Shall I go ahead?"

She debated. Once she had finally fled the hospital and fled Dr. Nicholas, nothings could compel her to come back. Still, she knew that the time would come when she could no longer live in seclusion, she must go into the world again and must be equipped to live in it; she banally acknowledged that she must be able to breathe. And finally, though the world to which she would return remained unreal, she gave the surgeon her permission.

He had now to penetrate regions that were not anesthetized and this he told her frankly, but he said that there was no danger at all. He apologized for the slip of the tongue he had made: in point of fact, he had not been near her brain, it was only a figure of speech. He began. The knives ground and carved and curried and scoured the wounds they made; the scissors clipped hard gristle and the scalpels chipped off bone. It was as if a tangle of tiny nerves were being cut dexterously, one by one; the pain writhed spirally and came to her who was a pink bird and sat on the top of a cone. The pain was a pyramid made of a diamond; it was an intense light; it was the hottest fire, the coldest chill, the highest peak, the fastest force, the furthest reach, the newest time. It possessed nothing of her but its one infinitesimal scene: beyond the screen as thin as gossamer, the brain trembled for its life, hearing the knives hunting like wolves outside, sniffing and snapping. Mercy! Mercy! cried the scalped nerves.

At last, miraculously, she turned her eyes inward tranquilly. Dr. Nicholas had said, "The worst is over. I am going to work on the floor of your nose," and at his signal she closed her eyes and this time and this time alone, she saw her brain lying in a shell-pink satin case. It was a pink pearl, no bigger than a needle's eye, but it was so beautiful and so pure that its smallness made no difference. Anyhow, as she watched, it grew. It grew larger and larger until it was an enormous bubble that contained the surgeon and the whole room within its rosy luster. In a long ago summer, she had often been absorbed by the spectacle of flocks of yellow birds that visited a cedar tree and she remembered that everything that summer had been some shade of yellow. One year of childhood, her mother had frequently taken her to have tea with an aged schoolmistress upon whose mantelpiece there was a herd of ivory elephants; that had been the white year. There was a green spring when early in April she had seen a grass snake on a boulder, but the very summer that followed was violet, for vetch took her mother's garden. She saw a swatch of blue tulle lying in a raffia basket on the front porch of Uncle Marion's brown house. Never before had the world been pink, whatever else it had been. Or had it been, one other time? She could not be sure and she did not care. Of one thing she was certain: never had the world enclosed her before and never had the quiet been so smooth.

For only a moment the busybodies left her to her ecstasy and then, impatient and gossiping, they forced their way inside, slashed at her resisting trance with questions and congratulations, with statements of fact and jokes. "Later," she said to them dumbly. "Later on, perhaps. I am busy now." But their voices would not go away. They touched her, too, washing her face with cloths so cold they stung, stroking her wrists with firm, antiseptic fingers. The surgeon, squeezing her arm with avuncular pride, said, "Good girl," as if she were a bright dog that had retrieved a bone. Her silent mind abused him: "You are a thief," it said, "you are heartless and you should be put to death." But he was leaving, adjusting his coat with an air of vainglory, and the interne, abject with admiration, followed him from the operating room smiling like a silly boy.

Shortly after they took her back to her room, the weather changed, not for the better. Momentarily the sun emerged from its concealing murk, but in a few minutes the snow came with a wind that promised a blizzard. There was great pain, but since it could not serve her, she rejected it and she lay as if in a hammock in a pause of bitterness. She closed her eyes, shutting herself up within her treasureless head.

PIUS XII (1876–1958)

"The Prolongation of Life"

Eugenio Pacelli, born in Rome, Italy, reigned over the Catholic Church as
Pius XII from 1939 to 1958. Coming from a Tuscan family that had supplied the Vatican with lawyers since the beginning of the nineteenth century, Pacelli was ordained as a priest in 1899 and immediately enrolled in
the Apollinaire, where he obtained a degree in law. In 1901, he undertook
work in the Papal Secretariat of State, and some ten years later was appointed Secretary of the Commission for the Code of Canon Law. An adroit
negotiator of Papal affairs, Pacelli played a pivotal role in securing the
Vatican's neutrality and independent status during the two world wars, a task
that took on Machiavellian dimensions in his dealings with Fascist Italy and
Nazi Germany. In contemplating the sources of war, Pius XII concluded
that hostility among nations was brought on by social discontent within
them. In a number of encyclicals, he argued that no political order could
survive if it did not preserve the rights of the individual, which he believed
to be grounded in the principles of Christian theology and its emphasis on
the fundamental sacredness of the human soul and person. Although elaborated within the context of medical rather than political practice, these principles guided Pius's recommendations in "The Prolongation of Life," an
address delivered to an International Congress of Anesthesiologists that met
in Rome in 1957. Noting that medicine's specialized knowledge gives it the
authority to define the moment of death, Pius argued that the physician is
under no moral obligation to initiate or prolong artificial respiration if the
patient's vital functions, as "distinguished from the simple life of organs,"
have ceased. Within the context of Christian theology, death is the departure of the soul, and from the moment of that departure, sustaining the body
becomes an empty gesture.

Dr. Bruno Haid, chief of the anesthesia section at the surgery clinic of the University of Innsbruck, has submitted to Us three questions on medical morals treating
the subject known as "resuscitation" [la réanimation].

THE PRACTICE OF "RESUSCITATION"

In the practice of resuscitation and in the treatment of persons who have suffered
headwounds, and sometimes in the case of persons who have undergone brain surgery or of those who have suffered trauma of the brain through anoxia and remain
in a state of deep unconsciousness, there arise a number of questions that concern
medical morality and involve the principles of the philosophy of nature even more
than those of analgesia.

From *The Pope Speaks* 4 (4) (Spring 1958):393–398.

If the lesion of the brain is so serious that the patient will very probably, and even most certainly, not survive, the anesthesiologist is then led to ask himself the distressing question as to the value and meaning of the resuscitation processes. As an immediate measure he will apply artificial respiration by intubation and by aspiration of the respiratory tract; he is then in a safer position and has more time to decide what further must be done. But he can find himself in a delicate position, if the family considers that the efforts he has taken are improper and opposes them. In most cases this situation arises, not at the beginning of resuscitation attempts, but when the patient's condition, after a slight improvement at first, remains stationary and it becomes clear that only automatic artificial respiration is keeping him alive. The question then arises if one must, or if one can, continue the resuscitation process despite the fact that the soul may already have left the body.

The solution to this problem, already difficult in itself, becomes even more difficult when the family—themselves Catholic perhaps—insist that the doctor in charge, especially the anesthesiologist, remove the artificial respiration apparatus in order to allow the patient, who is already virtually dead, to pass away in peace.

THREE QUESTIONS

The problems that arise in the modern practice of resuscitation can therefore be formulated in three questions:

First, does one have the right, or is one even under the obligation, to use modern artificial-respiration equipment in all cases, even those which, in the doctor's judgment are completely hopeless?

Second, does one have the right, or is one under obligation, to remove the artificial-respiration apparatus when, after several days, the state of deep unconsciousness does not improve if, when it is removed, blood circulation will stop within a few minutes? What must be done in this case if the family of the patient, who has already received the last sacraments, urges the doctor to remove the apparatus? Is Extreme Unction still valid at this time?

Third, must a patient plunged into unconsciousness through central paralysis, but whose life—that is to say, blood circulation—is maintained through artificial respiration, and in whom there is no improvement after several days, be considered *"de facto"* or even *"de jure"* dead? Must one not wait for blood circulation to stop, in spite of the artificial respiration, before considering him dead?

BASIC PRINCIPLES

Natural reason and Christian morals say that man (and whoever is entrusted with the task of taking care of his fellowman) has the right and the duty in case of serious illness to take the necessary treatment for the preservation of life and health.

But normally one is held to use only ordinary means—according to circumstances of persons, places, times, and culture—that is to say, means that do not involve any grave burden for oneself or another. A more strict obligation would be too burdensome for most men and would render the attainment of the higher, more important good too difficult. Life, health, all temporal activities are in fact subordinated to spiritual ends. On the other hand, one is not forbidden to take more than the strictly necessary steps to preserve life and health, as long as he does not fail in some more serious duty.

THE FACT OF DEATH

It remains for the doctor, and especially the anesthesiologist, to give a clear and precise definition of "death" and the "moment of death" of a patient who passes away in a state of unconsciousness. Here one can accept the usual concept of complete and final separation of the soul from the body; but in practice one must take into account the lack of precision of the terms "body" and "separation."

A DOCTOR'S RIGHTS AND DUTIES

1. Does the anesthesiologist have the right, or is he bound, in all cases of deep unconsciousness, even in those that are considered to be completely hopeless in the opinion of the competent doctor, to use modern artificial respiration apparatus, even against the will of the family?

The rights and duties of the doctor are correlative to those of the patient. The doctor, in fact, has no separate or independent right where the patient is concerned. In general he can take action only if the patient explicitly or implicitly, directly or indirectly, gives him permission. The technique of resuscitation which concerns us here does not contain anything immoral in itself. Therefore the patient, if he were capable of making a personal decision, could lawfully use it and, consequently, give the doctor permission to use it. On the other hand, since these forms of treatment go beyond the ordinary means to which one is bound, it cannot be held that there is an obligation to use them nor, consequently, that one is bound to give the doctor permission to use them.

The rights and duties of the family depend in general upon the presumed will of the unconscious patient if he is of age and *"sui juris."* Where the proper and independent duty of the family is concerned, they are usually bound only to the use of ordinary means.

Consequently, if it appears that the attempt at resuscitation constitutes in reality such a burden for the family that one cannot in all conscience impose it upon them, they can lawfully insist that the doctor should discontinue these attempts, and the doctor can lawfully comply. There is not involved here a case of direct disposal of the life of the patient, nor of euthanasia in any way: this would never be licit. Even when it causes the arrest of circulation, the interruption of attempts at resuscitation is never more than an indirect cause of the cessation of life, and one must apply in this case the principle of double effect and of *"voluntarium in causa."*

EXTREME UNCTION

2. We have, therefore, already answered the second question in essence: "Can the doctor remove the artificial respiration apparatus before the blood circulation has

come to a complete, stop? Can he do this, at least, when the patient has already received Extreme Unction? Is this Extreme Unction valid when it is administered at the moment when circulation ceases, or even after?"

If, as in the opinion of doctors, this complete cessation of circulation means a sure separation of the soul from the body, even if particular organs go on functioning, Extreme Unction would certainly not be valid, for the recipient would certainly not be a man anymore. And this is an indispensable condition for the reception of the sacraments.

WHEN IS ONE "DEAD"?

3. "When the blood circulation and the life of a patient who is deeply unconscious because of a central paralysis are maintained only through artificial respiration, and no improvement is noted after a few days, at what time does the Catholic Church consider the patient "dead," or when must he be declared dead according to natural law (questions *'de facto'* and *'de jure'*)?"

(Has death already occurred after grave trauma of the brain, which has provoked deep unconsciousness and central breathing paralysis, the fatal consequences of which have nevertheless been retarded by artificial respiration? Or does it occur, according to the present opinion of doctors, only when there is complete arrest of circulation despite prolonged artificial respiration?)

Where the verification of the fact in particular cases is concerned, the answer cannot be deduced from any religious and moral principle and, under this aspect, does not fall within the competence of the Church. Until an answer can be given, the question must remain open. But considerations of a general nature allow us to believe that human life continues for as long as its vital functions—distinguished from the simple life of organs—manifest themselves spontaneously or even with the help of artificial processes. A great number of these cases are the object of insoluble doubt, and must be dealt with according to the presumptions of law and of fact of which We have spoken.

May these explanations guide you and enlighten you when you must solve delicate questions arising in the practice of your profession.

"A Definition of Irreversible Coma: Report of the Ad Hoc Committee of the Harvard Medical School to Examine the Definition of Brain Death"

In the 1960s, a Harvard committee of physicians, ethicists, and other experts redefined death. Rejecting the notion that death was signaled by the permanent cessation of heart activity, they reconceptualized it as an event contingent on massive irreversible brain damage that rendered the patient comatose. The committee argued that this new criterion was needed in the wake of innovative resuscitative and supportive technologies that had made the beating heart a false and untenable sign of life. What immensely complicated the issues surrounding brain death was the fact that, although the patient was no longer viable, the patient's organs were. The first physician to address the moral questions raised by such a situation was Henry Beecher, a pioneering voice in medical ethics, who was then chairman of Harvard's Standing Committee on Human Studies. An anesthesiologist, Beecher had wide experience with respirators and intensive care units, as well as daily contact with surgeons. Two in particular were to play a decisive role in Beecher's thinking: John Merrill, a kidney specialist who had helped develop renal dialysis, and Joseph Murray, a plastic surgeon whose pathbreaking work in kidney transplantation later won him the Nobel Prize. In October of 1967, Beecher wrote to Robert Ebert, then dean of the Harvard Medical School, to suggest that the Committee on Human Studies take up the ethical problems posed by the "decerebrated individual" sustained by artificial life support. "Every major hospital," wrote Beecher, "has patients stacked up waiting for suitable donors." Ebert endorsed the creation of a new committee, which deliberated from January through July of 1968, publishing its final report in the *Journal of the American Medical Association* on August 5, 1968. In addition to Beecher, Murray, and Merrill, the committee included the neurologists Raymond Adams, Derek Denny-Brown, and Robert Schwab; Jordi Folchi-Pi, a researcher in neurophysiology, and William Sweet, head of neurosurgery at Massachusetts General Hospital; Clifford Barger, a physiologist; Dana Farnsworth, a psychiatrist; William Curran, a lawyer; Everett Mendelsohn, a historian of science; and Ralph Potter, a theologian.

From *JAMA* 205 (6) (August 5, 1968):337–340. Copyright 1968 by the American Medical Association.

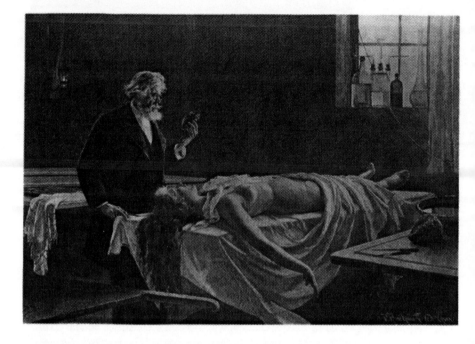

25. *Wood engraving after the painting* Ten!a Corazon *("She Has a Heart!") by Enrique Simonet y Lombardo, 1890. Wellcome Institute Library, London. The eroticization of death was a predominant theme in late-nineteenth-century European art, as the many representations of Shakespeare's Ophelia alone attest. Here, an anatomist contemplates the heart he has extracted from a prostitute's corpse. The body's languid pose, seductive drapery, and luxuriant hair seem to be at odds with the scene's moralistic overtones. The legs and feet of the crucified Christ are dimly visible to the left, while a collection of flasks and jars is illuminated on the upper right. Framed between icons of religion and science, death and sexuality nevertheless refuse to yield up their secrets.*

Our primary purpose is to define irreversible coma as a new criterion for death. There are two reasons why there is need for a definition: (1) Improvements in resuscitative and supportive measures have led to increased efforts to save those who are desperately injured. Sometimes these efforts have only partial success so that the result is an individual whose heart continues to beat but whose brain is irreversibly damaged. The burden is great on patients who suffer permanent loss of intellect, on their families, on the hospitals, and on those in need of hospital beds already occupied by these comatose patients. (2) Obsolete criteria for the definition of death can lead to controversy in obtaining organs for transplantation.

Irreversible coma has many causes, but *we are concerned here only with those comatose individuals who have no discernible central nervous system activity.* If the characteristics can be defined in satisfactory terms, translatable into action—and we believe this is possible—then several problems will either disappear or will become more readily soluble.

More than medical problems are present. There are moral, ethical, religious, and legal issues. Adequate definition here will prepare the way for better insight into all of these matters as well as for better law than is currently applicable.

CHARACTERISTICS OF IRREVERSIBLE COMA

An organ, brain or other, that no longer functions and has no possibility of functioning again is for all practical purposes dead. Our first problem is to determine the characteristics of a *permanently* nonfunctioning brain.

A patient in this state appears to be in deep coma. The condition can be satisfactorily diagnosed by points 1, 2, and 3 to follow. The electroencephalogram (point 4) provides confirmatory data, and when available it should be utilized. In situations where for one reason or another electroencephalographic monitoring is not available, the absence of cerebral function has to be determined by purely clinical signs, to be described, or by absence of circulation as judged by standstill of blood in the retinal vessels, or by absence of cardiac activity.

1. *Unreceptivity and Unresponsitivity.*—There is a total unawareness to externally applied stimuli and inner need and complete unresponsiveness—our definition of irreversible coma. Even the most intensely painful stimuli evoke no vocal or other response, not even a groan, withdrawal of a limb, or quickening of respiration.

2. *No Movements or Breathing.*—Observations covering a period of at least one hour by physicians is adequate to satisfy the criteria of no spontaneous muscular movements or spontaneous respiration or response to stimuli such as pain, touch, sound, or light. After the patient is on a mechanical respirator, the total absence of spontaneous breathing may be established by turning off the respirator for three minutes and observing whether there is any effort on the part of the subject to breathe spontaneously.

3. *No reflexes.*—Irreversible coma with abolition of central nervous system activity is evidenced in part by the absence of elicitable reflexes. The pupil will be fixed and dilated and will not respond to a direct source of bright light. Since the establishment of a fixed, dilated pupil is clear-cut in clinical practice, there should be no uncertainty as to its presence. Ocular movement (to head turning and to irrigation of the ears with ice water) and blinking are absent. There is no evidence of postural activity (decerebrate or other). Swallowing, yawning, vocalization are in abeyance. Corneal and pharyngeal reflexes are absent.

4. *Flat Electroencephalogram.*—Of great confirmatory value is the flat or isoelectric EEG. We must assume that the electrodes have been properly applied, that the apparatus is functioning normally, and that the personnel in charge is competent. We consider it prudent to have one channel of the apparatus used for an electrocardiogram. This channel will monitor the ECG so that, if it appears in the electroencephalographic leads because of high resistance, it can be readily identified. It also establishes the presence of the active heart in the absence of the EEG.

At least ten full minutes of recording are desirable, but twice that would be better.

It is also suggested that the gains at some point be opened to their full amplitude for a brief period (5 to 100 seconds) to see what is going on. Usually in an intensive care unit artifacts will dominate the picture, but these are readily identifiable. There shall be no electroencephalographic response to noise or to pinch.

All of the above tests shall be repeated at least 24 hours later with no change.

The validity of such data as indications of irreversible cerebral damage depends on the exclusion of two conditions: hypothermia (temperature below 90 F [32.2 C]) or central nervous system depressants, such as barbiturates.

OTHER PROCEDURES

The patient's condition can be determined only by a physician. When the patient is hopelessly damaged as defined above, the family and all colleagues who have participated in major decisions concerning the patient, and all nurses involved, should be so informed. Death is to be declared and *then* the respirator turned off. The decision to do this and the responsibility for it are to be taken by the physician-in-charge, in consultation with one or more physicians who have been directly involved in the case. It is unsound and undesirable to force the family to make the decision.

LEGAL COMMENTARY

The legal system of the United States is greatly in need of the kind of analysis and recommendations for medical procedures in cases of irreversible brain damage as described. At present, the law of the United States, in all 50 states and in the federal courts, treats the question of human death as a question of fact to be decided in every case. When any doubt exists, the courts seek medical expert testimony concerning the time of death of the particular individual involved. However, the law makes the assumption that the medical criteria for determining death are settled and not in doubt among physicians. Furthermore, the law assumes that the traditional method among physicians for determination of death is to ascertain the absence of all vital signs. To this extent, *Black's Law Dictionary* (fourth edition, 1951) defines death as

> The cessation of life; the ceasing to exist, *defined by physicians* as a total stoppage of the circulation of the blood, and a cessation of the animal and vital functions consequent thereupon, such as respiration, pulsation, etc [italics added].

Smith vs Smith (229 Ark, 579, 317 SW 2d 275) [was] decided in 1958 by the Supreme Court of Arkansas. In this case the two people were husband and wife involved in an auto accident. The husband was found dead at the scene of the accident. The wife was taken to the hospital unconscious. It is alleged that she "remained in coma due to brain injury" and died at the hospital 17 days later. The petitioner in court tried to argue that the two people died simultaneously. Later in the opinion the court said, " . . . [We] take judicial notice that one breathing, though unconscious, is not dead."

Arkansas Supreme Court considered the definition of death to be a settled, scientific, biological fact. It refused to consider the plaintiff's offer of evidence that "modern medical science" might say otherwise. In simplified form, the above is the state of the law in the United States concerning the definition of death.

In this report, however, we suggest that responsible medical opinion is ready to adopt new criteria for pronouncing death to have occurred in an individual sustaining irreversible coma as a result of permanent brain damage. If this position is adopted by the medical community, it can form the basis for change in the current legal concept of death. No statutory change in the law should be necessary since the law treats this question essentially as one of fact to be determined by physicians. The only circumstance in which it would be necessary that legislation be offered in the various states to define "death" by law would be in the event that great controversy were engendered surrounding the subject and physicians were unable to agree on the new medical criteria.

It is recommended as a part of these procedures that judgment of the existence of these criteria is solely a medical issue. It is suggested that the physician in charge of the patient consult with one or more other physicians directly involved in the case before the patient is declared dead on the basis of these criteria. In this way, the responsibility is shared over a wider range of medical opinion, thus providing an important degree of protection against later questions which might be raised about the particular case. It is further suggested that the decision to declare the person dead, and then to turn off the respirator, be made by physicians not involved in any later effort to transplant organs or tissue from the deceased individual. This is advisable in order to avoid any appearance of self-interest by the physicians involved.

It should be emphasized that we recommend the patient be declared dead before any effort is made to take him off a respirator, if he is then on a respirator. This declaration should not be delayed until he has been taken off the respirator and all artificially stimulated signs have ceased. The reason for this recommendation is that in our judgment it will provide a greater degree of legal protection to those involved. Otherwise, the physicians would be turning off the respirator on a person who is, under the present strict, technical application of law, still alive.

COMMENT

From ancient times down to the recent past it was clear that, when the respiration and heart stopped, the brain would die in a few minutes; so the obvious criterion of no heart beat as synonymous with death was sufficiently accurate. In those times the heart was considered to be the central organ of the body; it is not surprising that its failure marked the onset of death. This is no longer valid when modern resuscitative and supportive measures are used. These improved activities can now restore "life" as judged by the ancient standards of persistent respiration and continuing heart beat. This can be the case even when there is not the remotest possibility of an individual recovering consciousness following massive brain damage.

PAUL MONETTE (1945–1995)

Borrowed Time:
An AIDS Memoir

Author of the highly acclaimed *Becoming a Man: Half a Life Story* (1992), an account of his struggle to achieve his identity as a gay man, Paul Monette was a prolific writer, AIDS activist, and spokesperson for gay and lesbian issues. After graduating from Yale University in 1967, Monette began composing poetry while teaching at Milton Academy and Pine Manor College. The turning point of his life came at the age of twenty-eight when he met Roger Horwitz, who was to be his lover for over ten years. Diagnosed with AIDS in the early 1980s, Horwitz died from the disease in 1986; Monette himself died of AIDS in 1995. In *Borrowed Time* (1988) and *Love Alone: 18 Elegies for Rog* (1988), Monette wrote about his relationship with Horwitz, the social stigma and psychological devastation of AIDS, and the harrowing process of grieving the death of a loved one.

I don't know if I will live to finish this. Doubtless there's a streak of self-importance in such an assertion, but who's counting? Maybe it's just that I've watched too many sicken in a month and die by Christmas, so that a fatal sort of realism comforts me more than magic. All I know is this: The virus ticks in me. And it doesn't care a whit about our categories—when is full-blown, what's AIDS-related, what is just sick and tired? No one has solved the puzzle of its timing. I take my drug from Tijuana twice a day. The very friends who tell me how vigorous I look, how well I seem, are the first to assure me of the imminent medical breakthrough. What they don't seem to understand is, I used up all my optimism keeping my friend alive. Now that he's gone, the cup of my own health is neither half full nor half empty. Just half.

Equally difficult, of course, is knowing where to start. The world around me is defined now by its endings and its closures—the date on the grave that follows the hyphen. Roger Horwitz, my beloved friend, died of complications of AIDS on October 22, 1986, nineteen months and ten days after his diagnosis. That is the only real date anymore, casting its ice shadow over all the secular holidays lovers mark their calendars by. Until that long night in October, it didn't seem possible that any day could supplant the brute equinox of March 12—the day of Roger's diagnosis in 1985, the day we began to live on the moon.

The fact is, no one knows where to start with AIDS. Now, in the seventh year of the calamity, my friends in L.A. can hardly recall what it felt like any longer, the time before the sickness. Yet we all watched the toll mount in New York, then in

San Francisco, for years before it ever touched us here. It comes like a slowly dawning horror. At first you are equipped with a hundred different amulets to keep it far away. Then someone you know goes into the hospital, and suddenly you are at high noon in full battle gear. They have neglected to tell you that you will be issued no weapons of any sort. So you cobble together a weapon out of anything that lies at hand, like a prisoner honing a spoon handle into a stiletto. You fight tough, you fight dirty, but you cannot fight dirtier than it.

I remember a Saturday in February 1982, driving Route 10 to Palm Springs with Roger to visit his parents for the weekend. While Roger drove, I read aloud an article from *The Advocate*: "Is Sex Making Us Sick?" There was the slightest edge of irony in the query, an urban cool that seems almost bucolic now in its innocence. But the article didn't mince words. It was the first in-depth reporting I'd read that laid out the shadowy nonfacts of what till then had been the most fragmented of rumors. The first cases were reported to the Centers for Disease Control (CDC) only six months before, but they weren't in the newspapers, not in L.A. I note in my diary in December '81 ambiguous reports of a "gay cancer," but I know I didn't have the slightest picture of the thing. Cancer of the *what*? I would have asked, if anyone had known anything.

I remember exactly what was going through my mind while I was reading, though I can't now recall the details of the piece. I was thinking: How is this not me? Trying to find a pattern I was exempt from. It was a brand of denial I would watch grow exponentially during the next few years, but at the time I was simply relieved. Because the article appeared to be saying that there was a grim progression toward this undefined catastrophe, a set of preconditions—chronic hepatitis, repeated bouts of syphilis, exotic parasites. No wonder my first baseline response was to feel safe. It was *them*—by which I meant the fast-lane Fire Island crowd, the Sutro Baths, the world of High Eros.

Not us.

I grabbed for that relief because we'd been through a rough patch the previous autumn. Till then Roger had always enjoyed a sort of no-nonsense good health: not an abuser of anything, with a constitutional aversion to hypochondria, and not wed to his mirror save for a minor alarm as to the growing dimensions of his bald spot. In the seven years we'd been together I scarcely remember him having a cold or taking an aspirin. Yet in October '81 he had struggled with a peculiar bout of intestinal flu. Nothing special showed up in any of the blood tests, but over a period of weeks he experienced persistent symptoms that didn't neatly connect: pains in his legs, diarrhea, general malaise. I hadn't been feeling notably bad myself, but on the other hand I was a textbook hypochondriac, and I figured if Rog was harboring some kind of bug, so was I.

The two of us finally went to a gay doctor in the Valley for a further set of blood tests. It's a curious phenomenon among gay middle-class men that anything faintly venereal had better be taken to a doctor who's "on the bus." Is it a sense of fellow feeling perhaps, or a way of avoiding embarrassment? Do we really believe that only a doctor who's *our* kind can heal us of the afflictions that attach somehow to our secret hearts? There is so much magic to medicine. Of course we didn't know then that those few physicians with a large gay clientele were about to be swamped beyond all capacity to cope.

The tests came back positive for amoebiasis. Roger and I began the highly toxic treatment to kill the amoeba, involving two separate drugs and what seems in memory thirty pills a day for six weeks, till the middle of January. It was the first time I'd ever experienced the phenomenon of the cure making you sicker. By the end of treatment we were both weak and had lost weight, and for a couple of months afterward were susceptible to colds and minor infections.

It was only after the treatment was over that a friend of ours, diagnosed with amoebas by the same doctor, took his slide to the lab at UCLA for a second opinion. And that was my first encounter with lab error. The doctor at UCLA explained that the slide had been misread; the squiggles that looked like amoebas were in fact benign. The doctor shook his head and grumbled about "these guys who do their own lab work." Roger then retrieved his slide, took it over to UCLA and was told the same: no amoebas. We had just spent six weeks methodically ingesting poison for no reason at all.

So it wasn't the *Advocate* story that sent up the red flag for us. We'd been shaken by the amoeba business, and from that point on we operated at a new level of sexual caution. What is now called safe sex did not use to be so clearly defined. The concept didn't exist. But it was quickly becoming apparent, even then, that we couldn't wait for somebody else to define the parameters. Thus every gay man I know has had to come to a point of personal definition by way of avoiding the chaos of sexually transmitted diseases, or STD as we call them in the trade. There was obviously no one moment of conscious decision, a bolt of clarity on the shimmering freeway west of San Bernardino, but I think of that day when I think of the sea change. The party was going to have to stop. The evidence was too ominous: *We were making ourselves sick.*

How do I speak of the person who was my life's best reason? The most completely unpretentious man I ever met, modest and decent to such a degree that he seemed to release what was most real in everyone he knew. It was always a relief to be with Roger, not to have to play any games at all. By a safe mile he was the least flashy of all our bright circle of friends, but he spoke about books and the wide world he had journeyed with huge conviction and a hunger to know everything.

I wish of course we knew then what little we know now. That the Western Blot had been in place and we could have been tested for antibodies. That the antivirals had been sprung from the pharmaceutical morass. Then we would have slowed down and watched and monitored, the way I have myself. I wish my fellow warriors hadn't lost the first four or five years bogged down by homophobia and denial. When Larry Kramer tells Mathilde Krim in *Interview* about the closeted gay man at the National Institutes of Health who buried the AIDS data for two years, that's when I understand how doomed we were before we ever knew. It will be recorded that the dead in the first decade of the calamity died of our indifference.

Still, it would have taken a lot to slow us down. Our drive to be at the center of the lives we'd fashioned was far too urgent. By now we were starting to know more and more cases. . . . [W]e would hear it murmured about one and another: Michel

Foucault the philosopher, this actor, that dancer, all innuendo and secrecy. A distinguished and sweet-tempered producer we knew had been in the hospital for months now, but no, it wasn't AIDS. The disappearing had begun.

I'd convinced myself by this point that I was more than likely in the direct line of fire. I can't say what was hypochondriacal here. It was certainty born of dread: The glands in my neck and armpits were no bigger than almonds; they didn't hurt; they were nice and soft. Moreover, they didn't appear to be growing, but oh they were most definitely there.

My doctor's little speech about them, reiterated for two or three years now, came down to the same bland assertion that they could be anything. Dozens of things make the lymph nodes swell—stress, for instance, the blanket diagnosis of the age—but now the news was getting very specific about the lymph nodes being a flashing amber sign. *Pre-AIDS.* We still had that word then. Certain gay men I knew, in fact, were becoming obsessed with the notion. How deep exactly did *pre* go? Could you see it in a person's face? And how much time before *pre* burned down like a fuse on a keg of powder?

I tried not to talk nonstop about it; it sounded vain even then. I simply redoubled my efforts to mount a holding action. Lifecycle at the gym, vitamins, writing in bed, monitoring my almonds like a sort of DEW line. I vividly saw the process as a struggle to keep it from breaking through—a wall of water behind a dike, or the mangled son pounding on the door in Kipling's "The Monkey's Paw." "Breakthrough" was not then commonly used to describe the onset of full-blown infection, but the word has just the right edge, chilling and paranormal, like the breakthrough of alien life out of John Hurt's belly.

I knew all the warning signals now, rote as the seven danger signs of cancer that I carried on a card in my wallet in high school. Did I think I'd forget them? Night sweats, fevers, weight loss, diarrhea, tongue sores, bruises that didn't heal. None of the above. But I'd run through them every day, examining my body inch by inch as cowering people must have done in medieval plague cities, when X's were chalked on afflicted houses. I didn't even want to eat Asian food anymore, because it shot my bowels for a day after.

Any change, any slight modification . . . even a bruise you remembered the impact of, you'd watch like an x-ray till it started turning yellow around the purple. KS lesions do not go yellow. They also do not go white if you press them hard with your thumb. A whole gibberish of phrases and clues was beginning to gain currency. A canker sore in the mouth would ruin a day, for fear it was thrush—patches of white on the gums or the tongue. I read my tongue like a palmist before I went to bed at night.

At 2 A.M. on Sunday, the third of February, I finished the last lined page of my bound notebook, the type I use for a journal. I don't appear in a millennial mood as I close the volume.

> The dog is sleeping in a curl beside me. . . . May this house be safe from tigers. . . . R & I both struggling with viruses, and we had a heaping bowl of oatmeal after the ballet.

That is the first reference, right there, to the beginning of the end. But the twin flu is another sort of magic, homely as the oatmeal, for I felt safer that Roger and I were both under the weather. I knew deep down that all it was in me was a cold, ergo the same with him.

[On February 15, Roger] came home early from the office and went to bed. It was then I told him he really had to call Dr. Cope at UCLA. Not to panic, I quickly added as he winced apprehensively, but he could be harboring some sort of low-grade walking pneumonia that needed antibiotics. He agreed with a certain relief, comforted just to be talking about it as a concrete thing with beginning and end.

My memory of those weeks, back and forth to UCLA, is mostly shell-shock fragments. I can't even put them in chronological order, let alone weigh them. I know Roger spent three days in bed, then tried one at the office, only to wilt and crash with another fever.

Roger's blood was drawn fifteen different ways, but we had no test for antibodies yet, so none of the numbers led anywhere. Still there was no perceptible cough, and the general malaise and zigzag fever weren't in themselves conclusive, could still be that phantom flu, shimmering now like an oasis. During one of his consultations, Roger came out to the waiting room and said Dr. Cope wanted to meet me. The feeling was mutual.

As soon as we sat down with Dennis Cope I silently took back every idiot pun I'd ever made about his name. He's a bear of a man, seized with concentration yet extraordinarily mild by way of affect. Speaks carefully but not guardedly, and never to cover his ass. We were three ways blessed: that he was brilliant, that his reputation gave him power, and that Roger had been his private patient for five years going in. Dennis Cope and Roger already had each other's measure before they ever engaged in this battle together. Modest to a fault, incidentally; doesn't even hear praise. And not once in twenty months did he not have time.

He was perplexed the day I met him, but proceeded methodically and threw up no red flag that I could see. He said we had to keep probing these tentative symptoms, but no, whatever it was didn't present like AIDS at all. For one thing, Roger wasn't sick enough. If that sounds naive two years later, I have to remember the syndrome was defined then only by its direst fulminations—gasping on a respirator, lesions head to toe like shrapnel. Roger didn't exhibit the requisite pair of *pre* signs, or not sufficiently to chart a downward curve.

The blood-gas results proved to be in the normal range, which was a relief, yet there was clearly some kind of infection in the lung. The issue at week's end was whether or not that infection was "interstitial." Pneumocystis carinii—the deadly AIDS pneumonia, so-called PCP—is an interstitial infection, which means it invades the interstices between the lung sacs. A battery of x-rays seemed to indicate no interstitial involvement, and this was taken to be good news.

Despite the positive sign on the interstitial front, Roger still wasn't getting any better. Still not worse, but Cope decided it would only be prudent to have Roger come in for a bronchoscopy, in which a flexible tube is inserted in the lung for a specimen of tissue. The bronc has become such a fact of all our lives now, it's hard to recall there was a time I'd never heard of it. Roger would have to go into the hospital overnight to have it.

On the way to UCLA on Monday morning, driving along Sunset to the west side, Roger asked quietly: "What if it's really serious?"

Despite the positive talk all week—all month—and despite the fact that my last nickel was riding on denial, I don't know if I answered the right question, but I know my voice was steadier than I would've thought possible. Rog, I said, you have to understand how much everyone loves you. He had nobody out there even approaching enemy status; I'd never heard anyone say an unkind or quarrelsome word about him. The same could not be said of me, by a long shot. I gave a little encomium on his talent for friendship and loyalty, the idea being that everyone would be there for him if the going got rough.

I can't really separate the March 11 check-in on the tenth floor of the medical center from a dozen others. Amateurs still at the system, I expect we appeared like two meek refugees, with the overnight bag and a briefcase full of work.

We would both grow grimly accustomed to the first day of a hospitalization, with the interns sweeping in as if by revolving door, trying to look serious in spite of their comical youth, mad with backed-up things to do and racing like the White Rabbit. There would come a time when I would take over this phase, give the tedious history, answer the bald questions: Are you a homosexual? Are you or have you ever been an IV drug abuser? On March 11 I couldn't tell one intern from the next, intern from resident. I didn't realize that in a teaching hospital like UCLA every patient is one more unit to cover as they cram for the test of their budding careers. And here in the presence of a new disease, each kid doctor wanted an A. But remember, Roger was only supposed to be there overnight, so I held them all at arm's length and resisted differentiating.

Roger bore the process very well, and we seemed to be taking a proper stand of firmness in saying he was feeling not too bad. *Not sick enough, not sick enough*—I kept repeating Cope's phrase. It was still so, wasn't it? The pulmonary man came in to explain how the bronchoscopy worked. They would do it early in the morning, and we should probably have the results by noon. Home for lunch.

Dennis Cope was a welcome sight late in the day, because he at least knew who we were, and more to the point, the interns knew who he was. That is one of the shocking things about a hospital: its leveling of you to your body's weakest link. The Ph.D. in Comp Lit, the years in Paris, the wall of books—you do not wear these badges on your johnny gown. No wonder I was forever giving our résumés to doctors and nurses, as if to beg them to see us for real, see what happy lives we had left at the border, which waited still like a dog on the front stoop.

I was over at UCLA on Tuesday morning before the pulmonary team, and his parents and I gave Roger a bracing squeeze. I stayed with him till the doctor came in to administer the local anesthetic, and then I waited in the empty lounge with Al and Bernice, watching them as they dutifully read their books, refusing to leave my watch when the two of them went for coffee.

Altogether it took maybe twenty minutes. I was in Roger's room the second the team walked out. Roger was lying on his side, with an oxygen mask over his nose and mouth. They'd told us he would need it till the anesthetic wore off. What they hadn't said was that he would be coughing, almost without stopping and clearly in real discomfort. I patted him and talked a bit, but we really couldn't communicate. Even if this was a predictable reaction to the procedure and nothing more, the reality was jarring in the extreme. For this was the very cough we'd always said wasn't there. Could things have changed so fast? And who among my advisers would have me not worry now?

Finally it abated, and the oxygen mask came off. Roger was so debilitated from the trauma of the test that he lay back in an exhausted sleep. I don't know how much time went by. When the doctors came in—a pair of them, the intern and the pulmonary man—they stayed as close to each other as they could, like puppies. They stood at his bedside, for the new enlightenment demands that a doctor not deliver doom from the foot of the bed, looming like God. The intern spoke: "Mr. Horwitz, we have the results of the bronchoscopy. It does show evidence of pneumocystis in the lungs."

Was there a pause for the world to stop? There must have been, because I remember the crack of silence, Roger staring at the two men. Then he simply shut his eyes, and only I, who was the rest of him, could see how stricken was the stillness in his face.

"We'll begin treatment immediately with Bactrim. You'll need to be here in the hospital for fourteen to twenty-one days. Do you have any questions?"

Roger shook his head on the pillow. I wanted to kill these two ridiculous young men with the nerdy plastic pen shields in their whitecoat pockets. "Could you please leave us alone," I said.

And they tweedled out, relieved to have it over with. I ran around the bed and clutched Roger's hand. "We'll fight it, darling, we'll beat it, I promise. I won't let you die." The sentiments merged as they tumbled out. This is the liturgy of bonding. Mostly we clung together, as if time still had the decency to stop when we were entwined. After all, the whole world was right here in this room. I don't think Roger said anything then. Neither of us cried. It begins in a country beyond tears. Once you have your arms around your friend with his terrible news, your eyes are too shut to cry.

The intern had never once said the word.

Has anything ever been quite like this? Bad enough to be stricken in the middle of life, but then to fear your best and dearest will suffer exactly the same. Cancer and the heart don't sicken a man two ways like that. And it turns out all the certainties of health insurance and the job that waits are just a social contract, flimsy as the disappearing ink it's written in. Has anything else so tested the medical system and blown all its weakest links? I have oceans of unresolved rage at those who ran from us, but I also see that plague and panic are inseparable. And nothing compares. That is something very important to understand about those on the moon of AIDS. Anything offered in comparison is a mockery to us. If hunger compares, or Hamburger Hill or the carnal dying of Calcutta, that is for us to say.

My recollection of the two weeks Roger spent in 1028 is as fragmented as the weeks before the diagnosis. I'm not sure what preceded what, though I do have a sense of first week versus second, because the crisis took a turn midway that drove the panic off the graph. Roger was extraordinary in the days that followed the verdict, by which I mean he was utterly himself.

Still, by the third day of treatment he was feeling dreadful, coughing and feverish. The doctors said it was typical of PCP to get worse before it got better, which sounded as mean as an old wives' tale. In any case, he had to channel all his energy to fight the egregious symptoms, plus the drug made him nauseous. Now I wanted to be there all the time—fuck normalcy—to handle the dealings with doctors and staff, to man the phone. It was just as well, since I became totally unhinged when I left the hospital.

I went to my own doctor to get a prescription for sleeping pills, and I poured out the unspeakable news. "What do I do?" I said in desperation.

He shrugged his shoulders with a cavalier unconcern I can only attribute to his certainty that he was safe himself. I've seen that straight man's shrug a hundred times. "Burn the blankets," he replied facetiously, scribbling a prescription for Halcion.

I felt as if I'd just been run over by a truck, while he went on to give me the benefit of his own pain. His brother had died in a car crash while he was still in med school. "Sensitive as a toilet seat," as Holden Caulfield says. I guess it was there in that encounter that I came to revile the comparisons of others. Is this how a Jew feels when he hears "holocaust" appropriated to some other calamity? Yet I was still so wounded by the news itself, desperate for allies, that I didn't have the wit to slam out of his office. Besides, I needed him just as Roger needed Cope, didn't I? I told him in some defiance that Roger hadn't exhibited the two *pre* symptoms the way he'd said, for two months running. I never stopped feeling betrayed by all those phantom barriers that hadn't worked.

"You live alone, you die alone," my doctor said sententiously, serene as Pilate. A month later I would overhear him fretting about what color Ferrari he should get.

Not us, I thought, as the rage began to build like a boiling tsunami. My determination to be with Rog every minute I could, whatever happened, took stubborn form in the doctor's office. White-hot rage is the only thing that keeps you going sometimes.

It was sometime that week I had a nightmare that dragged me awake screaming and in a sweat: I walked into the bathroom and looked around the shower door, to see Roger sitting in the tub, the water to his waist. He was dead. Head lolled slightly to the side, he looked like a dreamer himself, fit and healthy, his skin beaded with water as if he'd just come in from swimming. It was only half a second before I was roaring in pain. I reached in and lifted him out of the water. His heaviness, actual as the weight of a man—my own dead self—pitched the scream to a howl like Lear's as I lurched out to the bedroom, full of nothing forever. I'd never had a dream so physical or so desolating. I'm still afraid it will come again, . . . and have to remind myself in the middle of naps that Roger is already gone—I never sleep below the surface anymore—so the bathtub dream won't engulf me.

So many monsters have haunted the darkness of AIDS. Only four thousand had died by March '85, but already we all knew stories of men left incoherent in their own excrement, abandoned overnight by friends, shipped back to a fundamentalist family to pay the wages of sin. They were chained to their beds with dementia in New York. They lost their houses and all their insurance. The most horrible death in modern medicine, people said.

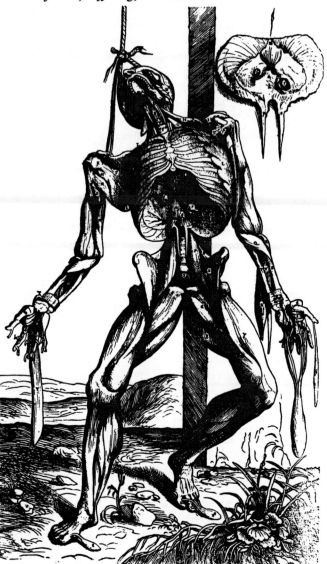

26. *The seventh plate of the muscles from Andreas Vesalius,* Suorum de Humani
Corporis Fabrica Librorum Epitome *(Basle: Johannes Oporinus, 1543). Wellcome
Institute Library, London. In his caption to this plate, Vesalius tells us that his "delin-
eation" of the corpse's muscles was done while it was still hanging from the rope. At
the time, it was commonplace for anatomists to dissect the bodies of executed prisoners. The diaphragm, which served as the early focus of Vesalius's disagreements with
Galen, is displayed to the right. With the "fabric" of the body stripped away, the
skeleton—the archetypal icon of death— is revealed at last. In a gruesome parody of
Renaissance iconography, it poses in the traditional stance of the resurrected Christ.*

PHILIP LARKIN (1922–1985)

"Aubade"

Philip Larkin's fame rests on a slender body of work—little more than one hundred pages—published in four volumes, one almost every decade, beginning with *The North Ship* in 1946. One of post–World War II England's preeminent poets, Larkin was born in Coventry and spent a painful and solitary youth there. Plagued by poor eyesight and stuttering, he was a lonely child who absorbed himself in reading and writing. In 1943, he graduated from Oxford with first-class honors in English literature and took the post of librarian in a small Shropshire town. This profession would support him for the rest of his life; he refused to profit from his poetry by holding lectures or readings. After serving as librarian for the University of Hull for thirty years, Larkin died following surgery for cancer of the throat. Distinguished by its avoidance of the stylistic experimentation typical of Modernism, Larkin's poetry is marked by its technical purity, lucidity, and flawless precision of expression; concerned with traditional metaphysical questions, it chronicles the dreary forms of unhappiness in a world where "the last rags of religious faith" can no longer lend meaning or hope to human suffering. As one critic has said, "a sense that life is a finite prelude to oblivion" pervades Larkin's poetry, which resists no opportunity to puncture the many self-deceptions we practice in the face of death.

I work all day, and get half-drunk at night.
Waking at four to soundless dark, I stare.
In time the curtain-edges will grow light.
Till then I see what's really always there:
Unresting death, a whole day nearer now,
Making all thought impossible but how
And where and when I shall myself die.
Arid interrogation: yet the dread
Of dying, and being dead,
Flashes afresh to hold and horrify.

The mind blanks at the glare. Not in remorse
—The good not done, the love not given, time
Torn off unused—nor wretchedly because
An only life can take so long to climb

From *Collected Poems*, ed. and intro. Anthony Thwaite (New York: Farrar, Straus & Giroux, 1989). Copyright 1988, 1989 by the estate of Philip Larkin. Reprinted by permission of Farrar, Straus & Giroux, Inc.

Clear of its wrong beginnings, and may never;
But at the total emptiness for ever,
The sure extinction that we travel to
And shall be lost in always. Not to be here,
Not to be anywhere,
And soon; nothing more terrible, nothing more true.

This is a special way of being afraid
No trick dispels. Religion used to try,
That vast moth-eaten musical brocade
Created to pretend we never die,
And specious stuff that says *No rational being
Can fear a thing it will not feel,* not seeing
That this is what we fear—no sight, no sound,
No touch or taste or smell, nothing to think with,
Nothing to love or link with,
The anaesthetic from which none come round.

And so it stays just on the edge of vision,
A small unfocused blur, a standing chill
That slows each impulse down to indecision.
Most things may never happen: this one will,
And realisation of it rages out
In furnace-fear when we are caught without
People or drink. Courage is no good:
It means not scaring others. Being brave
Lets no one off the grave.
Death is no different whined at than withstood.

Slowly light strengthens, and the room takes shape.
It stands plain as a wardrobe, what we know,
Have always known, know that we can't escape,
Yet can't accept. One side will have to go.
Meanwhile telephones crouch, getting ready to ring
In locked-up offices, and all the uncaring
Intricate rented world begins to rouse.
The sky is white as clay, with no sun.
Work has to be done.
Postmen like doctors go from house to house.

Index

ABOUT THE EDITORS

David J. Rothman is director of the Center for the Study of Society and Medicine at the College of Physicians and Surgeons of Columbia University. His latest book is *Strangers at the Bedside: A History of How Law and Bioethics Transformed Medical Decision Making.*

Steven Marcus is George Delacorte Professor in the Humanities at Columbia University. His books include *Engels, Manchester, and the Working Class* and *Freud and the Culture of Psychoanalysis.*

Stephanie A. Kiceluk is Master Teacher of the Humanities at New York University. She is currently writing a book on *Studies on Hysteria.*

CPSIA information can be obtained at www.ICGtesting.com
Printed in the USA
LVOW10s0113080815

449369LV00001B/103/P